Critical Car
Emergenci

What Do I Do Now?: Emergency Medicine

SERIES EDITOR-IN-CHIEF

Catherine A. Marco, MD, FACEP
Professor, Emergency Medicine & Surgery
Wright State University Boonshoft School of Medicine
Dayton, Ohio

OTHER VOLUMES IN THE SERIES

Pediatric Medical Emergencies
Pediatric Traumatic Emergencies
Legal and Ethical Issues in Emergency Medicine
Psychiatric Emergencies
Disaster Preparedness and Response
Critical Care Emergencies
Palliative Care in Emergency Medicine
Pediatric Emergency Radiology

Critical Care Emergencies

Edited by

Lillian Liang Emlet, MD, MS, CHSE, FCCM
Clinical Associate Professor
Department of Critical Care Medicine
Department of Emergency Medicine
University of Pittsburgh Medical Center
Pittsburgh, PA, USA

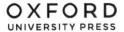
OXFORD
UNIVERSITY PRESS

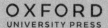

OXFORD
UNIVERSITY PRESS

Oxford University Press is a department of the University of Oxford. It furthers
the University's objective of excellence in research, scholarship, and education
by publishing worldwide. Oxford is a registered trade mark of Oxford University
Press in the UK and certain other countries.

Published in the United States of America by Oxford University Press
198 Madison Avenue, New York, NY 10016, United States of America.

Library of Congress Cataloging-in-Publication Data
Names: Emlet, Lillian Liang, editor.
Title: Critical care emergencies / [edited by] Lillian Liang Emlet.
Other titles: Critical care emergencies (Emlet) | What do I do now?. Emergency medicine
Description: New York, NY : Oxford University Press, [2023] |
Series: What do i do now? Emergency medicine |
Includes bibliographical references and index.
Identifiers: LCCN 2023006010 (print) | LCCN 2023006011 (ebook) |
ISBN 9780190082581 (paperback) | ISBN 9780190082604 (epub) |
ISBN 9780190082611 (online)
Subjects: MESH: Emergencies | Critical Care | Emergency Treatment | Case Reports
Classification: LCC RC86.7 (print) | LCC RC86.7 (ebook) | NLM WB 105 |
DDC 616.02/8—dc23/eng/20230313
LC record available at https://lccn.loc.gov/2023006010
LC ebook record available at https://lccn.loc.gov/2023006011

DOI: 10.1093/med/9780190082581.001.0001

Printed by Marquis Book Printing, Canada

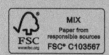

Contents

Contributors

David L. Allison, RRT, RRT-ACCS
Coordinator, Respiratory Therapy
Hartford Hospital
Hartford, CT, USA

Charles M. Andrews, MD, FACEP
Associate Professor Departments of
Emergency Medicine, Neurology,
and Neurosurgery
Medical University of South
Carolina
Charleston, SC, USA

Katrina Augustin, MD, BSN
Critical Care Fellow
Department of Anesthesiology,
Division of Critical Care Medicine
Emory University
Atlanta, GA, USA

**Jennifer Axelband, DO, FCCM,
FACOEP**
Clinical Associate Professor
(Adjunct)
Lewis Katz School of Medicine at
Temple University
Director Neurocritical Care
Department of Critical Care
Medicine
Department of Emergency
Medicine
St. Luke's University Health
Network
Bethlehem, PA, USA

Ani Aydin, MD, FACEP
Assistant Professor
Department of Emergency
Medicine
Department of Surgery, Division
of General Surgery, Trauma and
Surgical Critical Care
Medical Director, SkyHealth and
Adult Ground Critical Care
Transport
Associate Medical Director of
EMS, Critical Care
Yale University School of
Medicine
New Haven, CT, USA

**Torben Becker, MD, PhD,
RDMS, FAWM, FAEMS**
Associate Professor Department of
Emergency Medicine
University of Florida Health
Gainesville, FL, USA

Andrew J. Branting, MD
Emergency Medicine-Critical
Care Medicine Fellow
Department of Internal
Medicine
Division of Pulmonary, Critical
Care & Sleep Medicine
UC Davis Health System
Sacramento, CA, USA

John Bruno, MD
Neurocritical Care Fellow
Department of Anesthesia
Department of Emergency Medicine
Shands Hospital at University of
Florida
Gainesville, FL, USA

Michael Bux, MD
Department of Emergency
Medicine
University of Pittsburgh
Medical Center
Pittsburgh, PA, USA

Wan-Tsu Wendy Chang, MD
Departments of Emergency
Medicine and Neurology
Program in Trauma
University of Maryland School of
Medicine
Baltimore, MD, USA

Susan Cheng, MD, MPH
Clinical Associate Professor of
Emergency Medicine and Critical
Care Medicine
NYU Grossman School of
Medicine
NYU Langone Health
Brooklyn, NY, USA

Paul Crawford, MD
Clinical Instructor Department of
Emergency Medicine
University of Arizona College of
Medicine
Tucson, AZ, USA

Cassidy Dahn, MD
Clinical Assistant Professor
Department of Emergency
Medicine and Critical Care
NYU Langone Medical Center
NYC Health and Hospitals
Bellevue Hospital
New York, NY, USA

**James Dargin, MD,
FCCM, FCCP**
Assistant Clinical Professor of
Medicine
Tufts University School of
Medicine
Director, Medical Intensive Care Unit
Lahey Hospital & Medical Center
Burlington, MA, USA

Sagar B. Dave, DO
Assistant Professor
Department of Emergency
Medicine
Department of Anesthesiology,
Division of Critical Care
Medicine
Emory School of Medicine
Atlanta, GA, USA

Taylor M. Douglas, MD
Critical Care Medicine Fellow
Department of Medicine -
Division of Pulmonary and
Critical Care
University of Maryland School
of Medicine
Baltimore, MD, USA

Jessica Downing, MD
Emergency Medicine-Surgical
Critical Care Fellow
Program in Trauma/Surgical
Critical Care
R Adams Cowley Shock
Trauma Center
University of Maryland
Medical Center
Baltimore, MD, USA

**Marie-Carmelle Elie, MD,
FACEP, FAAEM**
Endowed Professor and Chair
Department of Emergency Medicine
University of Alabama at
Birmingham Heersink School
of Medicine
Birmingham, AL, USA

Timothy J. Ellender, MD
Associate Professor of Clinical
Emergency Medicine
Department of Emergency Medicine
Indiana University
Indianapolis, IN, USA

Christopher I. Eppich, DO
Utah Valley Emergency Physicians
Medical Director, Provo Fire &
Rescue
Affiliated Physician
Intermountain Health, Utah Valley
Hospital
Provo, UT, USA

**Roderick W. Fontenette, MD,
MHCM, CPE, Lt Col(ret), USAF,
MC, FS, FACEP, FCCM**
Emergency Medicine and Critical
Care Medicine
Assistant Professor, Uniformed
Services University
Volunteer Associate Professor, UC
Davis Department of Emergency
Medicine

Jessica Fozard, DO
Emergency Medicine/Critical Care
Medicine
WellSpan Health
York, PA, USA

Samuel Garcia, MD
Emergency Medicine Resident
Physician
Department of Emergency
Medicine
Mayo Clinic
Rochester, MN, USA

Jeremiah Garrison, MD
Clinical Instructor
Department of Emergency
Medicine
Department of Internal
Medicine
Division of Pulmonary, Allergy,
Critical Care and Sleep
University of Arizona
Tucson, AZ, USA

Alexandra June Gordon, MD
Clinical Assistant Professor
Department of Emergency Medicine
Stanford University
Palo Alto, CA, USA

John C. Greenwood, MD
Assistant Professor
Department of Anesthesiology
Department of Emergency
Medicine
University of Pennsylvania
Philadelphia, PA, USA

Daniel Haase, MD, FCCM, RDMS, RDCS
Medical Director, Critical Care
Resuscitation Unit (CCRU)
Program Director, EM-SCC and
ECLS Fellowships
Associate Professor, Departments of
Emergency Medicine and Surgery
Program in Trauma/Surgical
Critical Care
R Adams Cowley Shock
Trauma Center
University of Maryland School of
Medicine
Baltimore, MD, USA

Zachary J. Hernandez, MD
Faculty
Department of Emergency
Medicine
Department of Medicine
Division of Pulmonary, Allergy,
Critical Care and Sleep

University of Arizona College of
Medicine
Tucson, AZ, USA

Daniel Holt, MD
Faculty
Department of Critical Care Medicine
Virginia Mason Franciscan Health
Silverdale, WA, USA

Cameron Hypes MD, MPH
Assistant Professor
Department of Emergency Medicine
Department of Internal Medicine,
Division of Pulmonary, Allergy,
Critical Care and Sleep
University of Arizona College of
Medicine
Tucson, AZ, USA

Ashika Jain, MD, RDMS, FACEP, FAAEM
Associate Professor
Department of Emergency
Medicine
Trauma Critical Care
Emergency Ultrasound
NYU Langone Medical Center
NYC Health & Hospitals
Bellevue Hospital
New York, NY, USA

Meaghan Keville, MD
Emergency Medicine-Surgical
Critical Care Fellow
Program in Trauma/Surgical
Critical Care

R Adams Cowley Shock
Trauma Center
University of Maryland Medical Center
Baltimore, MD, USA

Josh Krieger, MD
Faculty
UCHealth Memorial Hospital
Colorado Springs, CO, USA

Skyler Lentz, MD
Assistant Professor
Department of Emergency
Medicine and Medicine
Larner College of Medicine at the
University of Vermont
Burlington, VT, USA

Fraser Mackay, MD
Faculty
Division of Pulmonary and Critical
Care Medicine
Beth Israel Lahey Health
Lahey Medical Center
Burlington, MA, USA

**Evie Marcolini, MD, FACEP,
FCCM**
Associate Professor of Emergency
Medicine and Neurology
Vice Chair of Faculty Affairs,
Department of Emergency Medicine
Geisel School of Medicine at
Dartmouth
Hanover, NH, USA

**Kusum S. Mathews, MD,
MPH, MSCR**
Clinical Research Physician

Chiesi USA, Inc.
Cary, NC, USA

Ashley Miller, MD
Assistant Professor of Critical Care
Medicine
Montefiore Medical Center
Bronx, NY, USA

Tim Montrief, MD, MPH
Assistant Professor
Department of Surgery
Department of Emergency
Medicine
University of Miami Miller School
of Medicine
Miami, FL, USA

Jarrod M. Mosier, MD, FCCM
Associate Professor
Department of Emergency
Medicine
Department of Medicine
Division of Pulmonary, Allergy,
Critical Care and Sleep
University of Arizona College of
Medicine
Tucson, AZ, USA

Shyam Murali, MD
Fellow
Division of Traumatology, Surgical
Critical Care, and Emergency
Surgery
Perelman School of Medicine
University of Pennsylvania
Philadelphia, PA, USA

Matthew T. Niehaus, DO
Faculty
Department of Emergency
Medicine
University Hospitals Case Western
Reserve University
Cleveland, OH, USA

Joseph Nobile, MD
Intensivist
Pulmonary and Critical Care
Consultants
Miami Valley Hospital
Dayton, OH, USA

Clark G. Owyang, MD
Assistant Professor
Division of Pulmonary and Critical
Care Medicine
New York-Presbyterian Hospital
Weill Cornell Medical Center
New York, NY, USA

Andrew W. Phillips, MD, MEd
Director of ECMO
Associate Medical Director of ICUs
DHR Health
Edinburg, TX, USA

April Jessica Pinto, MD
Faculty
Department of Emergency Medicine
University of Florida
Associate Medical Director
Haven Hospice
Gainesville, FL, USA

Mark M. Ramzy, DO, EMT-P
Clinical Assistant Professor of
Emergency Medicine
Core Faculty and Critical Care
Intensivist
Rutgers New Jersey Medical School
Newark, NJ, USA

Daniel J. Rowan, DO
Director of Education/Clinical
Affairs, Adult ECMO Program
Advocate Lutheran General
Hospital
Division of Critical Care
Department of Internal Medicine
Park Ridge, IL, USA

Krystle Shafer, MD
Faculty
Department of Emergency
Medicine
Department of Critical Care
Medicine
WellSpan York Hospital
York, PA, USA

Jesse Shriki, DO, MS, FACEP
Associate Professor
Department of Medicine and
Critical Care
The University of Arizona
Banner University Medical
Center
Phoenix, AZ, USA

Scott Simpson, DO
Faculty
Department of Critical Care
Department of Emergency
Medicine
Hendrick Medical Center
Abilene, TX, USA

**Aaron Skolnik, MD,
FAAEM, DABMT**
Faculty
Department of Critical Care
Mayo Clinic
Phoenix, AZ, USA

Samantha Strickler, DO, FACEP
Assistant Professor
Department of Emergency
Medicine
Emory University
Atlanta, GA, USA

Russell A. Trigonis, MD
Faculty
Department of Medicine, Division
of Pulmonary, Allergy, Critical
Care, and Sleep Medicine
Atrium Health
Charlotte, NC, USA

Tyler VanDyck, MD
Assistant Professor of Medicine and
Emergency Medicine

Drexel University College of
Medicine
Medical Director of ECMO
Services & Cardiothoracic
Intensivist
Department of Cardiovascular and
Thoracic Surgery
Division of Surgical Critical Care
Allegheny General Hospital
Pittsburgh, PA, USA

Danny VanValkinburgh, MD
Faculty
Critical Care Medicine
Sound Physicians
St. Louis, MO, USA

Maura W. Walsh, MD
Assistant Clinical Professor of
Emergency Medicine and Critical
Care
UCSF Fresno
Fresno, CA, USA

**Brian T. Wessman, MD,
FACEP, FCCM**
Associate Professor
Department of Anesthesiology
Department of Emergency
Medicine
Washington University in St. Louis
School of Medicine
St. Louis, MO, USA

PART 1

Airway

1 I can't breathe: Difficult intubations

Tim Montrief

A 64-year-old morbidly obese male presents to the ED for fever and shortness of breath. His past medical history includes obstructive sleep apnea and laryngeal cancer, for which he is scheduled to undergo surgical resection in 2 weeks. Upon initial evaluation, you notice he has a hoarse voice and his neck appears mildly swollen on the right side. His vitals are as follows: HR 125 bpm, RR 38 breaths/min, temperature 39°C, pulse oximetry saturation 95%, and BP 80/40 mmHg. It becomes apparent that he is worsening from severe sepsis despite appropriate resuscitation, and he may require intubation. You wonder what his laryngeal and upper airway anatomy looks like and how it may affect your airway management.

What do I do now?

anagement of the difficult airway remains one of the highest-risk procedures commonly performed by emergency medicine physicians.[1] Providers must have a thorough understanding of airway management, the anatomic and contextual predictors of a difficult airway, and best practices to manage these considerations. Preparation, planning, and familiarity with proper positioning and technique are essential to ensure that these challenging situations are managed successfully.

The awake fiberoptic intubation (AFOI) is an important yet clinically underutilized procedure in the ED.[2] Recent multicenter registry (NEAR III) data suggest that roughly 1% of all intubations in the ED involve AFOI as either the primary technique or a secondary rescue technique.[3,4] When AFOI was used as the initial technique, the first-attempt intubation success rate was only 51%, and the overall intubation success rate was 74%.[4] Similarly, when AFOI was used as a secondary rescue therapy, the successful intubation rate was 71%.[4] In comparison, meta-analyses of anesthesia-performed AFOI for anticipated difficult airways report an overall success rate of 99.4%, no deaths, and an incidence of severe adverse events of 0.34%.[5]

PATIENT SELECTION

The major benefit of AFOI is the clinician's ability to fully visualize the posterior pharynx, larynx, and supraglottic and subglottic structures without impacting the patient's hemodynamics, respiratory drive, or level of consciousness.[2] This is critically important in patients with acute, evolving, or asymmetric upper airway pathology, given the potential for loss of airway patency with depressed levels of consciousness.[6] AFOI is indicated when there is known or suspected difficulty with bag-valve mask ventilation or tracheal intubation for the patient who is able to maintain his or her own airway reflexes and ventilatory drive[2,7] (Table 1.1). Additionally, AFOI may be considered for management of an anticipated physiologically difficult airway.[8] Patients already experiencing some degree of respiratory or cardiovascular instability may not tolerate the impact on respiratory drive and hemodynamics that comes with rapid sequence intubation, so maintaining wakefulness can be desirable in these cases if time for appropriate preparation is available.[1]

TABLE 1.1 Predictors of difficult tracheal intubation and bag-valve mask ventilation

Difficult tracheal intubation	Difficult bag-valve mask ventilation
History of difficult intubation	Previous difficult bag-valve mask ventilation
BMI ≥30 kg/m²	BMI ≥30 kg/m²
Angioedema	Edentulous
History of head and neck tumors	Age >55 years
Cervical spine immobility or injury	Beard or facial hair
Small oropharyngeal orifice	History of obstructive sleep apnea
Mallampati ≥III	Mallampati ≥III
Mandibular retrusion (micrognathia or retrognathia)	Limited jaw protrusion

Infections
- Dental abscess
- Sublingual abscess
- Epiglottitis
- Croup

Cervical spine immobility or laxity
- Rheumatoid arthritis
- Ankylosing spondylitis
- Atlantoaxial instability

Iatrogenic causes
- Radiotherapy of the neck or airway
- Surgery of the neck or airway

Trauma
- Unstable cervical spine fractures
- Facial or mandibular fractures
- Upper airway or tracheal edema
- Airway or inhalational burns

Congenital abnormalities
- Pierre–Robin syndrome
- Treacher Collins syndrome
- Klippel–Feil syndrome
- Goldenhar syndrome
- Turner syndrome
- Mucopolysaccharidosis (MPS)
- Cystic hygroma
- Hemangioma

When AFOI is chosen as the airway management strategy, there must be adequate time to prepare and perform the procedure, which typically requires 10 to 15 minutes at minimum. For this reason, if a patient has any indication for urgent intubation, AFOI should not be considered. Relative contraindications to AFOI include uncorrectable hypoxemia, an inability of the patient to protect their airway, agitation or inability to participate in the procedure, active airway bleeding, hemoptysis or hematemesis, active vomiting, local anesthetic allergy, and hemodynamic instability.[2,9] Due to the fact that administration of topical anesthesia—and blunting of airway reflexes—may result in loss of airway patency, AFOI in patients presenting with stridor remains controversial, but it has been successfully used by experts in select cases.[2,10] Note that the requirement for supplemental oxygen is not a contraindication for AFOI.[7,11]

Clinicians must plan accordingly for any potential deterioration of hemodynamics, respiratory drive, oxygenation, or airway patency during the procedure.[1] The most experienced airway proceduralists available should be available to assist if possible, and potential need for emergent front-of-neck access must be considered.[7] Calm, clear communication and preparation of sequential airway plans as a team is essential in managing the difficult airway.

AIRWAY TOPICALIZATION

Preparation for AFOI includes achieving optimal airway anesthesia.[2,7] Antisialagogues, most commonly glycopyrrolate (0.2–0.4 mg IV), limit secretions, which facilitates absorption of local anesthetics and improves intubating conditions.[7] An alternative medication is atropine (0.4–0.6 mg IV).[9] Either of these should be given upon consideration of AFOI, ideally 15 to 30 minutes prior to initiation of the procedure.[2] Antisialagogues, especially antimuscarinics such as atropine, may cause unwanted side effects, most notably tachycardia, which may lead to increased patient anxiety and a more difficult intubation.[9] Vasoconstriction of the nasal passage using oxymetazoline or phenylephrine is recommended and has been shown to reduce epistaxis during the nasopharyngeal approach.[7] Ondansetron may also help decrease the gag reflex.[12]

The success of AFOI depends on effective delivery of topical anesthetics to the airway.[13,14] Attempts to manipulate the posterior pharynx and larynx without adequate topicalization will be highly uncomfortable for patients, leading to an unsafe level of stimulation during AFOI.[2] For AFOI, short-acting anesthetics such as lidocaine or tetracaine are preferred over long-acting agents such as bupivacaine.[7] Prepared benzocaine spray may be more familiar to EM physicians but should be avoided as it predisposes the patient to benzocaine overdose and resultant methemoglobinemia.[15,16] Lower concentrations of lidocaine (1–2%) are as effective as higher concentrations but have the benefit of allowing a greater volume to be given before toxicity.[7,17–19] The maximum dose for topical lidocaine administration is 9 mg/kg lean body weight, although this dose is rarely required in the majority of cases.[7] It is important to suction, then pat dry, the mouth with gauze prior to application of topical anesthetic; this may augment absorption and decrease the total dose of lidocaine.

There are a variety of methods to deliver local anesthetic, including mucosal atomization, spray-as-you-go through the fiberoptic scope, nebulization, ointment, and transtracheal injection.[7] Nebulized lidocaine is a pretreatment technique that anesthetizes the nasopharyngeal, oropharyngeal, and laryngeal spaces via larger droplet size, with variable absorption.[7] A superior method involves sequentially topicalizing each area of the path of intubation. Begin by having the patient gargle 4 mL of 1% lidocaine (total of 40 mg) for 1 to 2 minutes to provide dense anesthesia throughout the oropharyngeal and supraglottic structures.[2,20] Then, additional anesthesia can be provided by application of 4% to 5% lidocaine ointment (~5 mL) to the posterior tongue.[2] The patient should let this ointment sit on the posterior aspect of their tongue for a few minutes, after which they may swallow. Finally, 5 to 10 mL of 1% lidocaine is delivered via a mucosal atomizer. As the atomizer is advanced into the posterior oropharynx, the operator should begin to spray lidocaine (1–2%), starting with the uvula and soft palate, followed by the deeper structures of the supraglottis and larynx and onto the vocal cords.[2,21]

Nasal AFOI relies on vasoconstriction prior to topical anesthesia.[2] An optimal strategy includes placement of cotton-tipped applicators soaked in 2% to 4% lidocaine gel after application of oxymetazoline 0.05% solution introduced into the larger-sized patent naris.[2] An alternative is to place a nasal trumpet coated in lidocaine jelly into the naris, providing both topical anesthesia and dilatation of the nasal pathway.[2]

SEDATION

While AFOI can be accomplished using only topical anesthesia, some patients require a measure of sedation to facilitate the procedure by reducing patient anxiety and discomfort.[7,22] However, sedation should not be used as a substitute for adequate oral airway topicalization.[7] Sedation (and oversedation) carries with it an increased risk of respiratory depression, loss of airway patency, hypoxia, hemodynamic instability, and aspiration.[7,22] When sedation is used, clinicians should use a single agent and should have an alternative airway management strategy in place if the patient experiences apnea, hemodynamic collapse, or refractory hypoxia.[7]

During AFOI facilitated by sedation, the ideal medication should have a rapid onset, short half-life, and limited impact on respiratory drive and hemodynamics.[2] The three principal agents with these traits are ketamine, midazolam, and dexmedetomidine. Propofol, a commonly used sedative in the ED, carries a greater risk of oversedation, airway compromise, and hemodynamic collapse compared to other agents.[22,23] As such, it is not recommended for use during AFOI.[7]

Ketamine, a well-known agent for many emergency physicians, is commonly used for rapid sequence intubation, delayed sequence intubation, and moderate sedation.[24,25] A dissociative anesthetic, ketamine has several unique properties that make it an attractive option for AFOI, including preservation of cardiorespiratory tone and quick onset of action.[25] Ketamine may be given either as a slow bolus (0.5–1 mg/kg IV over 30–60 seconds) or as small aliquots (20 mg every 2 minutes) until the desired level of sedation is achieved.[2] Side effects of ketamine include increased salivation and bronchorrhea, which may be counteracted by glycopyrrolate.[2] When given IV as a "push," ketamine may cause a brief but undesirable period of apnea that is typically self-limiting.[26]

Midazolam, a benzodiazepine, is most useful as an anxiolytic during AFOI.[2,22] In the presence of adequate topical anesthesia, small boluses of 0.5 to 2 mg IV can reduce patient anxiety while facilitating patient cooperation.[2] It also provides some antiemetic effect, which can be helpful during AFOI.[2] The advantage of this approach lies in its simplicity, widespread experience, and predictable dosing pattern. Midazolam has no analgesic properties, and studies have shown that despite high doses of midazolam, a significant proportion of patients undergoing AFOI experience coughing or respiratory compromise.[22,27] Intermittent bolus administration of midazolam can be associated with overshoot and the risk of oversedation.[22]

Dexmedetomidine is associated with a low risk of oversedation and loss of airway patency when used for AFOI.[22] As an α2-adrenoceptor agonist, it produces deep sedation without impacting the patient's respiratory drive.[22] Respiratory compromise, if it occurs, is typically due to the patient receiving a large bolus of dexmedetomidine.[22] Dexmedetomidine also preserves patient cooperation throughout the procedure, while producing anterograde amnesia.[22] It may also have mild analgesic and antisialagogue properties.[28] Dexmedetomidine is typically started as a 1-μg/kg bolus given over 10 to 20 minutes, then an infusion of 0.3 to 1.2 μg/kg/hr.[22] This strategy helps avoid the drug's main adverse effects, bradycardia and hypotension.[22,29] Despite its favorable traits, there is currently no high-level evidence that dexmedetomidine outperforms ketamine or midazolam for AFOI.[9] A review of medications for AFOI is provided in Box 1.1.

TECHNIQUE

First, the procedure should be explained fully to the patient, as their cooperation and ability to provide feedback is essential to its success. The patient is generally placed upright in a sitting position with the bed at 45 to 90 degrees, facing the operator. Alternatively, the patient may be laid semirecumbent (30–45 degrees) with the operator at the head of the bed, so long as this positioning does not worsen obstruction.

The flexible bronchoscope has several benefits that make it ideal for AFOI, most notably its ability to easily be passed through the naris, as well as its ability to move in multiple planes of motion through distorted anatomy.[2,6] Compared to traditional videolaryngoscopy or direct laryngoscopy, AFOI provides a better view of the glottic inlet, although this technique requires more procedural time.[30] Compared to an oral approach, the nasal approach for AFOI naturally aligns the bronchoscope with the glottic opening, facilitating endotracheal tube passage and successful intubation.[2,31]

BOX 1.1 **Medications for awake fiberoptic intubation**

To inhibit oral secretions and facilitate local anesthesia:
- Glycopyrrolate 0.2–0.4 mg IV
  OR
- Atropine 0.4–0.6 mg IV

To provide vasoconstriction:
- Oxymetazoline 0.05% solution
  OR
- Phenylephrine 0.25% solution

To provide oral topical anesthesia:
- 4 mL of 1% lidocaine gargled (40 mg)
  AND
- 5 mL of 4–5% lidocaine ointment to posterior tongue (200–250 mg)
  AND
- 5–10 mL of 1% lidocaine via atomizer to posterior pharynx and supraglottis (50–100 mg)

To provide nasal topical anesthesia:
- 5 mL of 2–4% lidocaine gel on cotton-tipped applicators or nasal trumpet (200–250 mg)

For sedation (if necessary):
- Ketamine 20 mg IV bolus every 2 minutes until desired sedation achieved
  OR
- Midazolam 0.5–2 mg IV bolus PRN
  OR
- Dexmedetomidine 1 μg/kg over 10–20 minutes, then an infusion of 0.3–1.2 μg/kg/hr

The endotracheal tube is advanced over the bronchoscope—that is, the scope is placed within the lumen of the endotracheal tube to allow delivery after successful placement in the trachea at the carina. Optimal technique in bronchoscopy involves limiting the number of bends made in the flexible section of the bronchoscope, as an "S-shape" can impede the smooth advancement of the endotracheal tube over the scope.

In the case of the oropharyngeal route, it is best to use a bite block (e.g., Burman airway, Ovassapian airway) to protect the bronchoscope, as patients will reflexively bite down if inadequately anesthetized, and these devices facilitate placement of the bronchoscope into the laryngeal inlet.[2] The scope is advanced through the circular endoscopic bite block past the tongue to the posterior oropharynx, then down-flexed to visualize the glottic opening and advanced. After the bronchoscope has passed through the vocal cords and advanced to 2 cm above the carina, the endotracheal tube is passed over it, allowing confirmation of correct location during placement. Topicalization of the vocal cords with lidocaine sprayed through the bronchoscope channel is essential prior to advancing the scope through the cords, along with topicalization of the carina prior to advancing the endotracheal tube.[1]

If the nasal route is used, the bronchoscope should be placed in the larger, more patent naris, then advanced, parallel to the nasal floor.[2] When the naris is cleared, the posterior pharyngeal wall is encountered, and the bronchoscope should be down-flexed, then advanced through the glottic opening, similar to the oropharyngeal approach.[2,9] There are specialized nasotracheal tubes for this procedure (Parker Flex-Tip™), though endotracheal tubes may be used as well. The selected tube must be large enough to fit over the bronchoscope and small enough to be able to advance through the nasal passage, while also providing sufficient length. An endotracheal tube size 7.0 to 7.5 mm is acceptable.[6]

If a difficult airway is predicted, but the patient has adequate oxygenation and mental status, AFOI is the airway management technique of choice. Early preparation is key, focusing on airway desiccation with glycopyrrolate, nasal vasoconstriction, and adequate topicalization with lidocaine throughout the upper airway, with or without mild sedation. The decision to use an oral versus a nasal approach is dictated by the patient's airway anatomy, the clinician's experience, and the availability of equipment and resources in the department.

KEY POINTS TO REMEMBER

- Prepare for backup plans for ventilatory and airway control in the event of AFOI failure, including combining video and fiberoptic techniques with additional airway operators.
- Preparation for AFOI centers on achieving airway desiccation and optimal airway anesthesia. Give glycopyrrolate 0.2 to 0.4 mg IV at least 15 minutes prior to topicalization with 1% lidocaine.

- AFOI may be successful with topicalization only; sedation is not always required.
- During AFOI facilitated by sedation, the clinician should choose a medication characterized by its rapid onset, short half-life, ability to maintain respiratory drive, and limited impact on hemodynamics: dexmedetomidine, midazolam, or ketamine.
- Compared to an oral approach, the nasal approach for AFOI naturally aligns the bronchoscope with the glottic opening, facilitating endotracheal tube passage and successful intubation.

References

1. Cabrera JL, Auerbach JS, Merelman AH, Levitan RM. The high-risk airway. *Emerg Med Clin North Am.* 2020;38(2):401–417. doi:10.1016/j.emc.2020.01.008
2. Tonna JE, DeBlieux PMC. Awake laryngoscopy in the emergency department. *J Emerg Med.* 2017;52(3):324–331. doi:10.1016/j.jemermed.2016.11.013
3. Brown CA, Bair AE, Pallin DJ, Walls RM, NEAR III Investigators. Techniques, success, and adverse events of emergency department adult intubations. *Ann Emerg Med.* 2015;65(4):363–370. doi:10.1016/j.annemergmed.2014.10.036
4. Hayden EM, Pallin DJ, Wilcox SR, et al. Emergency department adult fiberoptic intubations: Incidence, indications, and implications for training. *Acad Emerg Med.* 2018;25(11):1263–1267. doi:10.1111/acem.13440
5. Cabrini L, Baiardo Redaelli M, Ball L, et al. Awake fiberoptic intubation protocols in the operating room for anticipated difficult airway: A systematic review and meta-analysis of randomized controlled trials. *Anesth Analg.* 2019;128(5):971–980. doi:10.1213/ANE.0000000000004087
6. Collins SR, Blank RS. Fiberoptic intubation: An overview and update. *Respir Care.* 2014;59(6):865–880. doi:10.4187/respcare.03012
7. Ahmad I, El-Boghdadly K, Bhagrath R, et al. Difficult Airway Society guidelines for awake tracheal intubation (ATI) in adults. *Anaesthesia.* 2020;75(4):509–528. doi:10.1111/anae.14904
8. Mosier JM, Joshi R, Hypes C, Pacheco G, Valenzuela T, Sakles JC. The physiologically difficult airway. *West J Emerg Med.* 2015;16(7):1109–1117. doi:10.5811/westjem.2015.8.27467
9. Leslie D, Stacey M. Awake intubation. *Continuing Education in Anaesthesia Critical Care & Pain.* 2015;15(2):64–67. doi:10.1093/bjaceaccp/mku015
10. Ho AMH, Chung DC, To EWH, Karmakar MK. Total airway obstruction during local anesthesia in a non-sedated patient with a compromised airway. *Can J Anaesth.* 2004;51(8):838–841. doi:10.1007/BF03018461

11. Badiger S, John M, Fearnley RA, Ahmad I. Optimizing oxygenation and intubation conditions during awake fibre-optic intubation using a high-flow nasal oxygen-delivery system. *Br J Anaesth*. 2015;115(4):629–632. doi:10.1093/bja/aev262

12. Kaviani N, Ranjbaran F. Evaluation of the efficacy of oral ondansetron on gag reflex in soft palate and palatine tonsil areas. *JIDS*. 2011;6(6):691–697.

13. El-Boghdadly K, Onwochei DN, Cuddihy J, Ahmad I. A prospective cohort study of awake fibreoptic intubation practice at a tertiary centre. *Anaesthesia*. 2017;72(6):694–703. doi:10.1111/anae.13844

14. Woodall NM, Harwood RJ, Barker GL. Complications of awake fibreoptic intubation without sedation in 200 healthy anaesthetists attending a training course. *Br J Anaesth*. 2008;100(6):850–855. doi:10.1093/bja/aen076

15. Abdel-Aziz S, Hashmi N, Khan S, Ismaeil M. Methemoglobinemia with the use of benzocaine spray for awake fiberoptic intubation. *Middle East J Anaesthesiol*. 2013;22(3):337–340.

16. Kern K, Langevin PB, Dunn BM. Methemoglobinemia after topical anesthesia with lidocaine and benzocaine for a difficult intubation. *J Clin Anesth*. 2000;12(2):167–172. doi:10.1016/s0952-8180(00)00113-6

17. Woodruff C, Wieczorek PM, Schricker T, Vinet B, Backman SB. Atomised lidocaine for airway topical anaesthesia in the morbidly obese: 1% compared with 2%. *Anaesthesia*. 2010;65(1):12–17. doi:10.1111/j.1365-2044.2009.06126.x

18. Wieczorek PM, Schricker T, Vinet B, Backman SB. Airway topicalisation in morbidly obese patients using atomised lidocaine: 2% compared with 4%. *Anaesthesia*. 2007;62(10):984–988. doi:10.1111/j.1365-2044.2007.05179.x

19. Xue FS, Liu HP, He N, et al. Spray-as-you-go airway topical anesthesia in patients with a difficult airway: a randomized, double-blind comparison of 2% and 4% lidocaine. *Anesth Analg*. 2009;108(2):536–543. doi:10.1213/ane.0b013e31818f1665

20. Chung DC, Mainland PA, Kong AS. Anesthesia of the airway by aspiration of lidocaine. *Can J Anaesth*. 1999;46(3):215–219. doi:10.1007/BF03012598

21. Leung Y, Vacanti FX. Awake without complaints: Maximizing comfort during awake fiberoptic intubation. *J Clin Anesth*. 2015;27(6):517–519. doi:10.1016/j.jclinane.2015.05.004

22. Johnston KD, Rai MR. Conscious sedation for awake fibreoptic intubation: A review of the literature. *Can J Anaesth*. 2013;60(6):584–599. doi:10.1007/s12630-013-9915-9

23. Rai MR, Parry TM, Dombrovskis A, Warner OJ. Remifentanil target-controlled infusion vs propofol target-controlled infusion for conscious sedation for awake fibreoptic intubation: A double-blinded randomized controlled trial. *Br J Anaesth*. 2008;100(1):125–130. doi:10.1093/bja/aem279

24. Weingart SD, Trueger NS, Wong N, Scofi J, Singh N, Rudolph SS. Delayed sequence intubation: A prospective observational study. *Ann Emerg Med*. 2015;65(4):349–355. doi:10.1016/j.annemergmed.2014.09.025

25. Merelman AH, Perlmutter MC, Strayer RJ. Alternatives to rapid sequence intubation: Contemporary airway management with ketamine. *West J Emerg Med.* 2019;20(3):466–471. doi:10.5811/westjem.2019.4.42753

26. Gao M, Rejaei D, Liu H. Ketamine use in current clinical practice. *Acta Pharmacol Sin.* 2016;37(7):865–872. doi:10.1038/aps.2016.5

27. Sidhu VS, Whitehead EM, Ainsworth QP, Smith M, Calder I. A technique of awake fibreoptic intubation: Experience in patients with cervical spine disease. *Anaesthesia.* 1993;48(10):910–913. doi:10.1111/j.1365-2044.1993.tb07429.x

28. Hall JE, Uhrich TD, Barney JA, Arain SR, Ebert TJ. Sedative, amnestic, and analgesic properties of small-dose dexmedetomidine infusions. *Anesth Analg.* 2000;90(3):699–705. doi:10.1097/00000539-200003000-00035

29. Abdelmalak B, Makary L, Hoban J, Doyle DJ. Dexmedetomidine as sole sedative for awake intubation in management of the critical airway. *J Clin Anesth.* 2007;19(5):370–373. doi:10.1016/j.jclinane.2006.09.006

30. Silverton NA, Youngquist ST, Mallin MP, et al. GlideScope versus flexible fiber optic for awake upright laryngoscopy. *Ann Emerg Med.* 2012;59(3):159–164. doi:10.1016/j.annemergmed.2011.07.009

31. Ezri T, Szmuk P, Evron S, Warters RD, Herman O, Weinbroum AA. Nasal versus oral fiberoptic intubation via a cuffed oropharyngeal airway (COPA) during spontaneous ventilation. *J Clin Anesth.* 2004;16(7):503–507. doi:10.1016/j.jclinane.2004.01.006

Further reading

Ahmad I, El-Boghdadly K, Bhagrath R, et al. Difficult Airway Society guidelines for awake tracheal intubation (ATI) in adults. *Anaesthesia.* 2020;75(4):509–528. doi:10.1111/anae.14904

Cabrera JL, Auerbach JS, Merelman AH, Levitan RM. The high-risk airway. *Emerg Med Clin North Am.* 2020;38(2):401–417. doi:10.1016/j.emc.2020.01.008

Collins SR, Blank RS. Fiberoptic intubation: An overview and update. *Respir Care.* 2014;59(6):865–880. doi:10.4187/respcare.03012

Cooper RM. Preparation for and management of "failed" laryngoscopy and/or intubation. *Anesthesiology.* 2019;130(5):833–849. doi:10.1097/ALN.0000000000002555

Tonna JE, DeBlieux PMC. Awake laryngoscopy in the emergency department. *J Emerg Med.* 2017;52(3):324–331. doi:10.1016/j.jemermed.2016.11.013

2 Breathing from the neck: Tracheostomy emergencies

Paul Crawford and Cameron Hypes

A 38-year-old man presents to your ED from a rehabilitation facility with bleeding from his tracheostomy. The patient's only significant past medical history is a recent discharge from the hospital after suffering a traumatic brain injury following a motorcycle accident. The patient's course was complicated by difficulty weaning from mechanical ventilation, dysphagia, and recurrent aspiration requiring a tracheostomy and gastrostomy tube. Today the patient presents ~1.5 weeks after tracheostomy placement with some bleeding from the tracheostomy site. The patient is no longer dependent on a ventilator. On presentation the patient's HR is 98 bpm, RR 36, and BP 127/83 mmHg, with oxygen saturations at 96% on room air. On examination the patient has clear breath sounds in all lung fields and a regular heart rate and rhythm, and the tracheostomy appears in place without any active bleeding on external exam.

What do I do now?

With an aging population and an increasing number of tracheostomies performed, there is a growing need for the emergency physician to understand the presentation and management of acute tracheostomy emergencies. Tracheostomy is generally performed when prolonged mechanical ventilation is expected or there is surgical or pathologic discontinuity or obstruction of the upper airway. The overall complication rate with tracheostomy placement is quite high (~40–50%), with a 30-day readmission rate of nearly 25%. Although the majority of complications are minor, almost 1% of tracheostomies will have catastrophic complications, and the mortality associated with these complications is ~50%.[1]

There are two main techniques by which tracheostomies are performed: open surgical technique in the operating room or percutaneously at the bedside in the ICU. Tracheostomies are placed generally between the second and fifth tracheal rings, with ideal placement being between the second and third tracheal rings, with lower tracheostomy placement being associated with a higher rate of complications. The left and right lobes of the thyroid lie laterally to the trachea and are connected by the thyroid isthmus, which crosses between the second and third tracheal rings. The thyroid veins are generally midline and course inferiorly to the thyroid isthmus. The innominate artery or the brachiocephalic trunk is the first major branch of the aorta and gives rise to the subclavian artery and right carotid artery. Generally, the innominate crosses anterior to the ninth tracheal ring, but this can range from the sixth to the 13th tracheal ring.[2] Be aware that some patients who present with tracheostomies also have had laryngectomies, therefore providing no route for orotracheal reintubation. Key history on initial exam requires determining laryngectomy status.

Tracheostomy emergencies can generally be separated into two main categories, emergent or urgent complications. Emergent presentations include hemorrhage, decannulation, and obstruction. Urgent presentations include tracheoesophageal fistula, infection, and stenosis. In evaluation of a tracheostomy emergency, it is important to ascertain some background information on the patient's tracheostomy, including why it was placed, when it was placed, tube size, and if the tube is cuffed or uncuffed. It is also very important to know if the patient has a continuous (patent) upper airway (laryngectomy status) and whether the patient is able to be ventilated orally should that become necessary.

In patients such as this patient who presents with tracheostomy bleeding, one of the first things to consider is the timing of the bleed. Bleeding within the first 48 hours of placement is usually perioperative and is largely self-limited, responding to correction of coagulopathy and direct topical hemostatic agents (Surgicel oxidized regenerated cellulose, thrombin). The most feared bleeding complication is the development of a tracheo-innominate artery fistula (TIAF). Seventy-five percent of TIAF hemorrhages will occur within the first 3 weeks of placement, but they can occur at any time. The mortality associated with a TIAF hemorrhage is >90%. Up to 50% of TIAF bleeds will have a sentinel or herald bleed, generally presenting as transient tracheostomy site bleeding or hemoptysis. This can occur up to 24 to 48 hours prior to the development of massive hemorrhage.[1] Risk factors for the development of TIAF include low tracheostomy placement, high cuff pressure, high-riding innominate artery, tracheostomy infection, and a thoracic deformity such as scoliosis.[2]

Initial evaluation and treatment of tracheostomy site bleeding should include several considerations, starting with large-bore IV access in anticipation of possible large-volume resuscitation. All bleeding should be evaluated by a surgical specialist and is considered a TIAF hemorrhage until proven otherwise, given the significant mortality. If there is no active bleeding, evaluation begins with an external exam. If there is oozing from the stoma, control can be attempted by direct pressure or with topical hemostatic agents such as silver nitrate. Internal tracheal mucosa can be evaluated at the bedside with a fiberoptic nasopharyngoscope or bronchoscope, and this can be used to evaluate for mucosal irritation and bleeding as well as differentiating tracheal versus lower respiratory sources of bleeding and hemoptysis.[3]

Patients who present with active tracheostomy site bleeding or hemoptysis should be treated as TIAF hemorrhage until proven otherwise. The first question is whether the patient has an upper airway that is contiguous with the oropharynx or a discontinuous oropharynx and trachea. This is crucial to ascertain, as asphyxiation is a frequent cause of death in these patients and maintaining a patent airway is vitally important. Frequent suctioning of blood from the airway should be performed. The next maneuver in a patient with a cuffed tracheostomy is overinflation of the tracheostomy balloon (Figure 2.1). The balloon can be filled with up to 50 mL air to provide pressure against the TIAF in an attempt to tamponade the bleeding. Cuff

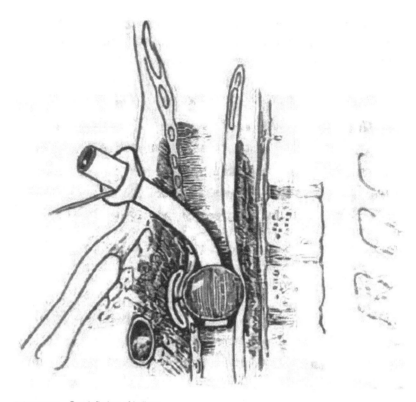

FIGURE 2.1 Overinflation of balloon

Reprinted from *Chest Surgery Clinics of North America*, 13/2, Allan JS & Wright CD,
Tracheoinnominate fistula: diagnosis and management, 331–341, Copyright 2003, with
permission from Elsevier.

overinflation is successful in temporizing bleeding about 85% of the time.[1]
If the patient does not have a cuffed tracheostomy and one is not immediately available, the patient can be intubated orally, should the patient have a
contiguous upper airway. The tracheostomy tube should be maintained in
place during oral intubation until the endotracheal tube has been successfully passed through the vocal cords. The endotracheal balloon can then be
overinflated in an attempt to tamponade bleeding and achieve hemostasis.
If the patient continues to bleed, the next maneuver is manual compression of the innominate artery. This is achieved by inserting a finger through
the stoma and extending downward, just anterior to the trachea. Pressure is

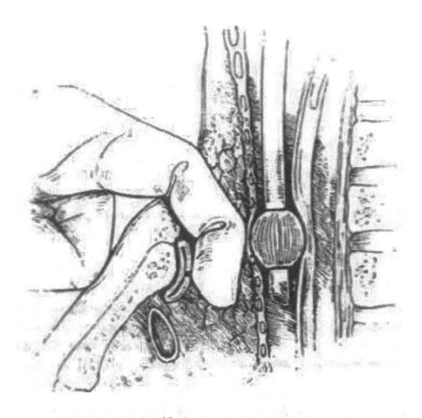

FIGURE 2.2 Manual compression of fistula

Reprinted from *Chest Surgery Clinics of North America*, 13/2, Allan JS & Wright CD, Tracheoinnominate fistula: diagnosis and management, 331-341, Copyright 2003, with permission from Elsevier.

then applied anteriorly against the manubrium (Figure 2.2). Digital compression must be maintained until definitive repair is undertaken in the operating room.

Another specific population is patients with a noncontiguous upper airway. These patients may have previously undergone laryngectomy or laryngotracheal separation. Laryngectomy is typically a consequence of laryngeal malignancy or other head or neck malignancy that has involved the larynx. Tracheolaryngeal separation is an intervention indicated for the prevention of severe and intractable aspiration, typically in the setting of severe motor and intellectual disabilities. This population cannot be ventilated orally and an airway must be maintained through the tracheostomy stoma.[4]

The disposition of a patient presenting with TIAF hemorrhage is the operating room. It is important to mobilize the appropriate surgical services early in the patient's care as this is a time-sensitive disease process. TIAFs are generally managed operatively by either otolaryngology, oral and maxillofacial surgery, or vascular surgery, possibly in conjunction with cardiothoracic surgery, as sternotomy and cardiopulmonary bypass is often required. Occasionally a TIAF will be amenable to embolization by an interventional radiologist; however, this is highly dependent on the patient's aortic arch anatomy and cerebral circulation. It is not available at all medical facilities and is sometimes thought of as a salvage procedure for a TIAF that cannot be repaired operatively.[3]

Tracheostomy placement is an increasingly common procedure with a high complication rate of which every emergency physician needs to be aware. TIAF hemorrhage is a rare complication with an exceptionally high mortality rate. All emergency physicians must appropriately appreciate the potential severity of any late tracheostomy bleeding and understand the acute management and resuscitation of a TIAF hemorrhage.

KEY POINTS TO REMEMBER

- TIAF hemorrhage is an uncommon but life-threatening complication of tracheostomy, with a mortality of >90%.
- All late (>48 hours after tracheostomy placement) bleeding should be evaluated carefully for TIAF. A surgical specialist should be involved.
- Hemorrhage concerning for TIAF should be initially managed by hyperinflation of a cuffed tracheostomy or by oral endotracheal intubation with hyperinflation of the endotracheal tube.
- Should balloon hyperinflation fail to control hemorrhage, a finger can be inserted just anteriorly to the trachea with pressure against the posterior aspect of the manubrium in an attempt to tamponade bleeding, with definitive repair undertaken in the operating room.

- Resources and an algorithm for the management of tracheostomy emergencies can be found at the National Tracheostomy Safety Project.[5] (https://www.tracheostomy.org.uk/storage/files/NTSP_GREEN_ Tracheostomy_Algorithm.pdf).

References
1. Bontempo LJ, Manning SL. Tracheostomy emergencies. *Emerg Med Clin North Am*. 2019;37(1):109–119.
2. Kornas R. Neck and upper airway disorders. In: Cydulka RK, Fitch MT, Joing SA, Wang VJ, Cline DM, Ma OJ, eds. *Tintinalli's Emergency Medicine Manual* (8th ed.). McGraw Hill; 2018:845–850.
3. Bradley PJ. Bleeding around a tracheostomy wound: What to consider and what to do? *J Laryngol Otol*. 2009;123(9):952–956.
4. Sato H, Kawase H, Furuta S, Shima H, Wakisaka M, Kitagawa H. Tracheoinnominate artery fistula after laryngotracheal separation: Prevention and management. *J Pediatr Surg*. 2012;47(2):341–346.
5. McGrath BA, Bates L, Atkinson D, Moore JA. Multidisciplinary guidelines for the management of tracheostomy and laryngectomy airway emergencies. *Anesthesia*. 2012;67:1025–1041.

Further reading
Allan JS, Wright CD. Tracheoinnominate fistula: Diagnosis and management. *Chest Surg Clin North Am*. 2003;13(2):331–341.
Bontempo LJ, Manning SL. Tracheostomy emergencies. *Emerg Med Clin North Am*. 2019;37(1):109–119.
Bradley PJ. Bleeding around a tracheostomy wound: What to consider and what to do? *J Laryngol Otol*. 2009;123(9):952–956.
Kornas R. Neck and upper airway disorders. In: Cydulka RK, Fitch MT, Joing SA, Wang VJ, Cline DM, Ma OJ, eds. *Tintinalli's Emergency Medicine Manual* (8th ed.). McGraw Hill; 2018:845–850.

3 The challenge down under: Subglottic airway access issues

Christopher I. Eppich and

Jarrod M. Mosier

A 63-year-old female arrives to the ED by ambulance in respiratory distress. She has a past medical history of hypertension and heart failure with reduced ejection fraction. Two years prior, the patient was admitted for ARDS due to influenza, required tracheostomy for prolonged mechanical ventilation, and was later decannulated. On examination, she is tripoding and speaking in one-word sentences, and she denies recent fever or cough. She is afebrile and has a pulse oximetry of 94% on a non-rebreather mask at 15 LPM, RR 35 breaths/min, HR 111 bpm, and BP 178/71 mmHg. Exam demonstrates equal and clear bilateral breath sounds as well as accessory muscle use and a small surgical scar on the anterior neck. There are no murmurs, jugular venous distention, or pedal edema. Venous blood gas analysis demonstrates a pH of 7.02, pCO_2 of 95, and HCO_3 of 31. She was placed on noninvasive positive-pressure ventilation (NIPPV), but her acidosis and mentation continued to worsen.

What do I do now?

Due to the patient's worsening mental status and work of breathing despite NIPPV, she required intubation, and the decision was made to intubate her in the ED via rapid sequence intubation. The vocal cords were visualized without difficulty using videolaryngoscopy. However, passage of an endotracheal tube (ETT) was difficult. She required multiple intubation attempts, and the procedure was complicated by profound hypoxemia resulting in a brief period of pulseless electrical activity. Ultimately, a pediatric bougie was advanced below the vocal cords and a 5-0 pediatric ETT was placed over the bougie, which restored ventilation. After a single round of chest compressions and epinephrine administration, return of spontaneous circulation was achieved. She was admitted to the ICU, where a pediatric bronchoscope was used to assess the airway and showed severe subglottic stenosis (Figure 3.1).

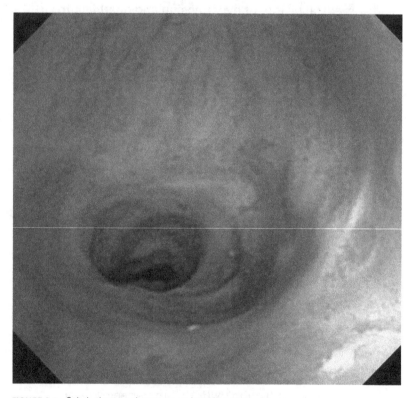

FIGURE 3.1 Subglottic stenosis as seen on bronchoscopy

In patients presenting in the ED with severe respiratory distress, immediate action is needed to identify the appropriate respiratory support to maintain gas exchange. This often involves tracheal intubation to initiate mechanical ventilation. While simultaneously placing the patient on cardiac monitoring, obtaining intravenous access, and providing supplemental oxygen, a targeted assessment of the patient should be performed. Obtaining an accurate and complete history is also essential; information should be obtained whenever possible from the patient, family, friends, prehospital personnel, and the electronic health record.

In this patient's case, a careful examination of the airway, including the oropharynx, sublingual space, peritonsillar space, and neck, should be performed to evaluate for any source of upper airway obstruction. In this patient, the exam was normal. Inspection and palpation of the chest and neck looking for equal chest rise, crepitus, swelling, masses, or signs of trauma is also helpful. In this case, abnormalities were demonstrated besides her prior tracheostomy scar. Auscultation of the lungs, neck, and heart showed no wheezing, rhonchi, rales, or stridor. She was tachypneic with a regular, tachycardic heart rate. The lower extremities were of equal size and without edema.

Chest imaging should augment the physical examination and narrow the differential diagnosis. X-ray and bedside ultrasound are useful to rapidly assess and exclude other causes of respiratory failure, including pneumonia, large pleural effusions, pulmonary embolism, pericardial tamponade, pneumothorax, and pulmonary edema. In this case, a portable chest x-ray did show findings concerning for subglottic narrowing. Focused bedside cardiac ultrasound can be helpful to quickly assess left and right ventricular function and the pericardial space as well, but in this case it showed no clear etiology for the patient's symptoms.

Ideally, specialty support teams (e.g., anesthesia, interventional pulmonology, thoracic surgery, otolaryngology) should be mobilized if subglottic stenosis is identified or suspected. If at all possible, these patients should be taken to the operating room, where rapid operative intervention is possible if the patient can't be intubated or oxygenated during attempts to secure the airway. If the patient must be intubated in the ED, or if the stenosis is an unexpected encounter during rapid sequence intubation, ensure the appropriate equipment (including progressively smaller ETT sizes), and supraglottic airways are immediately available. The most experienced operator should perform the intubation to increase the likelihood of first-pass success, and difficulty should not be met with trying to force a tube past as it will likely result in a complete airway obstruction from supra-stenotic edema. As this patient was in extremis with an airway obstruction (physiologic and anatomic difficult airway), rapid sequence intubation is an unsafe choice. Using paralytics could potentially place the airway operator into the "cannot intubate, cannot ventilate/oxygenate" scenario. Awake flexible endoscopic intubation would provide the safest means to visualize the airway and intubate the patient without removing the patient's respiratory drive.

Awake flexible endoscopic intubation allows the operator to visualize the entire airway past the subglottic level as well as ensure proper ETT passage and appropriate ventilation prior to paralysis. First, the airway should be anesthetized with atomized lidocaine and/or topically using lidocaine ointment or aqueous gel. Glycopyrrolate and atropine act as antisialagogues and are useful in decreasing oral and airway secretions, thereby improving views and increasing the likelihood of first-pass success. Finally, using medications such as ketamine, dexmedetomidine, remifentanil, or midazolam will allow for light to moderate sedation with minimal respiratory depression, and will allow the operator to visualize ETT passage prior to paralysis. The ETT or an airway exchange catheter (e.g., Aintree catheter) is preloaded onto the endoscope scope, and the scope is introduced into the oropharynx. The use of a bite block or intubating oral airway is also helpful in keeping the mouth open and preventing damage to the scope from biting. Once the scope has passed the cords, the ETT can then be passed and the scope withdrawn. Only when the tube position is confirmed by end-tidal CO_2 waveform and the patient can easily be ventilated should deeper sedation and paralysis be considered.

Airway obstructions can be divided into upper (mouth, nasopharynx, and larynx), lower (bronchioles and alveoli), and central (trachea and bronchi) obstructions. The central airway compromises the area from below the vocal cords to the tracheal and mainstem bronchi. Central obstructions may be caused by infections, airway edema, foreign bodies, stenosis, strictures, congenital malformations, tumors, or hematomas. Among these, malignancy is the most common cause of central airway obstruction, but it is usually accompanied by signs of jugular venous obstruction (face and upper extremity swelling, headache, papilledema, jugular venous distention). Unfortunately, tracheal stenosis is an uncommon but potentially life-threatening cause of airway obstruction and is generally not associated with specific physical exam findings.

Tracheal stenosis is a rare (roughly 5%) but known complication of endotracheal intubation, lung transplant, previous tracheostomy, and radiation therapy to the neck. Post-extubation airway injuries are common. Studies that performed endoscopic exams after extubation have shown that up to 80% of patients have a laryngeal injury, most commonly edema (70%), with nearly 30% having granulation tissue and nearly 20% having glottic or subglottic stenosis; the number of injuries increased dramatically with prolonged intubations.[1,2] Post-intubation tracheal stenosis is caused by pressure necrosis of the tracheal mucosa from the ETT balloon, resulting in stricture. Tracheal edema may be noted when initially weaning from the ventilator, but stenosis typically does not become symptomatic for several weeks, depending on the degree of stenosis and other contributing factors such as illness, patient exertion, or other comorbidities. The size of the stenotic lumen as well as the time over which it develops determines the severity of the symptoms. Patients with severe tracheal stenosis will present with signs of hypoxia, tachypnea, wheezing, tachycardia, or stridor, while others may be completely asymptomatic until enough stenosis is present (usually at least 30% of the tracheal lumen size).

Diagnosis of tracheal stenosis requires a high degree of suspicion as it can be easily misdiagnosed as another disease process. Chest radiography can be easily performed in the patient's room but is neither sensitive nor specific for tracheal stenosis; however, special care should be taken to examine the tracheal air column. CT imaging of the chest can be useful in identifying compressive tumors, hematoma, and infectious processes of the trachea and surrounding tissues. Direct visualization by bronchoscopy is the best diagnostic tool to assess for subglottic stenosis. This may be done at bedside in the ED if equipment is available, although early consultation with appropriate specialists is prudent. Using flexible endoscopy to examine the airway also provides the added benefit of being combined with awake intubation.

The mainstay of treatment for subglottic stenosis in the ED is improving ventilation to prevent further decompensation. Heated high-flow nasal cannulas can reduce upper airway resistance, reduce work of breathing, and improve CO_2 clearance. Heliox can be useful to improve laminar flow around an upper airway obstruction and thus reduce work of breathing. Endotracheal intubation can bypass the obstruction, but the intubation itself can be very dangerous. The difficulty and the success rates of the intubation differ depending on the location and length of the stenotic area. If the lesion is proximal, securing the airway may be done by rigid oral laryngoscopy, often requiring a smaller ETT than would be typically used to allow passage of the tube past the stenotic area. If the lesion is distal, severely stenotic, or several centimeters in length, however, tube placement may be impossible by conventional means. Patients can be difficult to mask ventilate by either face mask or supraglottic airway device due to the subglottic restriction, and emergent front-of-neck access is likely to fail as it remains above the stenotic lesion. There has been success in using a supraglottic airway in the operating room on patients with known tracheal stenosis. These were found to be effective in providing adequate oxygenation and ventilation in 96.4% of cases, with 90.7% placed on first attempt.[3] If the stenosis is due to a previous tracheostomy and there is a patent stoma, an ETT or tracheostomy tube could be passed under endoscopic guidance, ensuring the lumen is beyond the stenotic lesion. Specialist consultation is highly recommended if the diagnosis is known or suspected prior to respiratory decline so that the airway may be secured in the controlled environment of the operating room. In some cases, identification of the lesion prior to intubation can lead to alternative methods of airway management, such as cannulation for veno-venous extracorporeal membrane oxygenation (ECMO) to permit bronchoscopic or surgical repair of the lesion without the need for a dangerous attempt at intubation.[4]

Patients with a history of laryngectomy provide a unique and uncommon challenge to airway management. These patients are obligate "neck breathers" with an end stoma, and any attempt to ventilate, oxygenate, or intubate orally will be impossible. Special care should be taken to obtain a good patient history when possible. McGrath et al. developed management guidelines and algorithms[5] for these uncommon airway emergencies, which are summarized here. If a stoma is present in a patient with hypoxia or respiratory distress and the patient history cannot be obtained, oxygen should be placed on both the face and stoma until more information can be obtained. Any buttons or inner cannulas should be removed from the devices (which are often not present in laryngectomy patients) and a suction catheter should be passed to clear any obstruction and to assess the patency of the tube or stoma. If the catheter does not pass, deflate the cuff (if present), feel for air movement, and use waveform capnography if available. If there is continued concern for obstruction, then the tube should be removed from the stoma. If there is a need to manually ventilate the patient, a bag-valve mask with a pediatric mask can be placed over the stoma. Finally, intubation of the stoma in adults with a small ETT (6.0 cuffed) using a fiberoptic scope, bougie, or exchange catheter may be necessary.

Montgomery T-tubes (T-tubes) are T-shaped silicone devices whose internal branches are placed within both the proximal and distal trachea while the external branch exits a stoma or tracheostomy site; this is used to secure the device externally (Figure 3.2). Indications for placement include tracheal stenosis, tracheal reconstruction, laryngotracheal injuries, or

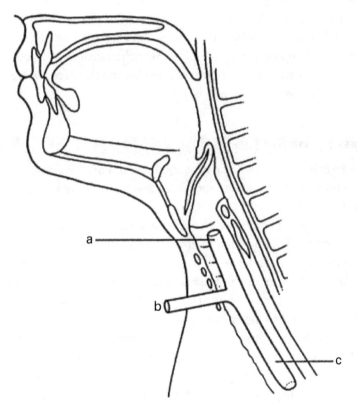

FIGURE 3.2 Artist's rendering of differences between tracheostomy, laryngectomy, and Montgomery T-tube

bridging to corrective surgery. There are potential complications of T-tubes, including mucous plugging and dislodgment. Proximal plugging is typically not life-threatening as the distal and external branches are generally sufficient for respiration. If there is obstruction in the distal tracheal or external branch and suctioning is not sufficient to restore patency, the T-tube can be removed through the stoma by using forceps and pulling the external branch firmly away from the neck.[6] If at all possible, this should be performed by the surgeon or service who placed the device unless the patient is in severe respiratory distress or cardiopulmonary arrest and the patency of the device is in question. After the device is removed, a non-rebreather mask or bag-valve mask may be applied at the stoma site and/or to the face. Attempts to ventilate the patient orally with a bag-valve mask may be inadequate if the stoma is not occluded or the T-tube external branch is not capped. Also, if a bag-valve mask is placed over the T-tube external branch, air leak from the proximal limb may prevent adequate ventilation. Additional care should be taken as tracheal stenosis and reconstruction is an indication for placement of a T-tube, and therefore passage of an ETT or tracheostomy tube may be difficult.

KEY POINTS TO REMEMBER

- A high index of suspicion is needed to diagnose tracheal stenosis in the ED and to recognize that endotracheal intubation may be difficult or even impossible.
- In patients with a potentially difficult airway, awake fiberoptic intubation could be used to prevent an "unable to intubate and unable to ventilate" situation.
- Signs and symptoms of tracheal stenosis are neither sensitive or specific but may include hypoxia, wheezing, tachypnea, tachycardia, and inspiratory stridor.
- Laryngectomy patients cannot be ventilated or oxygenated via the oropharynx, so the airway must be secured via the stoma.
- Montgomery T-tubes are T-shaped devices with internal branches in the proximal and distal trachea and an external branch exiting a stoma, which are used as either temporary or permanent airway stents.

· Early consultation with surgery or anesthesia is recommended in patients with complications of laryngectomies, Montgomery T-tubes, or tracheal stenosis.

References

1. Brodsky MB, Levy MJ, Jedlanek E, et al. Laryngeal injury and upper airway symptoms after oral endotracheal intubation with mechanical ventilation during critical care. *Crit Care Med.* 2018;46(12):2010–2017.

2. Tadié J-M, Behm E, Lecuyer L, et al. Post-intubation laryngeal injuries and extubation failure: A fiberoptic endoscopic study. *Intensive Care Med.* 2010;36(6):991–998.

3. Krecmerova M, Schutzner J, Michalek P, Johnson P, Vymazal T. Laryngeal mask for airway management in open tracheal surgery: A retrospective analysis of 54 cases. *J Thorac Dis.* 2018;10(5):2567–2572.

4. Natt B, Knepler J, Kazui T, Mosier JM. The use of extracorporeal membrane oxygenation in the bronchoscopic management of critical upper airway obstruction. *J Bronchology Interv Pulmonol.* 2017;24(1):e12–e14.

5. McGrath BA, Bates L, Atkinson D, Moore JA. Multidisciplinary guidelines for the management of tracheostomy and laryngectomy airway emergencies. *Anaesthesia.* 2012;67(9):1025–1041.

6. Touma O, Venugopal N, Allen G, Hinds J. Emergency airway management in a patient with a Montgomery T-tube in situ. *Br J Anaesth.* 2011;107(1):107–108.

Further reading

McGrath BA, Bates L, Atkinson D, Moore JA. Multidisciplinary guidelines for the management of tracheostomy and laryngectomy airway emergencies. *Anaesthesia.* 2012;67(9):1025–1041.

Touma O, Venugopal N, Allen G, Hinds J. Emergency airway management in a patient with a Montgomery T-tube in situ. *Br J Anaesth.* 2011;107(1):107–108.

Wain JC. Postintubation tracheal stenosis. *Semin Thorac Cardiovasc Surg.* 2009;21(3):284–289.

4 Physiologically difficult airways

Zachary J. Hernandez and Jarrod M. Mosier

A 52-year-old female with a history of pulmonary arterial hypertension (PAH) presents to a rural ED with a chief complaint of shortness of breath. The patient reports 5 days of increasing dyspnea on exertion and progressively worsening abdominal pain and now a fever for the past 2 days. Vital signs are HR 131 bpm, RR 43/min, O_2 saturation 64%, BP 96/63 mmHg, temperature 39.5°C. The patient is diaphoretic with intercostal retractions and in obvious extremis, but there are no anatomic predictors of a difficult intubation. Labs are notable for an ABG with pH 7.01, pCO_2 28, pO_2 45, bicarbonate 8, lactate 15, and WBC 24. The patient's partner reports that the patient follows regularly with a pulmonologist at a tertiary care center a few hours away and is compliant with all PAH medications.

What do I do now?

This is a classic presentation of a patient who is on the verge of cardiorespiratory arrest (i.e., walks in and codes). Several of the patient's characteristics signal the need for intubation and mechanical ventilation. The patient has very high work of breathing apparent on exam as diaphoresis, tachypnea, and intercostal retractions. This work of breathing cannot be maintained unassisted for much longer, and failure to intervene expeditiously will result in the patient's death. The patient's labs also show ominous signs. First, the patient's metabolic acidosis is inadequately compensated by their respiratory rate, leading to an accumulating respiratory acidosis. Second, the patient has hypoxemia (PaO_2 of 45 mmHg) that corresponds to their SpO_2 of 64%. However, the patient's pulmonary hypertension presents a unique challenge in terms of their cardiovascular pathophysiology creating a mixed shock state that must be handled with great care. While this patient needs to be intubated for impending respiratory failure, and has no signs of a difficult intubation, they present a high risk of peri-intubation cardiac arrest because of these physiologic abnormalities. We offer a methodologic approach to a physiologically difficult airway with emphasis on cardiovascular and metabolic optimization to avoid peri-intubation hemodynamic collapse in this patient.

This particular patient is in acute right ventricular (RV) failure secondary to decompensated PAH. Similar pathophysiology can be seen with acute massive pulmonary embolism, so the principles we set forth may be applied in that scenario as well. The right ventricle and pulmonary circulation is a low-pressure, high-compliance system. In high-afterload states, the RV adapts by increasing both contractility and preload, eventually progressing from dysfunction to overt failure characterized by RV dilation, tricuspid regurgitation, increased right atrial pressure, reduced cardiac output, and coronary perfusion, which in turn further decreases contractility. This process is often referred to as the RV death spiral.

The presence of hypoxemia during intubation confers an odds of cardiac arrest four times that of patients without hypoxemia. Thus, preoxygenation in this patient becomes critical for preventing desaturation resulting in cardiac arrest. A curious and unique characteristic of the lungs is that alveolar hypoxia results in vasoconstriction of the associated blood vessels, preserving a survivable ventilation/perfusion (V/Q) mismatch but also increasing pulmonary artery vasoconstriction and RV afterload. The extreme ends of the V/Q mismatch spectrum are shunt and dead space. V/Q mismatch generally responds to oxygen supplementation through autoregulatory mechanisms, and any atelectatic alveoli that can be recruited can reduce V/Q mismatch and thus reduce hypoxemia and RV afterload. This patient has also progressed to such severe respiratory failure that they are now unable to adequately blow off CO_2 and are now hypercapnic, which also further worsens pulmonary vascular resistance. The standard preoxygenation methods prior to intubation of a non-rebreathing mask will be inadequate in this patient. Peak inspiratory flows generated by patients in acute respiratory failure average between 30 and 40 L/min and in some instances mentioned in the literature, can even be as high as 120 L/min.[1,2] This means that there will likely be significant admixing of ambient air around the mask with the oxygen from the reservoir, reducing the effective FiO_2. A high-flow nasal cannula (HFNC) is the optimal way to address these issues in the patient with acute RV failure because it supplies sufficiently high flow and concentration of oxygen while avoiding positive intrathoracic pressure, which decreases preload. Ideally, the patient is placed on maximum flow rate (40–80 L/min) and FiO_2 (100%); then it can be titrated down or kept on until intubation (should it be necessary), depending on the patient's response. It should be said that the only potential disadvantage to this method of preoxygenation is that it may not be as effective as noninvasive ventilation in regards to CO_2 removal, but in this instance the sum total of the advantages provided by the therapy outweighs the disadvantage.[3,4]

If HFNC is unavailable, noninvasive positive-pressure ventilation (NIPPV) may be carefully administered when right-sided volume overload is considered or suspected. Ideally it is initiated with modest settings of 5/5 to avoid large shifts in preload but is best utilized in a scenario where the physician has determined that the patient has right-sided volume overload. In patients with severe hypoxemia (but not concurrent RV failure), NIPPV has been shown to potentially be better than HFNC, although robust data are lacking.[5] Additionally, preoxygenation with NIPPV will provide some insight into necessary ventilatory demand after intubation in patients with metabolic acidosis by evaluating the minute ventilation generated on NIPPV while spontaneously breathing.[6] If inhaled nitric oxide, epoprostenol, or milrinone is available, it can be added to dilate the pulmonary vasculature, thereby decreasing the afterload the RV is working against.

Next, attention must be given to assessing the patient's intravascular volume status. As mentioned before, the RV is not like the left ventricle (LV). The RV free wall is thin, with a low volume-to-surface ratio, which makes it poorly tolerant to acute elevations in afterload. RV systolic function occurs in three phases: papillary muscle contraction, inward movement of the free wall, and finally contraction of the LV, causing medial displacement of the interventricular septum toward the RV. In acute RV failure this displacement is reversed and the septum bows toward the LV, decreasing left-sided diastolic filling/function and decreasing the systemic arterial pressure. Point-of-care ultrasound (POCUS) at the bedside has become a common skill that most emergency physicians are trained in and is extremely valuable in determining whether decreased or increased right-sided preload is needed. A qualitative assessment of the inferior vena cava (IVC) is the quickest and easiest data point to obtain. A plethoric and full IVC with little to no respiratory variation signals that a patient could benefit from diuresis rather than volume resuscitation, which is a common, almost reflexive, response of the clinician to hypotension. In these cases, decreasing preload by means of diuresis or NIPPV brings the patient's RV "back on" to the Starling curve and actually improves right-sided cardiac output. More advanced measurements may be obtained to further quantify and characterize volume responsiveness of the RV if the physician is trained and feels comfortable interpreting them (see Chapter 15). Doppler velocity–time integral may be done very cautiously at the RV outflow tract before and after a small fluid challenge of either 250 mL crystalloid or a passive leg raise. Tricuspid annular plane systolic excursion is a commonly known measurement of RV systolic function but is load-dependent. A better measurement is isovolumic contraction velocity using tissue Doppler of the RV lateral wall, which can predict contractile reserve. McConnell's sign (akinesia of the mid-free RV wall) can be seen in patients with an acute massive pulmonary embolism and is a sign of previously healthy but now failing RV—in this instance, administration of systemic thrombolytics or transfer to a center capable of catheter-directed thrombolysis/thrombectomy should be considered.

After a decision is made regarding volume status and the appropriate intervention is started (either diuresis or fluid bolus), attention can be paid to more directly supporting the actual systolic function of the RV pharmacologically. The patient in our vignette is in a mixed shock state from RV failure and presumably sepsis (fever, tachycardia, leukocytosis, elevated lactate, abdominal pain). In this case the patient's systemic mean arterial pressure (MAP) is low due to decreased LV preload and decreased peripheral arterial resistance. There is some debate in the literature regarding the effects of various vasoactive drugs on pulmonary vascular resistance, but in our experience it is best to start a norepinephrine infusion at low doses and carefully titrate upward to an acceptable MAP of at least 65 in a floridly septic patient with RV failure. Other pure inotropes such as dobutamine would augment the contractility of the myocardium but come with the unwanted side effect of peripheral arterial vasodilation, which, again, would lower the systemic MAP. It should be emphasized that these therapies are merely to bridge the patient while the underlying mechanism of decompensation is addressed.

Once the initial resuscitation is done and the patient is optimized hemodynamically, a reassessment of the need for intubation and mechanical ventilation can be performed. If the patient continues to be hypoxic and repeat blood gases demonstrate non-improved acidosis incompatible with life, then this measure must be undertaken but with great care. When performed by a skilled operator, awake fiberoptic intubation (AFOI) is the preferred method to rapid sequence induction/intubation (RSI) because it avoids induction agents, which themselves can precipitate cardiovascular collapse in an already hypotensive patient, and the apnea that accompanies paralysis, which facilitates successful endotracheal intubation but may exacerbate hypoxemia and hypercarbic acidosis to the point of cardiac arrest. While a full discussion of AFOI is beyond the scope of this chapter, we still will emphasize a few key points here. First, maintaining HFNC therapy throughout the entire procedure is paramount and indeed one of the main advantages of the technique. Second, topical anesthesia of the naso/oropharynx is critical to successful AFOI. We prefer the use of 5% lidocaine ointment self-administered by the patient to the base of the tongue, followed by 4% aqueous lidocaine applied directly to the epiglottis and vocal cords via nebulization or flexible atomizer. Finally, if anxiolytics are required, we administer small serial doses of IV ketamine (10–20 mg) titrated to desired level of effect, or a low-dose dexmedetomidine infusion.

Ketamine is ideal in this situation because it has minimal negative effect on respiratory drive and in most cases has minimal negative effect on hemodynamics. If ketamine is unavailable, very small doses of midazolam could be considered, but this is not the first-line agent. If a fiberoptic scope is unavailable or the physician feels uncomfortable with this skill, then awake intubation with a video or direct laryngoscope may still be considered with similar pharmacologic adjuncts while maintaining spontaneous respiration and ideally with the patient in an upright or reclined position of no more than 45 degrees. Not all emergency physicians are comfortable with awake intubation as it does require some practice to maintain the technique, so if RSI is chosen as the method of attempted intubation, discussion of risks should be explained to the patient's surrogate decision-makers. In these cases, maximal optimization of the physiologic abnormalities prior to intubation become even more paramount to avoiding peri-intubation arrest, and preparation for peri-intubation arrest medications and team preparation communication are necessary. Hemodynamically neutral sedatives such as etomidate should be used for induction. After apnea is achieved with the paralytic, the emergency physician must "race to the trachea" in order to minimize time without ventilation as much as possible.[7,8]

After successful intubation, ventilator management is important to continue avoiding cardiovascular collapse in the severely physiologically deranged patient. Of course, ensuring the patient continues to avoid hypoxemia and hypercapnia is important. Ideally, minute ventilation matches the patient's own intrinsic drive prior to intubation, and this is most safely achieved by means of a high set respiratory rate on the ventilator. Permissive hypercapnia is a principle of lung protective ventilation that cannot be applied to the patient in RV failure as it can increase the pulmonary vascular resistance—we recommend attempting to achieve respiratory alkalosis. Perhaps the most salient point of post-intubation ventilator management is minimizing large changes in intrathoracic pressure, so a volume control mode with a low set tidal volume is best. Again, a large intrathoracic pressure that significantly decreases preload could affect the relatively fragile RV to the point of collapse; therefore, avoid excessive use of positive end-expiratory pressure (PEEP). Atelectasis also increases pulmonary vascular resistance, so it should be avoided with judicious use of PEEP (5–8 cmH$_2$O). A high MAP increases pulmonary vascular resistance and RV afterload;

therefore, it would be useful to continue inhaled pulmonary vasodilators through the ventilator circuit. These directly decrease afterload on the RV and improve V/Q mismatch, thereby improving oxygenation.

In patients requiring intubation in the ED, special attention must be paid not only to anatomic abnormalities that make the intubation technically difficult but also to physiologic abnormalities that place the patient at extremely high risk for peri-intubation cardiac arrest. This requires some basic familiarity with several pathophysiologic states, including hypoxemia, metabolic acidosis, and right-sided heart failure, which may be due to pulmonary hypertension or an acute PE. Emergency physicians are well trained to utilize advanced technologies such as POCUS and AFOI to facilitate the successful intubation of the severely physiologically deranged patient.

KEY POINTS TO REMEMBER

- Critically ill patients may be at higher risk for peri-intubation cardiac arrest because of physiologic/metabolic abnormalities (i.e., RV dysfunction/failure, systemic hypotension, hypoxemia, hypercapnia, metabolic acidosis).
- Correcting or improving these abnormalities through resuscitation before intubation will decrease the risk of peri-intubation cardiac arrest.
- Use HFNC or NIPPV with modest settings to preoxygenate prior to intubation. If available, inhaled pulmonary vasodilators (iNO, epoprostenol, milrinone) are extremely helpful in improving RV function and V/Q matching.
- Volume status assessment/optimization through fluids or diuresis and early use of pressors (we suggest norepinephrine) are recommended given the relatively fragile nature and limited reserve of the RV and its generally poor tolerance of overdistention from fluid boluses.
- In some patients, the physiologic abnormalities are refractory to the above. In those patients, awake intubation is the safest path forward.

. Ventilator management after intubation should be focused on continuing to correct hypoxemia and hypercarbia while limiting large shifts in intrathoracic pressure in patients with RV failure.

References

1. Mosier JM. Physiologically difficult airway in critically ill patients: Winning the race between haemoglobin desaturation and tracheal intubation. *Br J Anaesth.* 2020;125(1):e1–e4.
2. De Jong A, Rolle A, Molinari N, et al. Cardiac arrest and mortality related to intubation procedure in critically ill adult patients: A multicenter cohort study. *Crit Care Med.* 2018;46(4):532–539.
3. Mosier JM, Hypes CD, Sakles JC. Understanding preoxygenation and apneic oxygenation during intubation in the critically ill. *Intensive Care Med.* 2017;43(2):226–228.
4. Frat JP, Ricard JD, Quenot JP, et al. Non-invasive ventilation versus high-flow nasal cannula oxygen therapy with apnoeic oxygenation for preoxygenation before intubation of patients with acute hypoxaemic respiratory failure: A randomised, multicentre, open-label trial. *Lancet Respir Med.* 2019;7(4):303–312.
5. Fong KM, Au SY, Ng GWY. Preoxygenation before intubation in adult patients with acute hypoxemic respiratory failure: A network meta-analysis of randomized trials. *Crit Care.* 2019;23(1):319.
6. Mosier JM, Sakles JC, Law JA, Brown CA, 3rd, Brindley PG. Tracheal intubation in the critically ill: Where we came from and where we should go. *Am J Resp Crit Care Med.* 2020;201(7):775–788.
7. Mosier JM, Joshi R, Hypes C, Pacheco G, Valenzuela T, Sakles JC. The physiologically difficult airway. *West J Emerg Med.* 2015;16(7):1109–1117.
8. Natt BS, Malo J, Hypes CD, Sakles JC, Mosier JM. Strategies to improve first attempt success at intubation in critically ill patients. *Br J Anaesth.* 2016;117(Suppl 1):i60–i68.

Further reading

Cutts S, Talboys R, Paspula C, Prempeh EM, Fanous R, Ail D. Adult respiratory distress syndrome. *Ann Royal Coll Surg Engl.* 2017;99(1):12–16.
Dalabih M, Rischard F, Mosier JM. What's new: The management of acute right ventricular decompensation of chronic pulmonary hypertension. *Intensive Care Med.* 2014;40(12):1930–1933.
Treacher DF, Leach RM. Oxygen transport 1: Basic principles. *BMJ.* 1998;317(7168):1302–1306.

5 Coughing up blood: Massive hemoptysis

Jeremiah Garrison and
Cameron Hypes

A 65-year-old man presents with a chief complaint of cough and shortness of breath. He notes a 10-lb weight loss, night sweats, and fatigue for the past month. Today his cough was productive of a moderate amount of bright-red blood. He has a history of COPD and alcoholic cirrhosis. He is currently homeless and has a history of IV drug use. On examination, he is disheveled with a continuous cough. His vital signs are notable for mild tachycardia and BP 100/60 mmHg. Between coughs he is breathing at a rate of 18/min and his oxygen saturation on room air is 92%. He is afebrile. He has mild bilateral expiratory wheezes with diminished breath sounds and rales on the left. As you finish your examination, his cough becomes productive of a cupful of bright red blood.

What do I do now?

Care for the patient presenting with hemoptysis first involves stratifying the patient's bleeding as mild, moderate, or massive. Massive hemoptysis has been variably defined in studies and texts, but its most important feature is the clinical effect on the patient's hemodynamics and gas exchange.[1,2] Thus, care revolves around airway management, with rapid diagnosis and mobilization of consultants. Patients with mild or moderate hemoptysis may require a nuanced workup for infection or autoimmune diseases. This patient is presenting with risk factors for mild hemoptysis, including COPD with likely chronic bronchitis and coagulopathy from his cirrhosis (Box 5.1). His social history, which included homelessness and IV drug use, puts him at risk for more significant causes of hemoptysis such as malignancy, tuberculosis, and necrotizing pneumonia, which is especially concerning given his worsening clinical picture.

Before initial management, it must be noted that precautions should be taken to prevent the spread of infectious disease from patients with uncontrolled hemoptysis. In most patients this means universal precautions with appropriate garb and facemasks due to the risk of HIV and hepatitis B and C transmission. In patients at high risk for tuberculosis, consider moving the patient to an appropriate negative-pressure room.

BOX 5.1 **Common causes of hemoptysis**

Malignancy
Infections (e.g., tuberculosis, fungal, necrotizing pneumonia)
Arteriovenous malformation
Iatrogenic (e.g., Swan–Ganz placement, airway stent, biopsy complication)
Aortic aneurysm
Trauma
Pulmonary embolism
Medications (e.g., cocaine, anticoagulants)
Autoimmune diseases (e.g., systemic lupus erythematosus, ANCA-associated vasculitides, anti-GBM disease)
Bronchiectasis (e.g., COPD, cystic fibrosis, sarcoidosis)
Hematologic disorders (e.g., von Willebrand disease, disseminated intravascular coagulation [DIC], idiopathic thrombocytopenic purpura [ITP])

Most likely causes of massive hemoptysis are bolded.

Initial management is to assess for airway patency, adequacy of gas exchange, and work of breathing; if these are unacceptable, the patient should be intubated. Patients otherwise should be allowed to assume a position of comfort and provided with a Yankauer suction catheter to maximize their ability to clear their own airway. Airway equipment should be brought to the bedside and the patient placed on the monitor. Two large-bore IVs should be placed, as with any other bleeding patient. A portable chest radiograph will often localize the bleed unless it is diffuse. The bleeding lung should then be placed in a dependent position. Supplemental oxygen should be provided, but many patients will only tolerate nasal oxygen. In intubated patients, many physicians practice using increased positive end-expiratory pressure (PEEP) with the thought that this may stanch bleeding, but this has not been systematically evaluated. The value of PEEP in non-intubated patients with noninvasive positive-pressure ventilation (NIPPV; e.g., BIPAP) is even less clear in patients with hemoptysis.[3]

If the patient is stable without the need for emergent intubation, a rapid focused workup should begin. In addition to chest imaging (CT angiography), a laboratory evaluation for anemia, thrombocytopenia, coagulopathy (e.g., PT, PTT, fibrinogen), and uremia (as it predisposes to platelet dysfunction) should be performed, and a type and screen should be sent. A focused history to evaluate for use of antiplatelet agents or anticoagulants should be taken. Anticoagulation should be stopped and coagulopathy corrected where possible, with consideration given to both risks and benefits in high-risk cases such as patients with mechanical aortic valves, fresh coronary stents, or mechanical circulatory support devices. Appropriate cultures and antibiotics should be ordered if there is concern for infection. Use of nebulized tranexamic acid has been suggested, although the efficacy has yet to be proven and the ideal patient population is unclear.[4,5] A focused physical exam should be performed to rule out mimics of hemoptysis (e.g., posterior epistaxis, hematemesis), evaluate for trauma in cases where the history is unclear, and assess for stigmata of liver failure (e.g., cirrhosis, caput medusae, telangiectasias).

While many patients with massive hemoptysis will need to be intubated, the cough reflex is an effective method of clearing the airway and will be sacrificed by intubation. Use of intubation should be limited to those who suffer respiratory failure or hemodynamic instability unless otherwise required for necessary workup or management. If intubation is considered, advanced airway equipment should be made available, including videolaryngoscopy (VL), flexible fiberoptic bronchoscope, and a surgical airway kit. Traditionally, direct laryngoscopy (DL) is recommended over VL for the bloody airway. Newer technology has improved the visibility of VL and data suggest equivalent first-pass success with VL or DL in hematemesis, but data are lacking for hemoptysis.[6,7] A VL blade with traditional, non-hyperangulated geometry that can be used for VL and DL is optimal. A backup intubating laryngeal mask airway (LMA) should be available in case of intubation failure as the patient could then be intubated without visual confirmation.

Beyond the choice of device, there are a few other considerations in the safe intubation of patients with hemoptysis. Adequate suction should be made available, either with two Yankauer suction catheters on maximum continuous suction or ideally a large-bore suction device. The advantage of some of these large-bore suction catheters (e.g., DuCanto catheter, SSCOR) is that they can be used to intubate by placing them into the trachea and passing a bougie through them. The type of endotracheal tube (ETT) used should be 8.0 or larger if possible to prevent clogging of the tube with clot and to facilitate bronchoscopy, which may be required depending on the cause of the hemoptysis.

Localizing the source of hemoptysis is a crucial step and is needed both for diagnosis and, in cases of large-volume hemoptysis, for guiding therapy. A basic idea as to localization can be obtained by chest radiograph. In cases where bleeding is more than trivial and not explained by a clinical diagnosis such as bronchitis or pneumonia, CT angiography should be performed as it can identify a wide variety of causes, such as pulmonary embolism (PE), tumors, infections, diffuse alveolar hemorrhage (DAH), and arteriovenous malformations. The contrast should be timed for the systemic arterial phase rather than the pulmonary arterial phase (e.g., CT for PE), as 90% of massive hemoptysis arises from the bronchial arteries due to the higher pressures involved.[8]

Definitive management will depend on the underlying cause of hemoptysis as well as the location and volume of the bleeding, in addition to the stability of the patient. Available interventions are highly variable depending on both the size of the hospital and the training of the specialists; some have suggested a multidisciplinary approach to managing massive hemoptysis with early consultation with interventional pulmonologists and radiologists as well as thoracic surgery in the most unstable patients.[9] Initial evaluation may be made with a rigid or flexible bronchoscope, with the objective being to better localize bleeding, and in cases of DAH or infection bronchoalveolar lavage can be diagnostic. Bronchoscopy may be necessary for airway clearance in patients with refractory hypoxemia due to impaired gas exchange.[10] In select cases bronchoscopic methods may be used to stop or temporize bleeding, such as by instilling epinephrine (1:10 dilution of 1 mL of 1 mg epinephrine 1:1,000 with 9 mL sterile saline, a for final concentration of 100 mcg/mL, and instilling 1 or 2 mL at a time), cauterizing bleeding airway masses, or placing bronchial blockers to tamponade bleeding and prevent the blood from flowing into the healthy lung. In cases of DAH treatment is determined by whether the hemorrhage is bland or a result of capillaritis and typically is focused on the underlying cause (e.g., coagulopathy, valvular pathology, rheumatologic condition, pulmonary-renal syndromes). In cases of localized bleeding an interventional radiologist should be contacted for consideration of bronchial artery embolization, and this has become the first-line intervention for most presentations of massive hemoptysis.[11] In the dire situations, a trauma surgeon or cardiothoracic surgeon may be able to control bleeding through thoracotomy with lobectomy.

The sequence of interventions and diagnostics will be highly variable depending on the severity of the hemoptysis, the available resources (e.g., CT, bronchoscopy, interventional radiology, pulmonology, thoracic surgery), and the patient's history and imaging findings in terms of the cause of hemoptysis, its severity, the ability to localize it, and the patient's prognosis with associated goals of care. Cases in which the history or imaging suggests a known localized source (e.g., lung malignancy) will generally be more amenable to intervention. While imaging and complex multispecialty consultation are occurring, temporizing measures such as placing the affected side down, selective mainstem intubation, and bronchoscopic methods buy time to plan and implement more definite management.

Once the hemoptysis has been risk stratified based on the suspected etiology and appropriate initial efforts to treat and stabilize the patient have been initiated, the patient will need to be dispositioned. Select low-risk patients with scant hemoptysis due to chronic bronchitis or mild pneumonia may be discharged with close follow-up by the pulmonary service, but most other patients will need to be admitted. Those with risk factors for or findings of massive hemoptysis should be admitted to an ICU, preferably at a center with interventional radiology services.

References
1. Benson A, Albert R. Chapter 57: Massive hemoptysis. In: Hall J, Schmidt G, eds. *Principles of Critical Care*. 4th ed. McGraw Hill Education; 2015.
2. Ibrahim W. Massive haemoptysis: The definition should be revised. *Eur Respir J*. 2008;32(4):1131–1132.
3. Flume P, Mogayzel P, Robinson K, Rosenblatt R, Quittell L, Marshall B. Cystic fibrosis pulmonary guidelines: Pulmonary complications: Hemoptysis and pneumothorax. *Am J Respir Crit Care Med*. 2010;82(3):298–306.
4. Solomonov A, Fruchter O, Zuckerman T, Brenner B, Yigla M. Pulmonary hemorrhage: A novel mode of therapy. *Respir Med*. 2009;103(8):1196–1200.
5. Wand O, Guber E, Guber A, Epstein Shochet G, Israeli-Shani L, Shitrit D. Inhaled tranexamic acid for hemoptysis treatment: A randomized controlled trial. *Chest*. 2018;154(6):1379–1384.
6. Carlson J, Crofts J, Walls R, Brown III C. Direct versus video laryngoscopy for intubating adult patients with gastrointestinal bleeding. *West J Emerg Med*. 2015;16(7):1052–1056.
7. Sakles J, Corn G, Hollinger P, Arcaris B, Patanwala A, Mosier J. The impact of a soiled airway on intubation success in the emergency department when using the Glidescope or the direct laryngoscope. *Acad Emerg Med*. 2017;24(5):628–636.
8. Gupta A, Sands M, Chauhan NR. Massive hemoptysis in pulmonary infections: Bronchial artery embolization. *J Thorac Dis*. 2018;10(Supp 28):S3458–S3464.
9. Sakr L, Dutau H. Massive hemoptysis: An update on the role of bronchoscopy in diagnosis and management. *Respiration*. 2010;1:38–58.
10. Radchenko C, Alraiyes AH, Shojaee S. A systematic approach to the management of massive hemoptysis. *J Thorac Dis*. 2017;9(Supp 10):S1069–S1086.
11. Kathuria H, Hollingsworth HM, Vilvendhan R, Reardon C. Management of life-threatening hemoptysis. *J Intensive Care*. 2020;8:23.

PART 2

Breathing

Problems outside the lung: Pneumothorax and pleural effusions

John Bruno and Jennifer Axelband

A 48-year-old male with a past medical history of current alcohol abuse and type 2 diabetes mellitus presents to the ED with dyspnea and altered mental status. He has been staying at a shelter, and the staff noted the patient to have abnormal breathing and mild confusion this morning. One week ago, he had been admitted for 24 hours for community-acquired pneumonia. He received IV ceftriaxone and was discharged on cephalexin. The patient states he feels unwell but does not offer any other acute complaints. He admits inconsistently taking his antibiotics but did finish most of them. The patient appears acutely ill and diaphoretic.

Vital signs: HR 130 bpm, BP 100/46 mmHg, RR 30/min, oxygen saturation 86% improving to 92% on nonrebreather mask, temperature 102.3°F

Physical exam

Cardiovascular: Tachycardia, regular rhythm, no murmur

Pulmonary: Tachypnea, decreased breath sounds right hemithorax with diffuse right-sided rhonchi with faint end-expiratory wheezing, basilar rales bilaterally

Neurologic: Confused to date and place, non-focal motor exam

Psychological: Anxious

What do I do now?

The differential diagnosis is quite broad for both sepsis and hypoxia. Considering his recent hospitalization for pneumonia, physical examination findings, vital signs, and past medical history, the greatest concern would be worsening of a partially treated infection. Significant findings on presentation include leukocytosis, elevated lactic acid, elevated glucose, low serum bicarbonate, and elevated creatinine, and CXR showed opacification of the right hemithorax.

Pleural effusions, defined as a collection of fluid in the pleural space, are caused by diseases of the lung or the pleura. The incidence may approach 1.5 million total cases annually, and pleural effusions are similarly prevalent in surgical, cardiac, and medical ICUs.[1,2] They are clinically important, as retrospective data suggest that patients with pleural effusion have a significantly higher in-hospital and 1-year mortality, and effusions are associated with longer ICU stays and longer durations of mechanical ventilation.[1] Therapeutic drainage of pleural effusion may alleviate symptoms—with the caveat that drainage is associated with a higher mortality, although this may simply represent a sicker patient population.[1]

Effusions can be further classified as transudative or exudative based on Light's criteria (Table 6.1), a categorization that has both diagnostic and therapeutic implications. Transudative effusions can be caused by congestive heart failure (CHF), cirrhosis, nephrotic syndrome, pulmonary embolus, and hypoalbuminemia. The etiology of exudative effusions can include malignancy, bacterial pneumonia, viral etiology, post-cardiothoracic surgery, collagen vascular disease, or pulmonary embolus. Malignancy, pneumonia, and CHF account for 75% of pleural effusions. The majority of effusions diagnosed in critically ill patients are exudative.[1,2] The etiology of up to 20% of effusions may remain unclear.[3]

The diagnosis of pleural effusion can be established with lung ultrasound (LUS), CXR, or a chest CT scan. An effusion on LUS will appear as an echo-free space between the visceral and parietal pleura. LUS can also be helpful in differentiating transudative from exudative effusion and in facilitating procedural drainage.[4] Sensitivity of LUS is superior to CXR in initial diagnosis, especially in critically ill or recumbent patients. Supine films often will miss sizeable effusions.[5] Chest CT is useful for complex effusions with obscured anatomy that cannot be fully appreciated on LUS or CXR, and can distinguish empyema from lung abscess.[2,3,5]

	Pleural fluid assessment	
	Transudate	Exudate
Light's criteria		
Protein (pleural/serum)	≤0.5	>0.5
LDH (pleural/serum)	≤0.6	>0.6
Pleural LDH	Less than or equal to two-thirds upper normal serum LDH	More than two-thirds upper normal serum LDH
Additional tests to assist in diagnosis		
Albumin (serum/pleural)	>1.2 g/dL	≤1.2 g/dL
NT-ProBNP >1,500 (serum)	>1,500 pg/mL	
WBC differential:		
Neutrophil		Pulmonary Emboli, pneumonia, parapneumonia, empyema pancreatitis
Lymphocyte		Cancer, TB pleuritis, post CABG, CHF
Eosinophils		Pneumothorax, hemothorax, asbestosis, malignancy
Mononuclear		Chronic inflammatory process

Once a pleural effusion is identified, pleural fluid should be obtained for sampling, and the results may change management in up to 56% of cases. Thoracentesis is recommended if effusion thickness is >2 cm on CT or LUS or >10 mm on lateral CXR; if pleural thickening or irregularity on imaging is present; or if the patient appears ill.[1,2] Pleural fluid should be sampled and evaluated with Light's criteria; pleural cell counts can also be helpful diagnostically (see Table 6.1).[2,5] Pleural pH should be obtained in a blood gas specimen collector. In the setting of parapneumonic effusion a pleural pH <7.2 is the most specific determinant of complicated, infected effusion requiring prompt therapeutic drainage.[5,6] Additional studies can be helpful in identifying the etiology of the effusion but need to be interpreted carefully. A high serum/pleural albumin ratio is associated with transudative effusions but can be misleading and result in overdiagnosis in some patients. Pleural amylase may indicate pancreatitis, but levels can also be elevated in esophageal rupture or ectopic pregnancy. The diagnostic utility of amylase is low, and obtaining this level is not routinely indicated.[5] Rheumatoid arthritis (RA) is an uncommon cause of pleural effusion that can mimic parapneumonic effusion. It is associated with very low pleural glucose levels, such that a pleural glucose value >29 is thought to exclude RA as an etiology.[5] Chylothorax is typically a right-sided effusion with a high pleural triglyceride content. Pseudochylothorax has a thick white effusion fluid similar to chylothorax but without triglyceride content and is usually secondary to chronic fibrotic effusions. It is diagnosed by identifying cholesterol crystals in the effusion. If there is concern for infected effusions, both aerobic and anaerobic cultures should be obtained, although as many as 70% of infected effusions will be culture negative.[4,7] Acid-fast cultures have a particularly low yield, if there is clinical concern for mycobacterium effusion, a biopsy may be indicated (Table 6.2).[2]

Indications for therapeutic, as opposed to diagnostic, drainage of a noninfected pleural effusion are more complex and require more insight into the etiology and pathophysiology of each effusion. Therapeutic thoracentesis is a method of temporary drainage with an overall low rate of complications and can be useful if continuous drainage is not required. Larger and malignant pleural effusions have 30-day recurrence rates as high as 98%. Repeat thoracentesis is typically not definitive for resolution and is rarely recommended as serial drainage can cause the development of adhesions that can complicate further attempts.[2,8,9] Bilateral effusions are often transudative and are commonly secondary to CHF. Thoracentesis is not routinely performed in CHF patients unless there is severe dyspnea or atypical features.[5]

If continuous drainage is indicated (e.g., in source control of an infected effusion), a chest tube should be placed. A small-bore chest tube is likely less

TABLE 6.2 **Other pleural findings that may help narrow the differential diagnosis of pleural effusion**

Common findings on pleural fluid analysis

Transudative effusion	NT-ProBNP > 1,500 Lymphocyte predominance
Esophageal perforation	Elevated amylase
Pancreatitis	Elevated amylase
Chylothorax	Right-sided effusion: elevated triglycerides
Pseudochylothorax	Cholesterol crystals absent triglycerides
Parapneumonic effusion	Neutrophil predominance pH < 7.2 (most specific) LDH > 1,000 Glucose < 60 Elevated CRP
Empyema	Grossly purulent effluent
Mycobacterium infection	Lymphocyte predominance pH > 7.3 Normal glucose
Malignancy	Lymphocyte predominance malignant cells
Ectopic pregnancy	Elevated amylase

painful and is the recommended modality of drainage for simple fluid. A larger-bore tube has no significant difference in successful drainage. Small-bore chest tubes are generally placed over a guidewire via the Seldinger technique.[2,5,10] Placement of large-bore chest tubes involves an incision, blunt dissection, and blunt penetration of the pleura. Benefits of the blunt technique include increased speed in skilled providers and the ability to perform a finger sweep to confirm appropriate placement. Use of trocars to guide placement is associated with a high rate of ectopic placement and therefore should never be used.[11] Large-bore thoracostomy can be considered in complex effusions, postoperative effusions, and hemothorax, as well as large bronchopleural fistula. Complications of chest tube placement include tube dislodgement, infection, ectopic tube placement, visceral injury, intercostal artery laceration, iatrogenic hemothorax, and re-expansion pulmonary edema (REPE).[9,11] Use of ultrasound to guide chest tube placement decreases the risk of complications by up to 50%, and in the case of thoracentesis, LUS significantly decreases the risk of iatrogenic pneumothorax (PTX).[2,5,7]

REPE is one of the more rare, serious side effects of pleural effusion drainage, with a mortality as high as 20%.[2] REPE is associated with poor baseline functional status, large volumes of drainage, and longer duration of lung collapse. Pain during effusion drainage is associated with excessive negative pressure and should signal termination of the procedure.[2] Total pleural drainage should be limited to <1.5 L during a single procedure. Once a collection chamber is connected to wall suction, negative pressures in excess of –20 mmHg should be avoided.[2,5,9] Continuous positive airway pressure (CPAP) may be considered in high-risk patients to reduce intrapleural negative pressure during drainage, though this has not been shown to prevent REPE or improve outcomes and therefore is not routinely recommended. Treatment of REPE is largely supportive and often includes positive-pressure ventilation (noninvasive or intubation).

Regardless of technique, chest tubes should be placed in the "triangle of safety," which is located in the region of the lateral chest bounded anteriorly by the pectoralis muscle, laterally by the latissimus dorsi, inferiorly by the inframammary fold or fifth intercostal space, and superiorly by the base of the axilla. Chest tubes should be placed immediately superior to the rib to avoid vascular injury. More posterior insertion sites may be dangerous as the neurovascular bundle may descend from the costal groove into the intercostal space at this location. Anterior sites, such as the midclavicular line, are less preferred due to the risk of visceral injury and visible scars. Also, penetrating the pectoralis muscle is not ideal and the intercostal space is more narrow anteriorly.[5,12] When placing a chest tube for pleural effusion the patient should be positioned slightly upright at 45 to 60 degrees with a slight rotation toward the side of placement and the patient's upper extremity elevated and behind the neck or head. The initial incision should be several centimeters below the desired upper rib edge to allow for tunneling, as this may prevent PTX when the chest tube is removed.[12] The sentinel hole should be positioned 2 cm deeper than the rib margin to ensure proper location in the pleura, as placement in the soft tissue can lead to subcutaneous emphysema.[12] The chest tube should be directed posteriorly and basilar for pleural effusion drainage, and directed superiorly and anteriorly for placement in PTX (Figure 6.1).

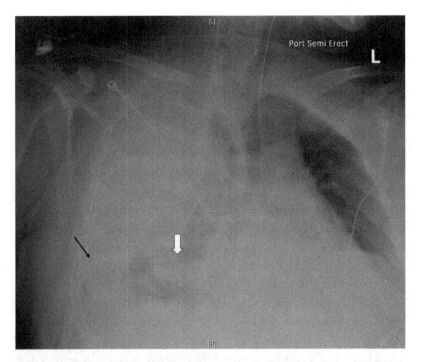

FIGURE 6.1 CXR with insertion of chest tube and incomplete drainage of effusion. Black arrow identifies chest tube. White block arrow identifies sentinel hole of chest tube.

Timing of removal of chest tubes varies in practice. A general recommendation for removal is when output is <100 to 200 mL in 24 hours. Some consider persistent air leak to be a contraindication to removal.[13] PTX recurrence is the most common complication of chest tube removal, yet routine CXR after chest tube removal rarely changes management and is not routinely recommended. There is currently no definitive evidence to provide a strong recommendation for the most effective method of removal; however, the majority of guidelines recommend chest tube removal during the expiratory phase of the respiratory cycle to minimize the recurrence rate.[13] Patients not appropriate for removal may be discharged with chest tubes in place with Heimlich valves, portable drainage devices, or digital drainage systems.

Despite conventional treatment as described above, treatment failure rates are quite high. In the case of empyema, the treatment failure rate approaches 33% and the patient will require further treatment modalities. Bronchopleural fistula and trapped lung are other examples unlikely to improve without surgical intervention.[7] Malignant effusions often require more definitive intervention, even if only for palliative purposes. Tunneled pleural catheters (TPCs) are indicated in cases of nonexpandable lung with persistent recurrent effusions and can be utilized in both benign and malignant effusions.[8] TPCs are useful in providing significant relief of symptoms, reducing rehospitalization rates, improving quality of life, and lowering complication rates compared to pleurodesis.[2,8] Talc pleurodesis involves administration of a chemical irritant into the pleural space, leading to adhesion of the visceral and parietal pleura and promoting lung re-expansion and effusion resolution. Talc has a 30% 1-month failure rate, and the rate increases with duration from the procedure date.[8]

Depending on the effusion etiology, treatment failures may respond to additional therapies. For infected effusions, antibiotic adjustments, additional drain placement, or pleural space instillation of dornase and tPA can be considered. In the MIST2 trial, instilling 5 mg DNase and 10 mg tPA mixed in 30 cc of sterile water twice daily for 3 days resulted in decreased effusion size and decreased need for surgery, and the hospital length of stay was shortened by a median of 6 to 7 days; however, it did not confer mortality benefit.[14] Video-assisted thoracoscopic surgery (VATS) may be required for definitive management, especially in the setting of bronchopleural fistula, trapped lung, or fibrothorax. VATS allows visualization of the pleural space, facilitates biopsy or sampling, and can also assist in therapeutic drainage and exploration of locules or pleurodesis.[2,5]

PTX, another commonly encountered pleural pathologic process, is managed somewhat similarly to pleural effusion, however with some unique nuances. The incidence of spontaneous PTX is ~24 in 100,000, with an overall low mortality. It is three times more common in males, and other risk factors include smoking/vaping and tall stature. Connective tissue disorders such as Marfan's disease and Ehlers–Danlos disease are also associated with increased risk of PTX. PTX can be subdivided into primary (in the absence of known lung disease) or secondary. Many patients with "primary" PTX are found to have previously undiagnosed lung disease and are eventually reclassified as secondary. Diagnosis of PTX on examination, confirmed with LUS, CXR, or CT, is common in hemodynamically stable patient presentations.

Management of primary PTX with minimal symptoms in young, healthy individuals should begin with supplemental O_2 and observation. The estimated rate of resorption is between 1.25% and 2.2% the volume of the PTX per day, which is accelerated up to four-fold with application of a high-flow nasal cannula or 100% nonrebreather. Many patients will not require ICU admission, and conservative management with oxygen and without chest tube placement, with improvement confirmed on repeat CXR in 4 to 6 weeks, requires no invasive interventions. A large PTX requires decompression, often via tube thoracostomy. However, the British Thoracic Society guidelines recommend an initial attempt at manual aspiration. This can be performed with or without ultrasound guidance. An 18g catheter is placed into the thoracic cavity; once air is aspirated, the catheter is advanced and secured to the skin. Air is manually aspirated with a 60-cc syringe and a three-way stopcock until resistance is met. If PTX does not improve on reimaging, then a tube thoracostomy (small bore (<14 French) Seldinger or large bore (28 French)) should be performed, with initial placement to low intermittent wall suction. This algorithm has a success rate similar to that of initial tube thoracostomy, with 60% of PTX cases successfully treated with aspiration alone. There is a decrease in hospitalization rates and a theoretical decrease in pain and complication rates.[14]

Secondary PTX often warrants surgical intervention after the first incident, given the high recurrence rate and presence of pulmonary disease. Interventions commonly performed include bullectomy, chemical pleurodesis, VATS with either chemical or mechanical pleurodesis, and open surgery. Chemical pleurodesis has a similar success rate with fewer incidences of complications compared to surgery.

Tension PTX, defined as complete unilateral PTX and associated hemodynamic collapse, is a clinical diagnosis based on high pretest probability of PTX and concomitant hemodynamic instability with classic exam findings such as tracheal deviation, jugular venous distention, and either severe tachycardia or bradycardia. It is immediately life-threatening and requires prompt intervention. If readily available, point-of-care LUS can aid in this diagnosis. Classically, management has been needle thoracostomy and decompression via the second intercostal space at the midclavicular line. This procedure is fraught with complications, including risks of pleural puncture and subsequent creation of pneumothorax, cardiac or large-vessel injury, and intrapulmonary placement. Therapeutic success is impacted by body habitus, which can limit ability to reach the pleural cavity with an angiocatheter.[15] Failure rates may approach 33%. Based on recent literature, Advanced Trauma Life Support now recommends decompression of the thoracic cavity in the fourth or fifth intercostal space in the mid-axillary line for adult patients. Finger thoracotomy at the mid-axillary line with pleural exploration can ensure adequate decompression and eliminate tension physiology rapidly, and is considered superior to needle thoracostomy for pleural decompression.[15] Tube thoracostomy can be performed at the same site after decompression, once the patient is stabilized.

The vignette at the start of the chapter describes a 48-year-old male with a history of alcohol abuse and likely incompletely treated pneumonia, now with worsening fevers and hypoxia. Given the patient's risk factors, this is concerning for empyema, a type of parapneumonic effusion. Parapneumonic effusions are a subtype of exudative effusions and may complicate as many as 20% to 57% bacterial pneumonias. The incidence of pleural infection is increasing globally due to increasing occurrence of *Staphylococcus aureus* and emerging serotypes of *Streptococcus pneumoniae* not covered by the pneumococcal vaccine.[7] Alcohol abuse is the most important risk factor; other risk factors include poor dental hygiene, IV drug abuse, malnutrition, and gastroesophageal reflux disease (GERD). These all confer increased aspiration risk.[4] Immunosuppressed patients and those with partially treated pneumonia are also at higher risk. The most common symptoms are fever, cough, fatigue, and weight loss as well as pleuritic chest pain and dyspnea. Persistent fever in pneumonia despite treatment with antibiotics should raise concern for development of a parapneumonic effusion. The most severe type of parapneumonic effusion is empyema, which is defined by the accumulation of pus in the pleural space, and carries a mortality rate of 15% to 30%.[2,4] Management requires drainage and is typically associated with prolonged hospital length of stay and courses of antibiotics. Conventional treatment of empyema carries a high rate of treatment failure, and successful management often requires a multidisciplinary team of intensivists, pulmonologists, and thoracic surgeons.[2,13]

· LUS and CT are both more sensitive and specific than CXR. LUS has a high sensitivity for detecting the presence of loculations, but CT may have more utility in characterizing details regarding complex effusions.

· A first episode of stable primary spontaneous PTX can be managed noninvasively if small. A larger primary spontaneous PTX can be managed conservatively using manual aspiration, with tube thoracostomy reserved for treatment failure.

· Management of tension PTX places priority on gaining access to the pleural cavity for thoracic decompression, which is best completed with finger thoracotomy and digital exploration. Needle decompression should be reserved as a last resort.

· Parapneumonic effusion and empyema effusions require prompt antibiotics and drainage to facilitate source control.

· Trapped lung, persistent air leak, recurrent primary PTX, secondary PTX, and infected effusions failing conservative therapy should be referred for definitive management with either chemical pleurodesis, VATS, or surgical intervention.

References

1. Bateman M, Alkhatib A, John T, Parikh M, Kheir F. Pleural effusion outcomes in intensive care: analysis of a large clinical database. *J Intensive Care Med*. 2019;35(1):48–54. doi:10.1177/0885066619872449

2. Aboudara M, Maldonado F. Update in the management of pleural effusions. *Med Clin North Am*. 2019;103(3):475–485. doi:10.1016/j.mcna.2018.12.007

3. Karkhanis V, Joshi J. Pleural effusion: Diagnosis, treatment, and management. *Open Access Emerg Med*. 2012;4:31–52. doi:10.2147/oaem.s29942

4. Marinkovic SP, Topuzovska IK, Stevanovic M, Anastasovska A. Features of parapneumonic effusions. *Pril (Makedon Akad Nauk Umet Odd Med Nauki)*. 2018;39(1):131–141. doi:10.2478/prilozi-2018-0033

5. Hooper C, Lee YCG, Maskell N. Investigation of a unilateral pleural effusion in adults: British Thoracic Society pleural disease guideline 2010. *Thorax*. 2010;65(Suppl 2):ii4–ii17. doi:10.1136/thx.2010.136978

6. Bhatnagar R, Maskell N. Pleural fluid biochemistry—old controversies, new directions. *Ann Clin Biochem*. 2014;51(4):421–423. doi:10.1177/0004563214531236

7. Rosenstengel D. Pleural infection—current diagnosis and management. *J Thorac Dis*. 2012;4(2):186–193.

8. Miller C, Bridges E, Laxmanan B, Cox-North P, Thompson H. Tunneled pleural catheter: Treatment for recurrent pleural effusion. *AACN Adv Crit Care*. 2018;29(4):432–441. doi:10.4037/aacnacc2018806

9. Hooper CE, Welham SA, Maskell NA. Pleural procedures and patient safety: A national BTS audit of practice. *Thorax*. 2015;70:189–191.

10. Mahmood K, Wahidi MM. Straightening out chest tubes: What size, what type and when? *Clin Chest Med*. 2013;34(1):63–71. doi:10.1016/j.ccm.2012.11.007

11. Kwiatt M, Tarbox A, Seamon MJ, et al. Thoracostomy tubes: A comprehensive review of complications and related topics. *Int J Crit Illn Inj Sci*. 2014;4(2):143–155. doi:10.4103/2229-5151.134182

12. Porcel JM. Chest tube drainage of the pleural space: A concise review for pulmonologists. *Tuberc Respir Dis*. 2018;81(2):106–115. doi:10.4046/trd.2017.0107

13. Noppen M, Alexander P, Driesen P, Slabbynck H, Verstraeten A. Manual aspiration versus chest tube drainage in first episodes of primary spontaneous pneumothorax. *Am J Respir Crit Care Med*. 2002;165(9):1240–1244. doi:10.1164/rccm.200111-078oc

14. Drinhaus H, Annecke T. Chest decompression in emergency medicine and intensive care. *Anaesthesist*. 2016;65(10):768–775.

15. Rahman NM, Maskell NA, West A, et al. Intrapleural use of tissue plasminogen activator and DNase in pleural infection. *N Engl J Med*. 2011;365(6):518–526.

7 Help me breathe: High-flow nasal cannula versus noninvasive ventilation troubleshooting

David L. Allison and James Dargin

A 55-year-old female with a history of chronic obstructive pulmonary disease presents to the ED with 2 days of dyspnea and a cough productive of purulent sputum. On physical examination, she has a temperature of 102.3°F, HR 125 bpm, RR 24 breaths/min, and oxygen saturation 82% on room air. There is no jugular venous distention. Lung exam reveals crackles in the left posterior chest without wheezing. There is no lower extremity edema. The patient is placed on supplemental oxygen at 15 L/min via a non-rebreather mask. A chest radiograph shows a dense left lower lobe consolidation. Broad-spectrum antibiotics are started. An arterial blood gas shows pH 7.48, pCO_2 30 mmHg, and PaO_2 59 mmHg. She remains in mild to moderate respiratory distress with an oxygen saturation of 89% on the non-rebreather mask.

What do I do now?

This patient has acute hypoxemic respiratory failure due to pneumonia. She remains hypoxic despite supplemental oxygen via a non-rebreather mask. A number of options for respiratory support could be considered in this case, including high-flow nasal cannula, noninvasive ventilation, or tracheal intubation. A growing body of evidence is now available to guide the provider in the use of different modalities of support for the patient with respiratory failure. Here we review the use of high-flow nasal cannula and noninvasive ventilation in the ED.

NONINVASIVE VENTILATION

Noninvasive ventilation is a form of respiratory support provided without the use of an endotracheal tube. There are two major forms of noninvasive ventilation: bilevel positive-pressure ventilation (BPAP) and continuous positive-pressure ventilation (CPAP). With CPAP, a single pressure is applied throughout the respiratory cycle. With BPAP, two levels of positive pressure are delivered: an inspiratory positive pressure administered when a breath is initiated and an expiratory positive pressure to assist with maintaining inflation once the patient exhales. Unlike CPAP, which provides support only for hypoxemic respiratory failure, BPAP augments tidal volume and therefore provides support for the patient with hypercapnic or hypoxemic respiratory failure. Noninvasive ventilation is provided for the patient with respiratory failure through any number of mask interfaces, including nasal prongs (pillows), nasal masks, oronasal masks, and full-face masks (covers the nose, mouth, and eyes). An appropriately fitting mask is important for patient tolerance while providing noninvasive ventilation. Nasal masks tend to result in a large leak from the patient's mouth, thus limiting the use of this interface in patients with acute respiratory failure. The oropharyngeal mask is fairly well tolerated and is the most commonly used interface for management of acute respiratory failure. The full-face mask provides similar gas exchange and improvement in respiratory parameters but is not as well tolerated as the oropharyngeal mask. The choice of interface often depends on availability at individual hospitals and provider and respiratory therapist preference.

For CPAP, common initial settings include a pressure in the range of 5 to 10 cmH$_2$O. The pressure can then be adjusted based on the target oxygen saturation. For patients on BPAP, most providers will typically start with a relatively low inspiratory pressure, in the range of 8 to 10 cmH_2O, and then titrate up to 12 to 20 cmH_2O as needed to meet the target tidal volume and reduction in work of breathing. The expiratory pressure is usually set in the range of 5 to 8 cmH_2O and titrated up to improve oxygenation. The fraction of inspired oxygen (FiO_2) is adjusted to achieve the target oxygen saturation goals in both CPAP and BPAP.

The patient should be closely monitored for several minutes immediately after initiating noninvasive ventilation to ensure ventilator synchrony and patient comfort. A leak from the mask interface can cause ventilator dyssynchrony, which can often be resolved by ensuring the use of a properly fitting mask with an adequate seal. Patient discomfort and anxiety can sometimes be reduced by trying a different mask interface (e.g., switching from a nasopharyngeal to full-face mask).

For patients who develop anxiety and do not tolerate the mask interface, the use of a sedative agent may help to improve tolerance of noninvasive ventilation. The use of sedative agents in patients with acute respiratory failure must be weighed against the risk of decreasing respiratory drive and precipitating the need for intubation. If sedation is utilized, dexmedetomidine may be preferred over midazolam for treating anxiety and improving tolerance of noninvasive ventilation with depressing respiratory drive.

Serious complications from noninvasive ventilation are fairly rare. Most commonly, patients may experience minor complications, such as eye irritation, mucosal dryness, or gastric insufflation leading to nausea and vomiting. Positive intrathoracic pressure from noninvasive ventilation can also cause hypotension, particularly in hypovolemic patients.

Once the patient appears to be tolerating noninvasive support, the respiratory rate, oxygen saturation, and mental status (especially in patients with hypercapnia) should be followed closely over the next 1 to 2 hours. Patients should demonstrate a reduction in work of breathing, a lower respiratory rate, and an improved level of consciousness after starting noninvasive ventilation. A repeat arterial blood gas sample can be helpful to confirm clinical findings and to monitor response to therapy. Patients not showing the expected improvement within the first hour or two after starting noninvasive ventilation may require intubation. Predictors of failure with noninvasive ventilation include older age, higher severity of illness, multiorgan failure, the need for vasopressors, and severe encephalopathy.

The evidence supporting the use of noninvasive ventilation is strongest for patients with acute exacerbations of congestive heart failure (CHF) and chronic obstructive pulmonary disease (COPD). Noninvasive ventilation has been shown to reduce intubation rates and mortality in patients with CHF exacerbations. CPAP and BPAP appear to be equally effective in the setting of cardiogenic pulmonary edema. Not only can noninvasive ventilation reduce the work of breathing and improve oxygenation in CHF, but it can also improve hemodynamics. Indeed, positive-pressure ventilation can help to reduce preload as well as augment cardiac output by reducing afterload in patients with decompensated heart failure. However, noninvasive ventilation is not commonly used in patients with cardiogenic shock as this population has been excluded from most trials and this condition is associated with a high risk of deterioration and subsequent intubation. Similar to CHF, noninvasive ventilation has been shown in multiple randomized trials to reduce intubation rates and mortality in moderate to severe COPD exacerbations (pH <7.35 with relative hypercarbia). BPAP rather than CPAP is used for COPD due to the more substantial ventilatory support provided with the former modality, including setting a mandatory respiratory rate.

The evidence supporting the use of noninvasive ventilation for conditions other than CHF and COPD is less robust. Pneumonia has generally been shown to be a predictor of noninvasive ventilation failure. However, there is some evidence that survival may be improved in patients with pneumonia and comorbid CHF or COPD. The evidence supporting the use of noninvasive ventilation in specific conditions, such as asthma and respiratory failure related to trauma is summarized in Table 7.1.

Perhaps the only absolute contraindication to the use of noninvasive ventilation is the presence of a clear indication for tracheal intubation (e.g., respiratory arrest). There are a number of situations that pose relative contraindications to noninvasive ventilation, and this form of respiratory support should be either avoided or used with caution in these circumstances (Box 7.1). Common clinical circumstances where noninvasive ventilation should be avoided (or at least used cautiously) include patients with difficulty clearing respiratory secretions and patients with a severely depressed level of consciousness. Patients with an impaired level of

TABLE 7.1 **Evidence supporting the use of noninvasive ventilation in specific causes of acute respiratory failure: Summary**

Indication	Evidence	Outcomes
Cardiogenic pulmonary edema	Multiple RCTs	Reduced intubation and mortality
Acute exacerbation of COPD	Multiple RCTs	Reduced intubation and mortality in moderate to severe cases
Pneumonia with respiratory failure	Small RCTs	Conflicting results
Immunosuppressed with respiratory failure	Small RCTs using BPAP	Reduced intubation and mortality
Chest trauma and respiratory failure	Small studies using BPAP or CPAP	Reduced mortality and intubation
Asthma	Small RCTs	Reduced work of breathing

RCTs = randomized controlled trials.

consciousness must be monitored closely when using noninvasive ventilation as they may not be able to remove the mask in the event of a vomiting episode, increasing the risk of aspiration.

HIGH-FLOW NASAL CANNULA

Conventional oxygen is delivered through a low-flow system (up to 15 L/min) via a nasal cannula or a face mask. The gas delivered is typically cold and dry

---

BOX 7.1 **Contraindications to the use of noninvasive ventilation**

Cardiac or respiratory arrest
Severely depressed level of consciousness
Difficulty clearing secretions
Agitation or poor cooperation
Hemodynamic instability
Airway obstruction
Epistaxis
Upper gastrointestinal bleeding
Facial fractures or recent facial surgery
Recent esophageal or gastric surgery

(or inadequately humidified), which is poorly tolerated by patients, particularly when higher liter flow rates are utilized. Patients with respiratory distress may have inspiratory flow rates in the range of 30 to >100 L/min. As a result, patients with respiratory distress entrain room air, and the FiO_2 delivered into the airways is reduced. A high-flow nasal cannula is a device that provides very high flow rates with the use of an active, heated humidifier. An air/oxygen blender is used to set an FiO_2 of 0.21 to 1.0 at a liter flow of up to 50 to 60 L/min.

There are many potential benefits to using high-flow nasal cannula oxygenation compared to conventional oxygen therapies. The high liter flow provided by this device helps to meet the patient's inspiratory demand, thus reducing the work of breathing. Furthermore, the high liter flow rate delivered prevents room air from being entrained, and the amount of oxygen delivered into the airways tends to closely match the actual FiO_2 prescribed (unlike traditional oxygen devices, where the FiO_2 is diluted). High-flow nasal cannula oxygenation may also provide a modest amount of positive end-expiratory pressure (PEEP), particularly when the mouth is closed (~0.8 cmH_2O for every 10 L/min of flow). The consistent and predictable FiO_2 delivery and the modest amount of applied PEEP may help to improve oxygenation when compared to conventional oxygen therapy. Finally, heating and humidifying the gas helps to improve patient comfort and improve mucociliary function and secretion clearance.

The high-flow oxygen is delivered via a large-bore nasal cannula, which is softer and more pliable than traditional nasal cannula devices and therefore improves patient comfort. Two parameters need to be set when initiating a high-flow nasal cannula: the liter flow and the FiO_2. The liter flow is often set to ~20 L/min and titrated up in increments of 5 to 10 L/min (as high as 60 L/min) as needed based on the patient's respiratory rate and work of breathing. The FiO_2 is adjusted from 0.21 to 1.0 to achieve the desired oxygen saturation. The patient should be monitored closely for clinical response immediately after initiation of high-flow nasal cannula oxygenation. Improvements in the oxygen saturation and work of breathing, as well as a reduction in the respiratory rate, are signs of improvement with the use of high-flow nasal cannula treatment.

Patients with persistent tachypnea or thoracoabdominal asynchrony after about 30 minutes of treatment with a high-flow nasal cannula may require intubation. The ROX index has been shown to be an accurate, objective measure to predict high-flow nasal cannula failure and the need for intubation. The ROX index is a ratio of the oxygen saturation as measured by pulse oximetry to the prescribed FiO_2, divided by the respiratory rate. For example, a patient with an oxygen saturation of 90% and a respiratory rate of 30 breaths/min on an FiO_2 of 1.0 would have a ROX index of 3:

$$\text{ROX index} = 90 \div 30 \div 1.0 = 3$$

A ROX index of <2.85 after 2 hours, <3.5 at 6 hours, or <3.85 after 12 hours of high-flow nasal cannula treatment all accurately predict the need for intubation. Thus, serial measurements of the ROX index over time may help with decision-making regarding the need for intubation. The presence of shock and a high severity of illness are also associated with high-flow nasal cannula failure, and close monitoring and reassessment for the need for intubation are required in these patient populations.

High-flow nasal cannula treatment is most commonly used for patients with hypoxemic respiratory failure, particularly due to pneumonia. A multicenter, randomized trial of adults with acute hypoxemic respiratory failure showed a significant reduction in mortality with use of a high-flow nasal cannula compared to either a non-rebreather mask or noninvasive ventilation. This study also showed a lower intubation rate with use of a high-flow nasal cannula in a subgroup of patients with more severe hypoxemia (PaO_2:FiO_2 <200). The majority of patients enrolled in this trial had pneumonia as the cause of respiratory failure, and patients were excluded if they had hypercapnia, asthma, or CHF as the underlying etiology. There is currently a lack of evidence supporting the use of high-flow nasal cannula oxygenation in patients with acute exacerbations of CHF and COPD. Given the high level of evidence for noninvasive ventilation in the management of COPD and CHF, high-flow nasal cannula oxygenation should not be a first-line therapy for these conditions. However, many patients do not tolerate the mask interface utilized for noninvasive ventilation, and a high-flow nasal cannula may be used cautiously in patients with CHF or COPD exacerbations who do not tolerate noninvasive ventilation.

A high-flow nasal cannula is generally well tolerated, and there are few contraindications to this device. As is the case with noninvasive ventilation, the only absolute contraindication is a clear indication for intubation. Patients supported with a high-flow nasal cannula should be monitored closely for signs of worsening gas exchange or work of breathing so as not to delay intubation. Use of a high-flow nasal cannula should be avoided in patients with recent facial or nasal surgery or with craniofacial abnormalities that prevent the cannula from fitting properly. Active epistaxis is also a relative contraindication to this therapy. The risk of serious complications, such as barotrauma or aspiration, is low.

CONSIDERATIONS FOR THE COVID-19 PANDEMIC

Patients with COVID-19 can develop a severe viral pneumonitis leading to the acute respiratory distress syndrome (ARDS). As patients with COVID-19 develop progressive hypoxemia, more aggressive respiratory support is often required, typically in the form of noninvasive ventilation or a high-flow nasal cannula. There are currently limited data to suggest benefit of one modality over the other in patients with COVID-19. However, data from patients with non-COVID-19 pneumonia suggest that a high-flow nasal cannula may be the preferred modality in patients who develop ARDS. It may be appropriate to use noninvasive ventilation in patients with COVID-19 who demonstrate increased work of breathing, have consolidated but potentially recruitable basal lung segments on imaging (CT or chest x-ray), or have acute exacerbations of COPD or CHF contributing to their respiratory failure. A high-flow nasal cannula and noninvasive ventilation are both generally considered aerosol-generating procedures, so airborne precautions should be maintained (negative-pressure room and N95 mask) in addition to standard PPE.

KEY POINTS TO REMEMBER

· Noninvasive ventilation has been shown to reduce intubation rates and mortality in patients with acute exacerbations of CHF and COPD.
· Oxygenation via a high-flow nasal cannula is primarily utilized in patients with acute hypoxemic, non-hypercapnic respiratory failure.
· The ROX index is an objective measure to help predict high-flow nasal cannula failure and the need for intubation.

Further reading

Allison MG, Winters ME. Non-invasive ventilation for the emergency physician. *Emerg Med Clin North Am*. 2016;34:51–62.Cuvelier A, Pujol W, Pramil S, et al. Cephalic versus oronasal mask for non-invasive ventilation in acute respiratory failure. *Intensive Care Med*. 2009;35:519–526.

Frat JP, Thille AW, Mercat A, et al. High-flow oxygen through nasal cannula for acute hypoxemic respiratory failure. *N Engl J Med*. 2015;372:2185–2196.

Groves N, Tobin A. High flow nasal oxygen generates positive airway pressure in adult volunteers. *Aust Crit Care*. 2007;20:126–131.

Hess DR. Non-invasive ventilation for acute respiratory failure. *Respir Care*. 2013;58:950–972.

Huang Z, Chen Y, Liu J. Dexmedetomidine versus midazolam for the sedation of patients with non-invasive ventilation failure. *Intern Med*. 2012;51:2299–2305.

Keenan SP, Sinuff T, Cook DJ, et al. Which patients with acute exacerbation of chronic obstructive pulmonary disease benefit from non-invasive positive pressure ventilation? *Ann Intern Med*. 2003;138:861–870.

Masip J, Roque M, Sanchez B, et al. Non-invasive ventilation in acute cardiogenic pulmonary edema: Systematic review and metaanalysis. *JAMA*. 2005;294:3124–3130.

Nishimura M. High-flow nasal oxygen therapy in adults: Physiologic benefits, indication, clinical benefits, and adverse effects. *Respir Care*. 2016;61(4):529–541.

Papazian L, Corley A, Hess D, et al. Use of high-flow nasal cannula oxygenation in ICU adults: A narrative review. *Intensive Care Med*. 2016;42:1336–1349.

Ritchie JE, Williams AB, Gerard H, et al. Evaluation of a humidified nasal high-flow oxygen system, using oxygraphy, capnography, and measurement of upper airway pressures. *Anaesth Intensive Care*. 2011;39:1103–1110.

Roca O, Caralt B, Messika J, et al. An index combining respiratory rate and oxygenation to predict outcome of nasal high-flow therapy. *Am J Respir Crit Care Med*. 2019;199:1368–1376.

Rochwerg B, Brochard L, Elliot MW, et al. Official ERS/ATS clinical practice guidelines: Noninvasive ventilation for acute respiratory failure. *Eur Respir J*. 2017;50:1–20.

Stefan MS, Priya A, Pekow PS, et al. The comparative effectiveness of noninvasive and invasive ventilation in patients with pneumonia. *J Crit Care*. 2018;43:190–196.

Vargas R, Saint-Leger M, Boyer A, et al. Physiologic effects of high-flow nasal cannula oxygen in critical care subjects. *Respir Care*. 2015;60:1369–1376.

8 Intubated and boarded in the ED: Ventilator 101

Jessica Fozard and Krystle Shafer

On the overnight shift, you get a notification from your local EMS for a 45-year-old male in cardiac arrest. Return of spontaneous circulation is achieved just prior to arrival. Your hospital is short-staffed this particular night, and your respiratory therapist and intensive care team are tied up with another critically ill patient upstairs. The EMS crew had successfully intubated the patient en route to the ED, and you confirm correct placement with auscultation of lung sounds bilaterally and continuous waveform capnography. Your team transfers the patient over to the stretcher, additional IV lines are started, an ECG shows no evidence of ischemia, and your patient's vital signs are adequate. One of the experienced ED nurses informs you that the ventilator is available in the department and asks if you would like to put the patient on it so that a provider can be relieved from bagging the patient.

What do I do now?

The mechanical ventilator can be intimidating, especially when providers are unfamiliar with the machine/circuit setup and initial settings. However, emergency physicians can be empowered by knowing the basics of how to safely ventilate patients with the mechanical ventilator. Generally, the strategy for ventilating should be individualized based on the patient's underlying disease process, by determining the minute ventilation (MV) and oxygen delivery required for the indication of mechanical ventilation. Settings will differ between patients who require a high MV and those who need a normal MV, and all patients should receive the lowest amount of oxygen (fraction of inspired oxygen, FiO_2) required to maintain adequate pulse oximeter saturations. Additionally, lung-protective strategies (e.g., limit tidal volume (V_T), maintain or improve lung parenchyma recruitment, limit airway pressures, and minimize hyperoxia/potential oxygen toxicity) are vital.

The first choice to make is between a pressure-based and a volume-based mode. Because every patient population benefits from lung-protective V_T ventilation (more about this topic later in the chapter), this is usually best accomplished by volume assist-control mode. Thus, for the purposes of this chapter, we will focus on this mode of ventilation initially. Once the mode is selected, four other ventilator variables must be set. To ventilate or encourage CO_2 removal and gas exchange, this is optimized via V_T and respiratory rate (RR). Additionally, to oxygenate the patient, this is titrated by the positive end-expiratory pressure (PEEP) and FiO_2.

In terms of the initial ventilator settings to use for most patients:

1. Choose volume-control mode, often called assist-control mode, volume-control mode, or control-mandatory ventilation mode.
2. Set V_T at 4 to 8 cc/kg ideal body weight (IBW); this would be lung-protective ventilation (low volumes). IBW is based on height.
3. Set the RR between 12 and 20 breaths/min to achieve the target MV; The higher the MV, the more CO_2 will be removed. Normal MV is ~8 L/min. This may be lower in patients with asthma or other obstructive lung diseases due to their need for a longer exhalation time.

4. Set FiO_2 at 100% initially, especially in patients with acute hypoxic respiratory failure. The goal is to titrate FiO_2 down to <60% as quickly as tolerated to avoid damage secondary to hyperoxia.
5. Set starting PEEP at 5 to 8 cmH_2O in the general non-chronic lung disease population.

These parameters can be particularly important with regard to limiting acute lung injury (ALI) or ventilator-associated lung injury (VALI). The ARDSNet ARMA trial showed mortality benefit in using a lung-protective strategy, primarily via low V_T.[1] Hence, the progression toward lower V_T ventilation should start early in the patient's course either to limit and/or to prevent VALI.

PRESSURE-CONTROL VENTILATION

Pressure-control ventilation is exactly as described by its name. The provider sets a pressure (airway pressure or driving pressure, Pi), inspiratory time, minimum RR, PEEP, and FiO_2. The patient therefore controls the V_T, flow rate, and total RR. The downside to this ventilation mode is that the volume delivered is variable. This variability can result in a decreased MV if the airway pressures are high as the breath delivered will be stopped when set pressure reached. Similarly, in patients with acute respiratory distress syndrome (ARDS), you will not be able to control V_T and they can be harmed by large and uncontrolled V_T. So why use this mode? The idea is that it may be more comfortable for patients and is more physiologically based on the decelerating flow, which is similar to the natural mechanics of breathing.

If this is the mode of choice for any reason, here are some initial settings:

1. Choose pressure control.
2. Set an initial pressure; this can be anywhere from 5 to 20 cmH_2O and can certainly vary.
3. Set RR between 12 and 20 breaths/min to achieve the target MV, ~8 L/min or a V_T of 6 cc/kg, ideally.
4. Set FiO_2 at 100% initially, especially in acute hypoxic respiratory failure.
5. Set starting PEEP at 5 to 8 cmH_2O in the general non-chronic lung disease population.

LUNG-PROTECTIVE VENTILATION

Volume targets

Why should ED physicians care about this? After all, the ED physician's main job is to manage patients while they are critically ill, stabilize them, then transfer to the ICU—consider that early ventilator management can make a difference. ARDSNet proved that using a low V_T and a lung-protective strategy decreases mortality, leading to its routine use in most mechanically ventilated patients, especially those with ARDS.[1] Additional studies since this landmark trial have confirmed that this strategy should be used in all patients placed on mechanical ventilation, no matter their age, comorbidities, or pathology requiring a need for ventilation. Fuller et al. demonstrated that starting lung-protective ventilation strategies in the ED is safe and effective and results in decreased ICU and hospital length of stay, as well as decreased length of time on the ventilator.[2] The care initiated in the ED setting will influence the trajectory of the patient's hospital stay, thus it is imperative to optimize the chance for recovery at the onset of mechanical ventilation.

Setting or selecting a V_T for obese patients can be prone to error, as some providers may be tempted to set a higher V_T initially. Do not be misled by a patient's body habitus—obese patients have the same underlying axial skeleton as their lean counterparts. Use IBW to calculate and choose an initial V_T. For example, for a 70-kg person (also their IBW), then 6 × 70 = 420 cc, which means a V_T of 6 cc/kg. For a 200-kg patient whose IBW is 100 kg, then 6 × 100 = 600 cc is their V_T. Additionally, do not assume that all patients have an IBW of 70 kg; for example, a 6-foot-6 man will have an appropriately larger 6 cc/kg V_T compared to a 5-foot-1 woman. PEEP may need to be adjusted to higher levels to effectively oxygenate and ventilate patients with a larger body habitus compared to patients who are closer to their IBW.

IBW is calculated as follows:

Males: IBW = 50 + [2.3 × (height in inches – 60)]
Females: IBW = 45.5 + [2.3 × (height in inches – 60)]

One way to avoid scrambling for this information is by posting reference cards on the ventilators, by the respiratory equipment storage area, or in

Lower PEEP/higher FiO$_2$

FiO$_2$	0.3	0.4	0.4	0.5	0.5	0.6	0.7	0.7
PEEP	5	5	8	8	10	10	10	12

FiO$_2$	0.7	0.8	0.9	0.9	0.9	1.0
PEEP	14	14	14	16	18	18–24

Higher PEEP/higher FiO$_2$

FiO$_2$	0.3	0.3	0.3	0.3	0.3	0.4	0.4	0.5
PEEP	5	8	10	12	14	14	16	16

FiO$_2$	0.5	0.5–0.8	0.8	0.9	1.0	1.0
PEEP	18	20	22	22	22	24

FIGURE 8.1 ARDSNet PEEP table

the resuscitation rooms, thus making it readily available to the providers/ physicians (Figures 8.1 and 8.2). A more accurate V$_T$ can be calculated if patients are routinely measured for their height as well. These are small measures that can be instituted up front to make determining ventilator settings easier when taking care of a critically ill patient.

Pressure targets

We cannot only focus on V$_T$ and ignore the pressure that is generated during mechanical ventilation. Setting a V$_T$ target allows the pressure to be determined based on the patient's lung compliance. It is important to limit barotrauma by monitoring plateau pressure (P$_{plat}$), peak inspiratory pressure (PIP), and driving pressure.

P$_{plat}$, which is measured during an inspiratory pause maneuver on the ventilator, refers to the pressure that is applied to the small airways and alveoli during mechanical ventilation. According to ARDSNet data, the goal P$_{plat}$ is <30 cm H$_2$O.[1] If P$_{plat}$ is above this target, the easiest way to drop it is to either drop the V$_T$ ventilation down, usually by increments of 1 cc/ kg of IBW at a time, and/or to decrease PEEP.

PIP includes both the small alveoli pressure and the pressure in the large airways. It is the highest pressure applied to the lungs during inhalation. High PIPs will result in barotrauma if not controlled.

Driving pressure is P$_{plat}$ minus PEEP. Research has indicated that physicians should likely target <15 cm H$_2$O. PEEP titration, sedation, and

MALE QUICK REFERENCE FOR TIDAL VOLUME

HEIGHT	INCHES	PBW	8 mL/KG	6 mL/KG	4 mL/KG
4'6"	54	36.2	290	220	150
4'7"	55	38.5	310	230	160
4'8"	56	40.8	330	250	170
4'9"	57	43.1	350	260	170
4'10"	58	45.4	370	270	180
4'11"	59	47.7	380	290	190
5'0"	60	50.0	400	300	200
5'1"	61	52.3	420	320	210
5'2"	62	54.6	440	330	220
5'3"	63	56.9	460	340	230
5'4"	64	59.2	480	360	240
5'5"	65	61.5	490	370	250
5'6"	66	63.8	510	390	260
5'7"	67	66.1	530	400	270
5'8"	68	68.4	550	410	280
5'9"	69	70.7	570	430	290
5'10"	70	73.0	590	440	290
5'11"	71	75.3	600	450	300
6'0"	72	77.6	620	470	310
6'1"	73	79.9	640	480	320
6'2"	74	82.2	660	500	330
6'3"	75	84.5	680	510	340
6'4"	76	86.8	700	520	350

KG = kilogram; mL = milliliter; PBW = predicted body weight

FEMALE QUICK REFERENCE FOR TIDAL VOLUME

HEIGHT	INCHES	PBW	8 mL/KG	6 mL/KG	4 mL/KG
4'6"	54	31.7	260	190	130
4'7"	55	34.0	270	210	140
4'8"	56	36.3	290	220	150
4'9"	57	38.6	310	230	160
4'10"	58	40.9	330	260	170
4'11"	59	43.2	350	260	180
5'0"	60	45.5	370	280	180
5'1"	61	47.8	380	290	190
5'2"	62	50.1	400	300	200
5'3"	63	52.4	420	320	210
5'4"	64	54.7	440	330	220
5'5"	65	57.0	460	340	230
5'6"	66	59.3	480	360	240
5'7"	67	61.6	500	370	250
5'8"	68	63.9	510	390	260
5'9"	69	66.2	530	400	270
5'10"	70	68.5	550	410	280
5'11"	71	70.8	570	430	290
6'0"	72	73.1	590	440	290
6'1"	73	75.4	610	450	300
6'2"	74	77.7	620	470	310
6'3"	75	80.0	640	480	320
6'4"	76	82.3	660	500	330

KG = kilogram; mL = milliliter; PBW = predicted body weight

FIGURE 8.2 IBW card

neuromuscular blockade, as well as prone ventilation, are early considerations for possible strategies to help lower the driving pressure. At this time, driving pressure management should be considered a complementary tool to determine safe ventilation parameters.

Monitoring excessive airway pressures is important in order to limit ventilator-induced lung injury (VILI) or VALI. Examples of barotrauma VILI include pneumothorax, pneumomediastinum, bronchial rupture, and excessive alveolar distention. Over time, barotrauma perpetuates the cellular injury that later develops into ARDS. Mechanical ventilation can injure the lung through trauma derived from excess pressures, volumes, and atelectasis reopening of collapsed lung segments.

Permissive hypercapnia

Patients who undergo mechanical ventilation should not have a V_T of >8 cc/kg. However, in ARDS patients, starting at 8 cc/kg is acceptable, with a target of achieving 6 cc/kg within 2 hours of initiation of mechanical ventilation.[1] To account for this decrease in MV, the easiest way to maintain this is by increasing RR. However, in some patients, dropping V_T will result in hypercapnia even with a compensatory RR increase. Because V_T control is of utmost importance, ARDSNet allows for permissive hypercapnia and a lower pH target as a result.[1] If a patient has a pH of 7.3 or above, no changes need to be made to increase the patient's MV. If pH is between 7.15 and 7.3, it is recommended to increase the RR, to a maximum of 35 unless breath stacking is created prior to a rate of 35, until a pH target of 7.3 or a pCO_2 of <25 is achieved. For patients with a pH of <7.15, then V_T is recommended to be increased by 1 cc/kg up to 8 cc/kg to increase pH, and bicarbonate supplementation may also be considered. As long as the pH is >7.15, do not change the V_T from a 6-cc/kg strategy; instead, focus on optimizing RR, allowing for permissive hypercapnia and mild respiratory acidosis.

PEEP titration

Patients should be started at a PEEP minimum of 5 cmH_2O, with the only exception being in patients with asthma, in whom a PEEP of 0 may be appropriate. PEEP refers to the pressure that is left within the alveoli at end-expiration to prevent their collapse and assists with oxygenation as noted above. Preventing the alveoli from opening and then collapsing during expiration is the primary goal to maintain alveolar recruitment to participate in gas exchange. PEEP that is too high for some lung unit areas can cause barotrauma and pneumothorax. Excess intrathoracic positive pressure during inhalation and exhalation can increase the afterload seen by the right ventricle and can reduce preload, often seen as hypotension and decreased cardiac output. In a patient with severe ARDS, excess PEEP can overdistend the healthier alveoli, causing worsening oxygenation and damage to these alveoli. Finally, in diseases such as asthma and chronic obstructive pulmonary disease (COPD) where the patient already has difficulty with air trapping and resulting prolonged exhalation time, higher PEEP can worsen this process.

To aid in decision-making about where to target PEEP, ARDSNet offers two PEEP titration tables, one with a lower PEEP strategy and one with a higher PEEP strategy. Patients with obstructive lung disease, right ventricular dysfunction, and uncontrolled shock, for example, should be placed on a lower PEEP titration. For the majority of newly intubated patients, it is recommended to start at levels between 5 and 8 cm H_2O and to increase based on the ARDSNet table, keeping an eye on the patient's BP, PIP/P_{plat}, and oxygenation parameters to help guide the titration process (Figure 8.1).

FIO_2 titration

FIO_2 should be titrated down as quickly as tolerated to avoid cellular injury from hyperoxia. According to ARDSNet, the oxygen saturation goal is 88% to 95% and the partial pressure of oxygen (PaO_2) goal is 55 to 80 mmHg. This is a good rule of thumb to use for most intubated patients. However, some patient populations may require higher oxygenation goals, such as pregnant patients. Similarly, COPD patients can have a goal of 88% to 92% to avoid diminishing their respiratory drive.

Patient positioning

Unless contraindicated, simple measures such as elevating the head of the bed at least 30 degrees can also aid in ventilation, alveolar recruitment, and prevention of ventilator-associated pneumonia (VAP). Elevating the head of the bed can be easily overlooked in the ED setting. Ensuring there are no other barriers to ventilation such as a distended abdomen may also be helpful; this can be remedied with a nasogastric tube. There are few absolute contraindications to prone positioning (proning), and in the event you are still caring for an ICU patient in the ED, this may be a life-saving maneuver. Involving the ICU team and nursing staff to assist with initiating proning in the ED sounds extreme but may be necessary in some circumstances.

COVID-19 CONSIDERATIONS

It is worth mentioning special circumstances regarding mechanical ventilation in COVID-19 patients. Essentially, the first steps in management regarding the decision to intubate will be the same, as well as the initial ventilator settings. Continue to use a ventilator mode that you feel comfortable with and can safely use rather than trying advanced settings that are unfamiliar. However, the needs of these patients may quickly escalate, and they are at high risk to deteriorate and may require proning emergently, which may or may not help. They tend to desaturate quickly and profoundly as they have little reserve and take an uncomfortable amount of time to recover, even with recruitment maneuvers. These patients are challenging; They are still subject to barotrauma and can easily develop pneumothoraces, pneumomediastinum, and other negative effects of high-pressure ventilation or aggressive recruitment maneuvers.

SEDATION, ANALGESIA, AND MONITORING

After the airway is secured, it is important to keep patients safe and essentially take their abnormal physiology out of the equation during this acute time period. Ensure pain control and sedation as needed to allow for adequate oxygenation/ventilation, ideally while using a lung-protective strategy. Freeman et al. did a thorough review of the literature regarding sedation in mechanically ventilated patients in the ED in the setting of ICU crowding. Further analysis of what we already know about these patients shows that what happens in the ED matters regarding patient mortality, length of stay, and overall ICU course.[3] Generally, controlling pain first is a reasonable approach, followed by additional sedation if the patient remains uncomfortable or agitated despite appropriate measures.[3] In most cases, patients will require a paralytic and sedation prior to intubation; therefore, it is extremely important to ensure pain medications are ordered and available for nursing staff to give up front and then based on the patient's respiratory mechanics and/or a validated pain scale (e.g., the Critical Care Pain Observation Tool). Reassessment is usually performed quite frequently, every 10 to 30 minutes as needed, and infusions are titrated for scale-based (common validated scales include RIKER and RASS) levels of sedation. It is also very important to have good communication as a team (nursing, respiratory therapy, provider, physician) regarding the patient's responses to medications and potential adjustments to sedation regimens. This will usually require a continuous infusion with intermittent boluses as needed based on the sedation score and goal. Having available push-dose vasopressors (e.g., phenylephrine 80–100 mcg) to counteract immediate post-intubation hypotension is important preparation. An example of an ED-oriented algorithm for sedation is shown in Figure 8.3.

If medications are needed immediately and staff are awaiting infusions, it may be helpful to have quick orders for fentanyl (50–100 mcg) and midazolam (2–4 mg) to maintain analgesia and sedation in the immediate period following intubation. These are often readily available and familiar to most ED physicians and nurses no matter the resources available or ED location. Typical infusion dose ranges to maintain sedation are propofol 10 to 50 mcg/kg/min and fentanyl 50 to 200 mcg/hr. Patients with depressed mental status prior to intubation will still benefit from sedation for ventilator synchrony and to prevent awareness. Midazolam is slowly metabolized by end-stage renal patients on dialysis and can promote delirium in elderly patients; therefore, avoid excessive use of midazolam when possible.

MONITORING VENTILATION MANAGEMENT

Monitoring ventilation management has been alluded to frequently in this chapter but not explicitly discussed. We have mentioned goals and parameters, but how can this be achieved in a busy ED with boarded ICU patients? Consider what is available. Sometimes this will be an i-STAT; other times it will be assessing serial arterial blood gasses (ABGs) every time the ventilator is adjusted. This can be as often as every 30 minutes or as infrequent as once per shift, depending on the patient, reason for intubation,

Post-Intubation Sedation Protocol in Adult ED Patients

Notes

(1) If you are concerned about hypotension, have vasopressors ready to be administered (for example, phenylephrine 100mcg IV push).

(2) While it can still occur, propofol drips are less likely to cause pronounced hypotension than propofol boluses. Propofol boluses of 0.5 to 1 mg/kg can be considered in patients who are not hypotensive and continue to have agitation despite fentanyl and propofol drips.[24]

(3) Dosing propofol requires an estimated or measured patient body weight for entering mcg/kg/min dosing into pumps. Fentanyl dosing is usually entered into pumps as mcg/hr (not weight-based).

(4) Typical dosing to maintain appropriate sedation in ED:
Propofol 10 to 50 mcg/kg/min.
Fentanyl 50 to 200 mcg/hour.

(5) If the patient does not tolerate propofol, midazolam (Versed) is a second-line option for sedation by continuous infusion. The starting dose is: midazolam 2 mg IV push, then 1 mg/hr continuous infusion. Avoid midazolam in dialysis patients.

(6) Patients with a depressed mental status prior to intubation may not arouse to verbal stimuli or make eye contact after intubation, but still may benefit from sedation in the ED.

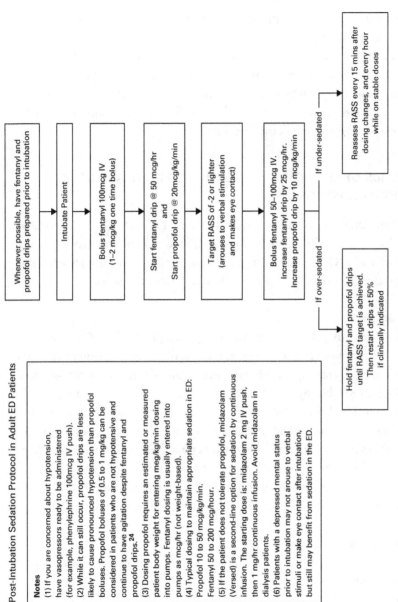

Whenever possible, have fentanyl and propofol drips prepared prior to intubation

↓

Intubate Patient

↓

Bolus fentanyl 100mcg IV
(1–2 mcg/kg one time bolus)

↓

Start fentanyl drip @ 50 mcg/hr
and
Start propofol drip @ 20mcg/kg/min

↓

Target RASS of -2 or lighter
(arouses to verbal stimulation
and makes eye contact)

↓

Bolus fentanyl 50–100mcg IV.
Increase fentanyl drip by 25 mcg/hr.
Increase propofol drip by 10 mcg/kg/min

— If over-sedated → Hold fentanyl and propofol drips until RASS target is achieved. Then restart drips at 50% if clinically indicated

— If under-sedated → Reassess RASS every 15 mins after dosing changes, and every hour while on stable doses

FIGURE 8.3 ED sedation algorithm for intubated patients boarding in the ED

From reference 3.

and staffing. In the immediate period, if frequent adjustments are being made, generally scheduled ABGs every 2 to 4 hours will be reasonable, especially in a patient with ARDS. This provides a frequent reassessment and, in the average ED, less of an opportunity to forgo reassessment while attending to other ED patients. If oxygenation is adequate and SpO_2 monitoring is reliable, then ABGs/i-STATs are not necessary and the ventilator, specifically FiO_2, can be weaned as long as saturation remains adequate. We cannot stress enough that this will vary between patients and their specific reasons for intubation in the first place.

BASICS OF ADJUSTING VENTILATOR SETTINGS AND BASIC TROUBLESHOOTING

When adjusting settings, consider the goal: gas exchange (CO_2 removal by increasing or decreasing MV using RR and V_T) and oxygenation (using PEEP and FIO_2). This may be a reactionary move, but consider ventilator adjustments based on the goal and feedback from the patient.

Example 1

The initial ABG shows an elevated CO_2 and a pH of 7.22. First, maximize the RR and then second, if needed, increase the V_T to a maximum safe level of 8 cc/kg. Increasing the RR will increase the MV and allow for increased CO_2 removal, but by less of a multiplicative rate than by increasing the V_T first. The idea behind this is that 12 breaths/min × 500 cc (V_T) = 6 L/min, so this is the starting point. If the V_T is increased first, 12 breaths/min × 750 cc (for example) = 9 L/min. On the other hand, if the RR is increased first, such as 16 breaths/min × 500 cc = 8 L/min, much less of a rise in MV will be observed compared to the original 6 L/min. Keep this in mind when deciding how much to increase the RR to achieve ideal pH and pCO_2 targets.

Example 2

What if the CO_2 is too low? Unlike the issues noted above, consider either decreasing the RR or decreasing the V_T to remove less CO_2. Inadequate sedation, pain, and agitation may cause the patient to over-breathe the ventilator set rate and the patient will require more sedative/analgesic medications.

Example 3

What if oxygenation is unsatisfactory? The starting FiO_2 is usually 100%, which is then decreased as PaO_2 or oxygen saturation values allow. If inadequate oxygenation is the issue, first increase the FiO_2. When this is persistently 100% and oxygenation is still an issue, then incremental increases in the PEEP may allow for additional recruitment of lung parenchyma and improved oxygenation. Be sure to assess for other issues that would prevent adequate oxygenation, such as tube displacement, obstruction, pneumothorax, or equipment malfunction.

Example 4

What if bronchospasm occurs? Give these patients enough time to exhale, as the primary issue can be air trapping, and on a ventilator this can become life-threatening. Air trapping occurs when full exhalation does not occur, resulting in unintended residual air left in the lungs that steadily increases with each breath. Unchecked, this can lead to hypotension, pneumothorax, and even death. Breath stacking is a patient/ventilator synchrony problem and can be combated by decreasing the RR and the V_T, by adjusting the inspiratory/expiratory ratio to allow for a longer expiratory time, adjusting the sensitivity of the flow or pressure triggers, or providing adequate sedation to allow synchrony with the ventilator. Continue to treat the underlying issue with bronchodilators while appropriately supporting the patient/ventilator interaction.

Example 5

What if there is sudden oxygen desaturation? Consider causes of hypoxia while on a ventilator as mentioned earlier—the tube may be displaced or obstructed, for example. Confirm the tube is in place by looking directly or by using other means such as x-ray or continuous waveform end-tidal CO_2 monitoring. If you are concerned about obstruction, attempt to pass a suction catheter through the tube. Another sudden cause of hypoxia, especially if the patient is on positive-pressure ventilation, could be pneumothorax, so have a low threshold to suspect this and treat it immediately with needle decompression, finger thoracostomy, or a chest tube. Lastly, consider faulty equipment as the cause: Disconnect from the ventilator, ventilate the patient with a bag-valve mask, and reassess. Other potential causes of hypoxia could be mucous plugging, mainstem intubation or displacement, and pulmonary embolism. Beyond this, refer to Chapter 9 for advanced strategies for managing the refractory hypoxic patient.

Example 6

What if peak airway pressures are high? The first step is to determine what type of issue is causing the high pressures. In the instance of elevated PIP, check an inspiratory pause or an inspiratory hold maneuver to check the P_{plat}. When this pressure is elevated or near the PIP, the issue is with lung compliance. Consider ARDS, pulmonary edema, atelectasis, pneumothorax, or mainstem intubation as most likely culprits. If the P_{plat} is low in the setting of elevated PAP, this is likely a resistance issue. Check the endotracheal tube to ensure it is not kinked, evaluate for mucous plugs, or treat bronchospasm if present.

KEY POINTS TO REMEMBER

- If things are not going well with managing the ventilator and none of the troubleshooting methods are working, go back to bagging the patient.
- Use references for ventilator settings, especially when it comes to V_T and PEEP settings.
- Monitor P_{plat} to limit lung injury.
- Decrease FiO_2 early and as tolerated by the patient.
- Look out for breath stacking, especially in patients with obstructive lung pathologies.

References

1. Acute Respiratory Distress Syndrome Network. Ventilation with lower tidal volumes as compared with traditional tidal volumes for acute lung injury and the acute respiratory distress syndrome. *N Engl J Med.* 2000;342:1301–1308.
2. Fuller B, Ferguson I, Mohr N, et al. Lung-protective ventilation initiated in the emergency department (LOV-ED): A quasi-experimental, before-after trial. *Ann Emerg Med.* 2018;70(3):406–418.
3. Freeman C, Evans C, Barrett T. Managing sedation in the mechanically ventilated emergency department patient: A clinical review. *J Am Coll Emerg Physicians Open.* 2020;1:263–269.

Further reading

Aoyama H, Yamada Y, Fan E. The future of driving pressure: A primary goal for mechanical ventilation? *J Intensive Care*. 2018;6:64.

Garbarini P, Grooms D. Driving pressure in ARDS patients. Hamilton Medical. February 4, 2020. Accessed October 7, 2020. https://www.hamilton-medical.com/en_US/Resource-center/Article-page~knowledge-base~09161a01-6223-4668-8fa8-d906319d64f9~.html

Meier A, Sell RE, Malhotra A. Driving pressure for ventilation of patients with acute respiratory distress syndrome. *Anesthesiology*. 2020;132(6):1569–1576.

Owens W. *The Ventilator Book*. First Draught Press; 2012.

Spiegel R, Mallemat H. Emergency department treatment of the mechanically ventilated patient. *Emerg Med Clin North Am*. 2016;34(1):63–75.

Weingart S. Managing initial mechanical ventilation in the emergency department. *Ann Emerg Med*. 2016;68(5):614–617.

9 I still can't breathe: ARDS and advanced ventilation strategies

Ashley Miller and Cassidy Dahn

A 65-year-old man with diabetes presents to the ED complaining of 2 days of trouble breathing, also noting fever, productive cough, and generalized fatigue. On arrival, his vitals are BP 95/50 mmHg, HR 110 bpm, oxygen saturation 83% on room air, RR 35 breaths/min, and core temperature 102.1°F, with a weight of 90 kg and height of 178 cm.

COVID-19 rapid testing is negative. The patient is treated empirically for sepsis with antibiotics and fluids, but he eventually progresses from hypoxemic respiratory insufficiency to hypoxemic respiratory failure, resulting in intubation via rapid sequence intubation with low-dose etomidate and a paralytic. His workup reveals multilobar pneumonia on chest x-ray (Figure 9.1), leukocytosis, and lactic acidosis. He is placed on volume-assist-control ventilation (tidal volume [V_T] 550 mL, rate 20, PEEP 5 cmH$_2$O, FiO$_2$ 100%) with initial arterial blood gas (ABG) results of 7.30 (pH)/33 (PaCO$_2$)/105 (paO$_2$). The ventilator "high peak airway" alarm is insistent, and the patient's oxygen saturation is slowly dropping to the high 80s.

What do I do now?

An alarming ventilator with a persistently hypoxic patient is a nightmare situation for many emergency medicine providers. While many of us consider ourselves airway experts, our comfort does not always extend to complicated ventilator management. However, in patients with acute respiratory distress syndrome (ARDS), following some simple management principles, especially when it comes to early ventilator management before the patient reaches the ICU, can make the difference between life and death.

Recognizing ARDS is the first step. ARDS is an acute, generalized inflammatory process in the lungs associated with hypoxemia, decreased lung compliance, and ultimately a very high mortality. It can be subtle and non-specific with an insidious onset, so a high index of suspicion in critically ill patients is crucial. It should be considered in patients with progressive dyspnea, increasing hypoxia, and bilateral alveolar infiltrates on chest imaging. The patient can appear tachypneic and/or in respiratory distress, can be tachycardic, and can have diffuse crackles on lung auscultation. The patient can progress to cyanosis, diaphoresis, and confusion. In patients already intubated and on the ventilator, ARDS can present with high pressure ventilator alarms and a down-trending oxygen saturation or arterial partial pressure of oxygen (PaO_2).[1,2]

It is important to recognize that the presentation of ARDS often overlaps with other diagnoses, including those that can *cause* ARDS. Over 60 causes of ARDS have been identified, but the majority of cases are attributed to sepsis, aspiration, and pneumonia. Other major inciting incidents include trauma (especially in those patients with bilateral lung contusions or fat emboli), transfusion, transplant, and medications or drugs (both illicit and prescribed). An additional diagnostic dilemma is differentiating ARDS from cardiogenic pulmonary edema. Point-of-care echocardiography can help to assess cardiac function; however, pulmonary B lines can be seen in both cardiogenic pulmonary edema and ARDS. It is best to err on the side of caution and include ARDS in your differential if the diagnosis is unclear, as a missed diagnosis and lack of early appropriate treatment may lead to poor outcomes.[1,3,4]

This patient has septic shock secondary to pneumonia. The presentation, labs, and chest x-ray (see Figure 9.1) meet the criteria for moderate ARDS based on the Berlin Definition for ARDS.[4] These criteria include respiratory failure not secondary to cardiac failure within 1 week of an inciting

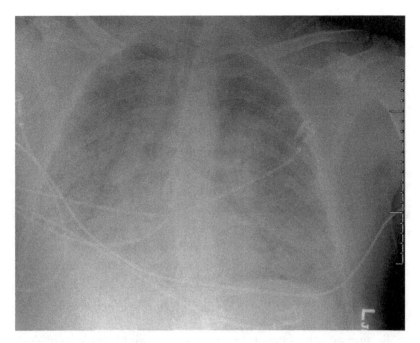

FIGURE 9.1   Chest x-ray with ARDS

clinical insult noted by bilateral opacities on chest imaging. The final criterion to be classified as having ARDS is the PaO_2/FiO_2 (P:F) ratio. The P:F
ratio divides patients into mild (≤300 mmHg), moderate (≤200 mmHg),
and severe (≤100 mmHg) categories based on the degree of hypoxemia.
These categories are relevant to ED providers because certain management
strategies apply to different categories of hypoxemia (e.g., consideration of
prone positioning ["proning"]). Of note, the more severe forms of ARDS
are associated with higher mortality.[5]

The mainstay of treatment for ARDS, apart from addressing the inciting
source, is appropriate ventilator management with lung-protective strategy.
Most critical is ventilation with low V_T (4–8 cc/kg ideal body weight [IBW]).
Studies have demonstrated that low V_T ventilation is associated with better
mortality: ARDS patients ventilated with 6 cc/kg IBW showed improved
survival and more ventilator-free days than those ventilated with higher V_T.[6]
Low V_T ventilation strategies initiated in the ED have been shown to improve
mortality. This strategy may be effective by decreasing the risk of alveolar

overdistention and lung injury. It simply requires providers to measure (or estimate) a patient's height to determine their ideal or predicted body weight. Starting at 6 cc/kg is reasonable, and providers can go slightly up or down based on the patient's ventilatory needs. If time allows, clinicians can even calculate a patient's predicted body weight (PBW) prior to intubation so that an appropriate V_T is set before even placing the patient on the ventilator (see Chapter 8).

In addition to setting appropriate lung-protective V_T based on PBW, providers can help their patients with ARDS by monitoring plateau pressure (P_{plat}). This is checked by performing an inspiratory hold on patients who are paralyzed or at least well sedated and synchronous with a ventilator. P_{plat} is related to the compliance of the lungs. The LUNG SAFE study noted that patients with lower P_{plat} values (in addition to lower peak and driving pressures, higher PEEP, and lower RR) had improved survival.[3] This means that as you titrate up your PEEP, you should be checking associated P_{plat} values, because if they are increasing well beyond a level of 30, you may want to avoid further increasing PEEP, consider proning, or consider other ARDS therapies.

Because we know lung-protective ventilation with lower V_T provides a mortality benefit, most providers use the volume-control mode on the ventilator, as you can then control this critical variable. However, if you cannot ventilate and oxygenate your patient on volume-control mode you can consider trialing pressure-control mode to see if your patient tolerates it better. Please note that with this setting, you cannot control for the volume, and thus if you are not monitoring the ventilator closely, your patient could be taking much larger V_T than ideal. In addition, if your patient's compliance suddenly changes, V_T could decline and contribute to a profound respiratory acidemia.

Figure 9.2 depicts a PEEP:FiO_2 ladder. These ladders come from the ARDSNet database[6] and depict how one can titrate PEEP and FiO_2. In general, you want to avoid things such as a PEEP of 5 with a FiO_2 of 100%, or a PEEP of 15 and a FiO_2 of 40%. Use both aspects of the ventilator to improve oxygenation in patients. More recently, providers have been utilizing driving pressure for PEEP titration rather than the ARDSnet ladders. Driving pressure is a patient's plateau pressure-PEEP. Providers can assess what happens to a patient's plateau pressure at different PEEP levels. If the patient is benefiting from more PEEP, their plateau pressure will not

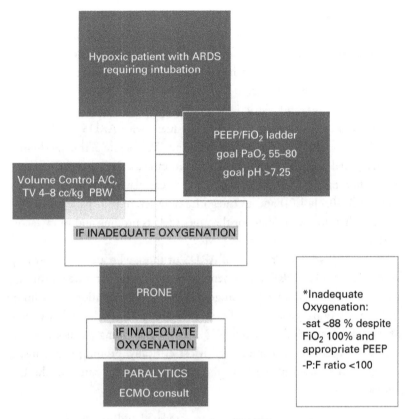

FIGURE 9.2 Summary flowchart for care of a patient with ARDS

increase or increase slightly. If the patient is being overdistended by more PEEP, the driving pressure and plateau pressure will rise notably. This pathway for PEEP adjustments allows for more specific, patient-tailored strategies that focus on a patient's own lung compliance. Providers should target driving pressures of <15.

Mechanical ventilation priorities are as follows:

1. Low V_T ventilation (4–8 cc/kg predicted body weight (PBW) based on height), goal pH >7.25
2. Monitor P_{plat} (goal <30).
3. Follow PEEP:FiO_2 ladders as a guide, with goals of PaO_2 55 to 80 and oxygen saturation >92%.

Lastly, consider the level of sedation and ventilator dyssynchrony. Recall that you can set your ventilator to the best settings possible, but if the patient is dyssynchronous, it is all for naught. Providers can use other adjuncts for patient care such as decreasing oxygen demands (via antipyretics, pain control), transfusing for a hemoglobin goal of 7 to avoid decreased oxygenation with anemia, and restrictive fluid strategies.[7–9]

Unlike most ED scenarios, having a patient with ARDS can be made slightly easier with ABGs and an arterial line. We tolerate permissive hypercapnia (usually aim for a pH of ≥7.25) and target a PaO_2 between 55 and 80. Obtaining this PaO_2 value allows you to calculate a P:F ratio (PaO_2 on ABG/FiO_2 [0.21–1.0]) and to categorize how severe your patient's disease is and if they are a candidate for therapies such as proning and/or extracorporeal membrane oxygenation (ECMO).

In patients with severe cases of ARDS or those who are not improving with other standard ARDS treatment, proning may be warranted. Proning, with the assistance of gravity, changes the pressure distribution in the lungs and can aid in oxygenation and preventing lung injury through a variety of mechanisms including better V:Q matching. Proning has been associated with a reduction in mortality. Most critically, proning is not just a modality to be used in the ICU and can be conducted safely in the ED with a few tips:

1. Ensure the patient is appropriately sedated and paralyzed if necessary before flipping.
2. Ensure you have conducted any procedures you anticipate might need to be accomplished in the next 12 to 18 hours, such as central lines, arterial lines, dialysis lines, and so forth; these will be significantly more challenging if not impossible while the patient is proned.
3. Ensure you and your team have a plan on how to flip the patient, including who will be managing the endotracheal tube and any drains/lines, adjusting where the vital sign monitors are, the direction of turning, and so forth. One person should stand at the foot of the bed to oversee the whole process.
4. Proning beds are infrequently used; all you need is some pillows and appropriate cushioning/padding for dependent areas.[10]

In general, early, consecutive proning should be considered in patients with moderate-severe ARDS (P:F ratio <100) if ventilatory techniques alone have not been successful.[2,11]

Other more controversial treatment modalities include ECMO and neuromuscular blockade. If you continue to have issues with ventilator synchrony despite adequate sedation, paralytics can be trialed, though the data supporting their use are mixed. We recommend trialing a push dose of a paralytic to see if it improves your patient's synchrony and your ability to oxygenate/ventilate the patient, and then considering a drip if effective.[12,13] If proning, paralytics, and lung-protective ventilation are ineffective, the next step to consider is ECMO, which, put simply, involves a machine to oxygenate/ventilate that bypasses the lungs, giving them time to recover. Providers can call an ECMO referral center to discuss their patient's case with an ECMO provider and see if their patient qualifies for transfer, usually after the patient has not improved despite lung-protective ventilation, appropriate PEEP, and proning. If you are not at an ECMO center, consider ECMO referral early so that if your patient is a candidate, the transfer process can be expedited.

In our patient, his V_T was decreased to 450 and his peak pressure alarms ceased. His PEEP was increased in intervals to 15 with an FiO_2 of 80%, but his P:F ratio remained <100. He was placed in prone position on hour 3 of his stay in the ED with almost immediate improvement in his oxygenation, with his PEEP down-titrated to 12 and a P:F ratio of 160. He ultimately received a bed in the ICU (10 hours later). He remained on the ventilator for a week and was ultimately extubated neurologically intact.

KEY POINTS TO REMEMBER

- ARDS is an underrecognized diagnosis associated with a variety of conditions leading to profound hypoxemia, decreased lung compliance, and high mortality.
- The mainstay of treatment for ARDS, aside from addressing the underlying cause, is appropriate oxygenation/ventilation techniques using low V_T, PEEP titration strategies, and maintaining low peak/plateau pressures.

- If lung-protective ventilation is not effective, the best next option for refractory hypoxemia is early proning. Other possible treatment modalities to consider include neuromuscular blockade and ECMO.

References

1. Bellani G, Laffey JG, Pham T, Fan E, Brochard L, Esteban A, et al. Epidemiology, patterns of care, and mortality for patients with acute respiratory distress syndrome in intensive care units in 50 countries. *JAMA*. 2016;315(8):788–800.
2. Papazian L, Aubron C, Brochard L, Chiche JD, Combes A, Dreyfuss D, et al. Formal guidelines: management of acute respiratory distress syndrome. *Ann Intensive Care*. 2019;9(1):69.
3. Laffey JG, Bellani G, Pham T, Fan E, Madotto F, Bajwa EK, et al. Potentially modifiable factors contributing to outcome from acute respiratory distress syndrome: The LUNG SAFE study. *Intensive Care Med*. 2016;42(12):1865–1876.
4. ARDS Definition Task Force. Acute respiratory distress syndrome: The Berlin definition. *JAMA*. 2012;307(23):2526–2533.
5. Rezoagli E, Fumagalli R, Bellani G. Definition and epidemiology of acute respiratory distress syndrome. *Ann Transl Med*. 2017;5(14):282.
6. Acute Respiratory Distress Syndrome Network. Ventilation with lower tidal volumes as compared with traditional tidal volumes for acute lung injury and the acute respiratory distress syndrome. *N Engl J Med*. 2000;342(18):1301–1308.
7. Fan E, Del Sorbo L, Goligher EC, Hodgson CL, Munshi L, Walkey AJ, et al. An official American Thoracic Society/European Society of Intensive Care Medicine/Society of Critical Care Medicine clinical practice guideline: Mechanical ventilation in adult patients with acute respiratory distress syndrome. *Am J Respir Crit Care Med*. 2017;195(9):1253–1263.
8. Goligher EC, Hodgson CL, Adhikari NK, Meade MO, Wunsch H, Uleryk E, et al. Lung recruitment maneuvers for adult patients with acute respiratory distress syndrome: A systematic review and meta-analysis. *Ann Am Thorac Soc*. 2017;14(S4):S304–S311.
9. National Heart, Lung, and Blood Institute Acute Respiratory Distress Syndrome (ARDS) Clinical Trials Network. Comparison of two fluid-management strategies in acute lung injury. *N Engl J Med*. 2006;354(24):2564–2575.
10. Hao D, Low S, DiFenza R, Shenoy ES, Ananian L, Prout LA, et al. Prone positioning of intubated patients with an elevated body-mass index. *N Engl J Med*. 2022;386(14):e34.
11. Guérin C, Reignier J, Richard JC, Beuret P, Gacouin A, Boulain T, et al. Prone positioning in severe acute respiratory distress syndrome. *N Engl J Med*. 2013;368(23):2159–2168.

12. Papazian L, Forel JM, Gacouin A, Penot-Ragon C, Perrin G, Loundou A, et al. Neuromuscular blockers in early acute respiratory distress syndrome. *N Engl J Med*. 2010;363(12):1107–1116.

13. National Heart, Lung, and Blood Institute PETAL Clinical Trials Network, Moss M, Huang DT, et al. Early neuromuscular blockade in the acute respiratory distress syndrome. *N Engl J Med*. 2019;380(21):1997–2008. doi:10.1056/NEJMoa1901686

10 Upside-down is best: Practical proning

Danny VanValkinburgh and Brian T. Wessman

A 50-year-old man presents to your community ED for shortness of breath. The patient's family states that 5 days ago he was diagnosed with influenza by his primary care physician. He has been at home since the diagnosis and has had persistent malaise with worsening shortness of breath. His family called EMS for difficulty breathing this morning. On arrival the patient is tachypneic, tachycardic, and in respiratory distress. On auscultation, there are crackles bilaterally in all lung fields. The initial oxygen saturation is 77% on room air. The patient requires intubation and the chest radiograph shows bilateral patchy infiltrates. Initial arterial blood gas values show persistent hypoxemia with a PaO_2 of 53 despite an FiO_2 of 100% and a positive end-expiratory pressure (PEEP) of 12.5. A bedside ultrasound shows normal cardiac function without evidence of volume overload. CT imaging of the chest reveals bilateral patchy opacities and no pulmonary embolism. Reviewing the Berlin criteria (occurring within 7 days of known insult, bilateral opacities on imaging, respiratory failure not fully explained by cardiac failure or volume overload, a PaO_2/FiO_2 (P:F) ratio <300 with a minimum of 5 cmH_2O PEEP) leads you to a diagnosis of acute respiratory distress syndrome (ARDS). The patient is to be admitted to the ICU; however, while boarding in the ED for several hours he continues to desaturate.

What do I do now?

This patient presents with signs and symptoms concerning for type 1 respiratory failure caused by ARDS. ARDS is a histologic diagnosis with diffuse alveolar damage dispersed through the lung parenchyma characterized by hyaline membrane formation and alveolar wall thickening. Physiologically, ARDS is an acute lung injury process causing inflammation of the alveoli with pulmonary infiltrates on imaging and the inability to oxygenate appropriately. The Berlin criteria, most recently reviewed in 2012, are accepted as defining ARDS. The four criteria are (1) an acute lung injury within 7 days of a known insult or worsening respiratory symptoms, (2) bilateral opacities seen on chest radiography, (3) pulmonary edema not fully explained by cardiogenic edema or volume overload, and (4) hypoxia, defined as a P:F ratio <300 while receiving support of PEEP or continuous positive airway pressure (CPAP) settings of at least 5 cm H_2O on invasive or noninvasive ventilation. The Berlin criteria can subsequently risk stratify patients with ARDS by their P:F ratios: mild, 201 to 300 mmHg; moderate, 101 to 200 mmHg; and severe, <100 mmHg. Mortality based on the P:F ratio is described as 27% (mild), 32% (moderate), and 45% (severe). The patient in the vignette has features consistent with ARDS likely due to his previous viral infection, has ongoing pneumonia, and would be classified as having severe ARDS.

Treatment of ARDS has evolved over the past several decades, with noted mortality improvements. The inflammatory changes of ARDS are typically exacerbated by mechanical ventilation–induced volutrauma, barotrauma, atelectrauma, hyperoxia, and volume overload. Current treatment strategies are aimed at minimizing further lung damage as well as improving oxygenation. Volutrauma is minimized by low tidal volume settings of 6 to 8 cc/kg of ideal body weight. Barotrauma is combatted by maintaining plateau pressures <30 mmHg. Atelectrauma is mitigated by appropriate stepwise PEEP levels corresponding to the level of hypoxia with at least 5 mmH$_2$O on initiation of mechanical ventilation. Hyperoxia is avoided by targeting PaO$_2$ levels of 55 to 80 mmHg or oxygen saturations >93%. Appropriate ventilator management is one of the cornerstones of the management of ARDS as well as being the most impactful treatment modality. Concurrently, the clinician needs to promote a balanced fluid resuscitation strategy and limit aggressive volume over-resuscitation; lungs don't like to be "wet." Other treatments such as neuromuscular blockade, glucocorticoid use, and extracorporeal membrane oxygenation (ECMO) have shown mixed results and may be beneficial in certain ARDS phenotypes. However, one of the more successful strategies for improving oxygenation has been prone positioning.

A large study by Guérin et al. in the *New England Journal of Medicine* was one of the first studies showing that prone positioning used early in the treatment of severe ARDS improved mortality.[1] Previous studies had shown improvement in oxygenation and reduced ventilator-induced lung injury; however, none had shown a mortality benefit. Prone positioning improves mortality due to redistribution of stress and strain of positive-pressure ventilation as well as improving ventilation/perfusion (V/Q) mismatch. When prone, there is improved lung tissue perfusion through dependent areas where there also is increased alveolar ventilation. Overall, patients have improved oxygenation and reduced lung injury when in the prone position. The protocol used by Guérin et al. was initiated early in the ARDS course and called for patients to be in the prone position for a minimum of 16 consecutive hours. Afterwards, the patients underwent daily trials of "de-proning" to evaluate for clinical improvement. Prone positioning is now seen as a viable treatment option in severe ARDS that leads to reduced mortality. It can be performed in the ED and should be a part of the treatment algorithm for refractory hypoxemia.

Although there are benefits to prone positioning, there are also potential adverse effects and limitations. Placing a patient in the prone position requires multiple people to safely and successfully change a patient from supine to prone without dislodging the endotracheal tube or venous access. Although multiple techniques exist, one method is described by Guérin et al. and shown in a video that can be seen online at the *New England Journal of Medicine* website.[2] A pre-procedure checklist may be helpful for safely repositioning the patient (Box 10.1). The process includes placing all lines and monitoring cables in a head-to-toe plane, rolling the patient to one lateral side, changing cardiac monitor leads to the back, sliding to

Standard pre-procedure checklist and steps for proning a patient

Standard method

- Explain to the family the plan and clinical benefits.
- Coordinate your ICU team.
- Gather team:
  - MD to supervise and monitor (should not be involved in the actual proning)
  - Respiratory therapist (RT) to hold the endotracheal tube during the full procedure
  - Two to four nurses to roll the patient (depending on the patient's body habitus)
  - One nurse to change sheets, replace monitoring equipment and leads, and so forth
  - Runner available outside of room to grab medications if needed
- Decide which way to roll.
- Line all IV tubing, ventilator tubing, and all other invasive lines/ devices in a head-to-toe (off the bed) configuration.
- Ensure there is enough slack in IV tubing, chest tubes, and ventilator tubing to turn the patient.
- Place adhesive padding on pressure points under the hips and chest wall.
- Remove unused monitoring leads/stickers on chest/abdomen to prevent skin breakdown.
- RT holds the tube in place and instructs the team on when to begin turning.
- Roll the patient in the agreed-upon direction, stopping when the patient is perpendicular to the floor.
- Transition current monitoring leads to similar physiologic locations along the back/posterior aspect of the patient (and remove the anterior chest wall/abdomen monitoring leads).
- Change out old/dirty sheets as needed, placing clean new sheets.
- Consider placing pressure pads under the hips and chest wall.
- On the RT's count, turn the patient all the way to the prone position.

Alternative approach: the "burrito" approach
- All steps are the same as above, aside from the roll modification.
- For the "burrito" approach, the existing top sheet is wrapped around the patient (pulled up on either side) to create a human "burrito."
- Roll the patient in the agreed-upon direction completely to the proned position in the "burrito" sheet wrapping, and remove the top sheet (which should now be over the patient's back).
- Transition current monitoring leads from the lateral aspects to similar physiologic locations along the back/posterior aspect of the patient.

For both approaches
- Ensure the patient's head in turned laterally and the endotracheal tube is still in the correct position (confirm with continuous capnography).
- "Swim" the patient's contralateral arm to above the head in the same direction the face is pointing. The other arm can remain down.
- Ensure all IV tubing, vascular access sites, tubes, and drains are in place, carefully avoiding pressure wounds under skin.
- Ensure ventilator compliance is acceptable. Check expected tidal volume and inspiratory pressures.
- Head and arms are moved every 2 hours (swimming position). Head is rotated to the other direction with the contralateral arm being positioned above the head and the ipsilateral arm remaining down (in the "swimming position").

the side of the bed, and then rolling on the patient's abdomen. The head is usually turned to the side with pillows or soft foam support. Pressure ulcers commonly occur in areas not normally expected like the face and extremities, and measures should be employed to reduce the likelihood of pressure wounds. Prophylactic hydrocolloid dressings to the face, chin, and shoulders are commonly used. Patients must also be moved several times a day to help redistribute skin pressure by placing the arms in the "swimmer's position." Eye drops and eye shields should also be considered for reducing ocular injury. In the event of significant deterioration while in the prone position, flipping to the supine position may not be able to be done quickly without sufficient help. In the case of cardiac arrest, compressions may be delayed while the patient is returned to supine. There are also data showing the potential benefit of "back compressions" while in the prone position (the authors of this chapter actually prefer this method to minimize lack of circulatory time).

Patients with moderate to severe ARDS (defined as a P:F ratio <150 mmHg) have high mortality rates. In addition to evidence-based ventilator management and fluid strategies, prone positioning has been shown to improve mortality by increasing oxygenation while mitigating ventilator-induced lung injury.

The patient in the vignette has severe ARDS with refractory hypoxia. After appropriate ventilator management and sedation, a decision was made to prone the patient while in the ED. Fortunately, the ED staff had recently had an in-service on proning patients, had reviewed online educational videos, and were familiar with the process. After appropriate personal were gathered and the patient was prepared, the patient was successfully proned. The patient was transported to the ICU in the prone position. Over the next 16 hours, improvement in oxygenation was noted. Ventilator adjustments were made to both the PEEP and FiO_2, and ultimately the patient required less support. The patient underwent a de-proning trial the next day and was extubated successfully 3 days later.

KEY POINTS TO REMEMBER

- Appropriate deep sedation with or without paralysis
- Empiric placement of central venous access and arterial monitoring (if not already done) before proning
- Prophylaxis of pressure ulcers, facial head and neck positioning, head-of-bed positioning
- Care when transferring supine to prone, prone to supine, and changing positions in "swimming" positions
- Close monitoring of airway and venous access sites
- Continued cardiopulmonary monitoring

References

1. Guérin C, Reignier J, Richard JC, Beuret P, Gacouin A, Boulain T, et al. Prone positioning in severe acute respiratory distress syndrome. *N Engl J Med*. 2013;368(23):2159–2168.
2. Hao D, Law S, Di Fenza R, Shenoy ES, Ananian L, Prout LA, et al. Prone positioning of intubated patients with an elevated body-mass index. *N Engl J Med*. 2022;386:e34.https://www.nejm.org/doi/full/10.1056/NEJMvcm2108494

Further reading

Acute Respiratory Distress Syndrome Network. Ventilation with lower tidal volumes as compared with traditional tidal volumes for acute lung injury and the acute respiratory distress syndrome. *N Engl J Med*. 2000;342(18):1301–1308.

Brower RG, Lanken PN, MacIntyre NR, Matthay MA, Morris AH, Ancukiewicz M, et al. Higher versus lower positive end-expiratory pressures in patients with the acute respiratory distress syndrome. *N Engl J Med*. 2004;351(4):327–336.

Fuller BM, Ferguson IT, Mohr NM, et al. Lung-protective ventilation initiated in the emergency department (LOV-ED): A quasi-experimental, before-after trial. *Ann Emerg Med*. 2017;70(3):406–418.

Kollef M. *The Washington Manual of Critical Care*. 3rd ed. Lippincott Williams & Wilkins; 2017.

Marino P. *The ICU Book*. 4th ed. Lippincott Williams & Wilkins; 2013.

11 It's getting harder to breathe: Refractory ARDS and VV-ECMO

Fraser Mackay

A 40-year-old female without past medical history presents to a community ED with 3 days of worsening dyspnea, cough, fevers, and diarrhea. Triage reveals tachycardia to 130 bpm, BP 135/90 mmHg, temperature 39.4°C, RR 28 breaths/min, and room air SpO_2 85%. She becomes increasingly hypoxemic and agitated, prompting emergent intubation. She is placed on volume assist control at 100% FiO_2, tidal volume 360 mL (predicted body weight is 60 kg), rate 24, and PEEP 12 cmH_2O. This yields a SpO_2 of 91%, plateau pressures of 30 to 32 cm H_2O. A chest x-ray reveals dense multifocal opacities with the endotracheal tube in a good position. Lab work shows a lactic acid of 3.8 mg/dL, WBC of 18, and a normal complete metabolic panel. Her viral PCR swab is positive for SARS-CoV-2.

A bedside echo shows a hyperdynamic left ventricle but mild-moderate right ventricular dysfunction/dilation. She is sedated on fentanyl and propofol, is passive on the ventilator (intubated with vecuronium), but her SpO_2 continues to fall. Up-titrating PEEP causes elevated plateau/driving pressures and hypotension, so her ventilator settings do not change. Her ABG results are now 7.23/51 mmHg /35 mmHg /14.8 mEq/L/ 89%. The consulting intensivist states that while an ICU bed is available, the patient may be too ill for what her ICU can support; the patient will need to be transferred. The nearest ECMO-capable center is 2 hours by ground transport and 40 minutes by helicopter transport. The patient's SpO_2 is now 86%.

What do I do now?

The scenario of severe viral pneumonia (with possible secondary bacterial infection) and acute respiratory distress syndrome (ARDS) has the patient in a precarious situation. She meets all criteria for severe ARDS (see Chapters 9 and 10). She was appropriately intubated, her ventilator settings exemplify evidence-based ARDS care, and she is sedated and paralyzed to maximize ventilator efficacy. Despite this, the patient's poor compliance (~20 mL/cmH$_2$O) and shunt physiology have exceeded the ventilator's ability to perform gas exchange. While diuresis and steroid administration may be appropriate to optimize the patient's condition further, her degree of hypoxemia suggests a level of acuity that is unlikely to improve in time for these measures to take effect. The next step is an emergent trial of prone positioning (see Chapter 10). However, her decreasing stability makes a transfer to the ICU risky, and the "available" ICU bed is not staffed to meet the demands that the patient requires of prone position care.

In this circumstance, the best chance of stabilization lies with prone positioning and possibly also with temporary administration of a pulmonary vasodilator (such as inhaled epoprostenol). Prone positioning likely needs to occur without delay and in the ED (possibly with help from in-house ICU staff or in consultation with the accepting center). The logistics of the case also imply this patient may require transfer in the prone position, something with which EMS systems since the 2009 influenza pandemic (and the more recent COVID-19 pandemic) have become increasingly familiar. While inhaled agents have been shown to provide no benefit (or possibly even to harm patients in the case of nitric oxide), they can be used for bridging therapy in cases of severe hypoxemia while more definitive care is arranged.

However, what if a trial of prone positioning results in no improvement? At that point, the patient would require evaluation for the implementation of emergent venovenous extracorporeal membrane oxygenation (VV-ECMO) at a capable tertiary care center.

CLINICAL AND HISTORICAL CONTEXT

Patients with severe, refractory ARDS rarely present in the ED, though severe ARDS certainly does occur every year (and with increased frequency in particularly virulent pandemics). Severe ARDS more typically presents several hours to days after initiating invasive mechanical ventilation, with delays in diagnosis and treatment weighing heavily on outcomes. VV-ECMO succeeds most often in ARDS cases when implemented early in the course of disease, with the largest success being in healthy patients with single-organ-system failure. This was best demonstrated by the CESAR trial in 2009, in which patients with severe ARDS were randomized to "conventional treatment" at local hospitals versus transfer to ECMO centers for consideration of ECMO.[1] In the end, most patients in the intervention arm simply required ventilator changes at experienced centers and avoided further support altogether. The more recent EOLIA study in 2018 randomized ARDS patients in more straightforward fashion, arguably showing a strong signal toward VV-ECMO benefit for sicker patients early in their course.[2]

Despite early consideration and initiation of VV-ECMO during the COVID-19 pandemic, outcomes and mortality have not changed. VV-ECMO mortality is approximately 40%, with median duration of therapy of 14–20 days. Mortality increases with the duration of mechanical ventilation before ECMO, and patients deteriorating in non-ECMO capable centers should be referred early for management and consideration of therapy.[4]

WHAT IS VV-ECMO AND "LUNG RESCUE" THERAPY?

Chapter 17 also covers ECMO, though with differing clinical context, components, and goals of therapy. VV-ECMO refers to the narrow application of a bypass circuit (cannulas, pump, and membrane oxygenator) to drain venous blood from the femoral vein/caval circulation, perform gas exchange, and then return oxygen-rich blood to the right heart via the right atrium. Oxygen-rich blood then flows through injured lungs, then into the left heart, then out to the rest of the body (Figure 11.1). As the patient's lungs recover, the medical team weans the circuit flow to gradually transition the function of gas exchange back to the lungs/ventilator. Cannulas range in size depending on the size and habitus of the patient, but they can range from 15 to 24 French and are typically inserted percutaneously with serial dilations (a procedure not much different than the process of placing a central line, dialysis catheter, or chest tube). The outflow cannula's output of blood is usually directed into the right atrium and directly at the tricuspid valve via transesophageal echocardiography or fluoroscopy to maximize oxygen delivery.

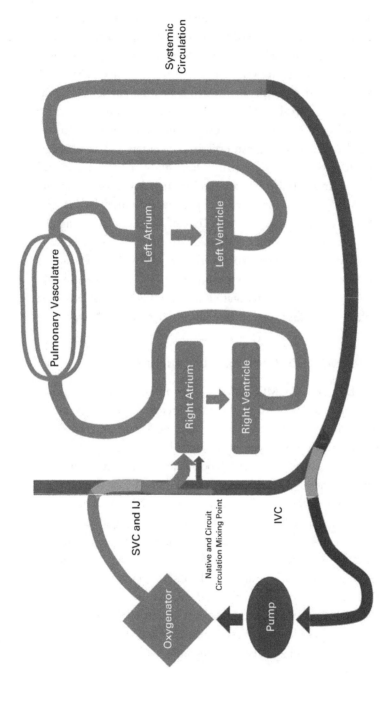

FIGURE 11.1 Schematic of a VV-ECMO circuit. Deoxygenated blood (blue) drains via the femoral vein and inflow cannula (gray) and is drawn into the centrifugal pump-head. Blood is then pushed into the membrane oxygenator and fully oxygenated (red). Oxygenated blood travels through the right and left heart, and then into the systemic circulation. In this two-cannula configuration, the circuit and native circulation may mix in the caval system, and can contribute to recirculation at higher flow rates.

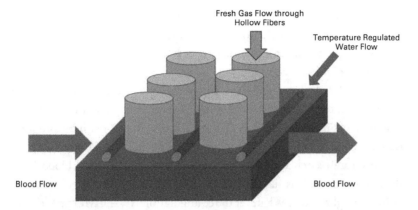

Fresh Gas Flow through
Hollow Fibers

Temperature Regulated
Water Flow

Blood Flow

Blood Flow

FIGURE 11.2 Schematic of the membrane oxygenator at a microscopic level. Gas, temperature-controlled water, and blood pass through the membrane at 90 degrees with respect to each other, maximizing temperature and countercurrent gas exchange.

With the circuit in place, the pump draws venous blood from the inflow cannula into the countercurrent membrane oxygenator, where gas, water, and blood flow interact to maximize countercurrent gas exchange and temperature regulation (Figure 11.2). CO_2 elimination takes place here also and is primarily modified with "sweep" gas, and the team can tailor gas flow to target a desired $PaCO_2$. The physics of CO_2 elimination versus oxygenation in the membrane lung differ significantly, resulting in CO_2 being much easier to eliminate than oxygen to infuse. This results in CO_2 elimination relying entirely on gas flow through the oxygenator, whereas oxygenation relies entirely on blood flow and through the oxygenator (as well as hemoglobin level). While this relationship can challenge teams for patients needing high circuit flows, it does make VV-ECMO an excellent salvage modality for critically ill status asthmaticus patients or transplant candidates with dangerous hypercapnia.

The blood exiting the oxygenator has a PaO_2 of ~400 to 500 mmHg, and the outflow or "return" cannula delivers oxygenated blood into the right atrium. This flow encounters some mixing with the native circulation (caval system, right atrium, and lungs) as shown in Figure 11.1, so the resulting peripheral PaO_2 will initially become 200 to 300 mmHg with 100% saturation. Flow can then be weaned to ensure normoxemia, and the ventilator settings are then usually set to a "lung rest" mode. Since the ventilator now contributes little to gas exchange, the circuit literally removes the need for the patient to "breathe" at all. Common "lung rest" modes have very low set respiratory rates, low tidal volume, and moderate PEEP to prevent atelectasis.

Figure 11.1 depicts a two-cannula system (one in the femoral vein and one in the internal jugular), but another common configuration utilizes a dual-lumen single catheter inserted in the neck. While neither configuration seems superior in terms of outcomes, the dual-lumen "Avalon" catheter may decrease recirculation (a phenomenon where oxygenated blood from the outflow cannula is sucked directly into the inflow cannula without entering the right heart). Whatever the configuration, VV-ECMO provides no boost to cardiac output and requires a functioning cardiac output to carry oxygenated blood to systemic circulation.[6] This key difference separates this type of extracorporeal life support (ECLS) from VA-ECMO (discussed in Chapter 17) or other devices that augment cardiac output. That having been said, it is also common for patients to require vasopressors treat the distributive shock seen in the setting of severe ARDS, which is entirely compatible with the use of VV-ECMO.[5]

VV-ECMO INDICATIONS AND PATIENT SELECTION

VV-ECMO registry data suggest that ECMO has the best chance of success at experienced centers, with a reasonable threshold of 50 total cases and/or 10 to 20 cases per year. As such, the most frequent and important exposure to VV-ECMO patients that most providers have is the time of initial evaluation prior to mechanical support. Both ED and ICU physicians should understand the indications and cautions associated with VV-ECMO salvage and endeavor to recognize potential candidates as early as possible. This not only avoids unnecessary transfers but also ensures early recognition/referral and intervention. Some centers even employ mobile cannulation and retrieval teams for patients who may emergently need ECLS (i.e., a team travels to the referring hospital and cannulates on site).[3]

The vignette beginning the chapter portrays the ideal VV-ECMO patient: She has few comorbid conditions, she is young, and her disease process thus far seems straightforward/reversible. She has no multiple-organ failure, which further improves the chances that VV-ECMO would be an appropriate escalation strategy. In fact, delay of transfer for evaluation by even a day could put her at risk for multiple-organ ischemia and dysfunction from impaired oxygen delivery and worsen chances of successful VV-ECMO salvage. Of course, nothing in clinical practice is ever truly "ideal," and depending on various centers' level of expertise and experience, riskier cases may or may not be ECMO candidates. In addition to some of the basic indications and contraindications shown in Box 11.1, some centers

---

BOX 11.1 **Summary of VV-ECMO considerations**

INDICATIONS FOR EMERGENT VV-ECMO CONSIDERATION

Severe, refractory ARDS (hypoxic respiratory failure with Murray score >3)[1]
 · pH $\leq$7.25 w/$PaCO_2$ $\geq$60 mmHg for >6 hours
 · PaO2:FiO2 < 80 mmHg for >6 hours
 · PaO_2 <60 mm Hg on FiO_2 1.0 and PEEP $\geq$10 cm H_2O for $\geq$3 hours
Refractory status asthmaticus
Refractory air leak syndrome (ex: bronchopleural fistula)
Bridge to lung transplant*

ABSOLUTE CONTRAINDICATIONS TO VV-ECMO

Recent/ongoing intracranial hemorrhage, large cerebrovascular accident, or brain injury
Active or high risk for GI bleed/inability to tolerate anticoagulation[Δ]
Need for significant cardiac output support[†]

RELATIVE CONTRAINDICATIONS TO VV-ECMO[‡]

Age $\geq$65, advanced dementia, and/or debilitated state at baseline
BMI $\geq$45 and/or significant obstacles to vascular access
Prolonged invasive mechanical ventilation (>7 days)

* Patients previously on hospice or undergoing palliative care are inappropriate for ECLS. Select cases of end-stage organ disease may be evaluated for VV-ECMO at advanced centers where transplant workups/plans can be executed.
Δ Circuits are increasingly heparin-bound, and some centers may initiate ECMO and then taper back or discontinue anticoagulation altogether.
† Patients can require vasopressors while on VV-ECMO, but VA-ECMO or other devices are more appropriate for patients with low cardiac output.
‡ Different centers have different levels of comfort with these obstacles on a case-by-case basis, but all are associated with worse outcomes.

incorporate various composite scores (e.g., RESP, PRESET, or ECMOnet) into patient evaluation.[7] However, most consider these tools mainly supplemental to clinical judgment.

CLINICAL OUTCOMES AND CONCLUSION

Severe ARDS has an accepted mortality of about ~45% to 50%, with prone positioning and other management strategies contributing to substantial mortality improvements. VV-ECMO should never take place without first maximizing those treatments, especially proning. However, VV-ECMO can salvage refractory cases and represents an important option once all other measures have failed. That said, clinicians should view VV-ECMO's benefit in the context of risk reduction. For the lowest-risk patients, ARDS salvage with VV-ECMO still results in mortality ranging from 25% to 35%. While this lowers the risk of death to less than a coin flip, it is by no means a panacea. It remains one of the most invasive of means of support to which a patient can be subjected: Average "pump runs" for ARDS average about 12–14 days (as long as 2–3 weeks without transplant), necessitate prolonged analgesia and sedation, and require invasive monitoring as well as anticoagulation. Prolonged mechanical ventilation with tracheostomy and long hospital and rehabilitation courses remain the norm after circuit discontinuation. While this is completely appropriate for some patients, initial evaluation must weigh the invasive nature and high resource utilization of the therapy against the patient's baseline quality of life/health and age and their goals of care. As with all life support, its purpose is to provide temporary stabilization and a bridge to definitive therapy, ultimately allowing for meaningful healing and a return to an acceptable quality of life. For young patients with potentially reversible single-organ lung failure, early recognition by the emergency medicine provider for referral consultation to ECMO centers is imperative.

KEY POINTS TO REMEMBER

- VV-ECMO is a salvage therapy for refractory ARDS and temporarily replaces the lung's ability to perform gas exchange.

- With appropriate patient selection, VV-ECMO can reduce the mortality of severe ARDS.
- ED and ICU providers should be familiar with the indications and contraindications for VV-ECMO, choosing expeditious stabilization as well as transport when required.
- VV-ECMO is a high-cost invasive therapy that requires a large amount of resources, and adverse events are common. It may not be appropriate for patients with comorbid conditions or other risk factors.

References
1. Peek GJ, Mugford M, Tiruvoipati R, et al. Efficacy and economic assessment of conventional ventilatory support versus extracorporeal membrane oxygenation for severe adult respiratory failure (CESAR): A multicentre randomised controlled trial. *Lancet.* 2009;374(9698):1351–1363.
2. Combes A, Hajage D, Capellier G, et al. Extracorporeal membrane oxygenation for severe acute respiratory distress syndrome. *N Engl J Med.* 2018;378(21):1965–1975.
3. Lucchini A, De Felippis C, Elli S, et al. Mobile ECMO team for inter-hospital transportation of patients with ARDS: A retrospective case series. *Heart Lung Vessel.* 2014;6(4):262–273.
4. Badulak J, Antonini MV, Stead CM, et al. Extracorporeal Membrane Oxygenation for COVID-19: Updated 2021 Guidelines from the Extracorporeal Life Support Organization. *ASAIO Journal.* 2021;67(5):485–495.
5. Brogan TV, Lequier L, Lorusso R, MacLaren G, Peek G. *Extracorporeal Life Support: The ELSO Red Book.* Extracorporeal Life Support Organization; 2017.
6. Jayaraman AL, Cormican D, Shah P, Ramakrishna H. Cannulation strategies in adult veno-arterial and veno-venous extracorporeal membrane oxygenation: Techniques, limitations, and special considerations. *Ann Card Anaesth.* 2017;20(Suppl):S11–S18.
7. Giordano L, Francavilla A, Bottio T, et al. Predictive models in extracorporeal membrane oxygenation (ECMO): a systematic review. *Systematic Reviews.* 2023;12:44.

Further reading
Acute Respiratory Distress Syndrome Network, Brower RG, Matthay MA, et al. Ventilation with lower tidal volumes as compared with traditional tidal volumes for acute lung injury and the acute respiratory distress syndrome. *N Engl J Med.* 2000;342(18):1301–1308.
Amato MB, Meade MO, Slutsky AS, et al. Driving pressure and survival in the acute respiratory distress syndrome. *N Engl J Med.* 2015;372(8):747–755.

Bellani G, Laffey JG, Pham T, et al. Epidemiology, patterns of care, and mortality for patients with acute respiratory distress syndrome in intensive care units in 50 countries [published correction appears in *JAMA*. 2016 Jul 19;316(3):350]. *JAMA*. 2016;315(8):788–800.

Ferguson ND, Fan E, Camporota L, et al. The Berlin definition of ARDS: An expanded rationale, justification, and supplementary material [published correction appears in *Intensive Care Med*. 2012 Oct;38(10):1731–2]. *Intensive Care Med*. 2012;38(10):1573–1582.

Gebistorf F, Karam O, Wetterslev J, Afshari A. Inhaled nitric oxide for acute respiratory distress syndrome (ARDS) in children and adults. *Cochrane Database Syst Rev*. 2016;2016(6):CD002787.

Guérin C, Reignier J, Richard JC, et al. Prone positioning in severe acute respiratory distress syndrome. *N Engl J Med*. 2013;368(23):2159–2168.

Huesch MD. Volume–outcome relationships in extracorporeal membrane oxygenation: Retrospective analysis of administrative data from Pennsylvania, 2007–2015. *ASAIO J*. 2018;64(4):450–457.

National Heart, Lung, and Blood Institute PETAL Clinical Trials Network, Moss M, Huang DT, et al. Early neuromuscular blockade in the acute respiratory distress syndrome. *N Engl J Med*. 2019;380(21):1997–2008.

Palmér O, Palmér K, Hultman J, Broman M. Cannula design and recirculation during venovenous extracorporeal membrane oxygenation. *ASAIO J*. 2016;62(6):737–742.

Papazian L, Forel JM, Gacouin A, et al. Neuromuscular blockers in early acute respiratory distress syndrome. *N Engl J Med*. 2010;363(12):1107–1116.

Roch A, Guervilly C, Papazian L. Fluid management in acute lung injury and ARDS. *Ann Intensive Care*. 2011;1(1):16.

Searcy RJ, Morales JR, Ferreira JA, Johnson DW. The role of inhaled prostacyclin in treating acute respiratory distress syndrome. *Ther Adv Respir Dis*. 2015;9(6):302–312.

Villar J, Ferrando C, Martínez D, et al. Dexamethasone treatment for the acute respiratory distress syndrome: A multicentre, randomised controlled trial. *Lancet Respir Med*. 2020;8(3):267–276.

Yeo HJ, Kim D, Jeon D, Kim YS, Rycus P, Cho WH. Extracorporeal membrane oxygenation for life-threatening asthma refractory to mechanical ventilation: Analysis of the Extracorporeal Life Support Organization registry. *Crit Care*. 2017;21(1):297.

Yeo HJ, Kim YS, Kim D; ELSO Registry Committee, Cho WH. Risk factors for complete recovery of adults after weaning from veno-venous extracorporeal membrane oxygenation for severe acute respiratory failure: An analysis from adult patients in the Extracorporeal Life Support Organization registry. *J Intensive Care*. 2020;8:64.

PART 3

Circulation

12 Hot and shocky: Distributive/septic shock

Ani Aydin and Kusum S. Mathews

A 65-year-old male with a past medical history
of hypertension, hyperlipidemia, and diabetes
presents to the ED with complaints of a cough,
fever, and generalized weakness. EMS providers
were called for complaints of shortness of
breath and fever, and upon arrival placed the
patient on a non-rebreather (NRB) mask for
significant hypoxemia on pulse oximetry (85%
on room air). The patient states that he has been
short of breath for the past 2 days and has a
gradually worsening cough with yellow sputum
production. He also complains of fever of 103°F
today and last took an antipyretic medication
1 hour prior to arrival. On physical examination,
he is tachypneic with an increased work of
breathing, speaking in one-word sentences, and
has coarse breath sounds bilaterally. His initial
vital signs are BP 74/48 mmHg, HR 132 bpm,
RR 34 breaths/min, pulse oximetry 94% on an
NRB, and temperature 102.4°F.

What do I do now?

This case is a classic presentation of septic shock, likely secondary to a pneumonia. Septic shock is a form of distributive shock, which is one of the most common forms of shock encountered in the ED.

Shock is a disease state characterized by organ hypoperfusion. It can be mediated by different mechanisms, including a low intravascular volume (hypovolemic/hemorrhagic shock), decreased cardiac output (cardiogenic shock) or pump failure (obstructive shock), or vasodilation (distributive shock). Distributive shock results from arterial or venous vasodilation, leading to an inadequate tissue perfusion. It can be due to anaphylaxis, neurologic injury, or drug overdose. However, the most common form of distributive shock is septic shock, which results in vasodilation and inadequate tissue perfusion due to an infectious etiology. While sepsis has been described since the time of the ancient Greeks, our definitions of these disease processes have changed over time, as has our management.

The management of sepsis and septic shock was revolutionized by early goal-directed therapy (EGDT), an algorithmic approach to the early identification and resuscitation of these patients. The original EGDT trial from 2001 was conducted at a time when sepsis and septic shock were not readily recognized, leading to a significant burden of disease at the time of diagnosis with higher associated mortality rates.[1] Many aspects of the EGDT algorithm have been incorporated into standard-of-care resuscitation bundles and quality metrics, leading to a significant reduction in mortality associated with sepsis and septic shock over the past 20 years, achieved through the implementation science of improving the quality of sepsis care and multiprofessional adult and pediatric sepsis guidelines and education initiatives. Sepsis protocols are now widely used in most hospitals to facilitate identification and treatment and measure adherence to the recommendations as a quality measure. More recently, a series of landmark trials (ProCESS, ProMISe, ARISE, and PRISM)[2-7] have evaluated the efficacy of different aspects of EDGT. These more contemporary trials compared EDGT to current standard or usual types of care, which often contain more contemporaneous protocolized sepsis resuscitation bundles. The findings of these studies show that EDGT did not result in better outcomes that usual care, and often the use of EDGT resulted in higher rates of ICU admissions and costs, as there are several invasive procedures associated with the original algorithm that are no longer used routinely.

To standardize our classifications of sepsis and septic shock, the Third International Consensus Definitions were updated in 2016,[8,9] and the Surviving Sepsis Campaign (SSC) diagnostic and treatment guidelines were updated in 2021.[10–13] Sepsis is defined as a life-threatening disease with organ dysfunction secondary to a dysregulated host response to an infection caused by a bacteria, virus, fungus, or parasite. Septic shock is a subset of sepsis, characterized by severe dysregulation of circulatory and cellular metabolism resulting in end-organ hypoperfusion. It can be associated with severe hypotension unresponsive to isolated crystalloid resuscitation. The goal of adequate resuscitation in sepsis and septic shock is to reverse any hypoperfusion in order to prevent further end-organ damage. Once sepsis is suspected, the SSC makes some recommendations about the diagnostic evaluation and treatment. These recommendations are tiered based on currently available supporting evidence and are updated to provide guidelines for the care of these critically ill patients. The 2021 SSC guidelines[10] outline the following as best practice in the care of patients with suspected sepsis or septic shock:

- Sepsis and septic shock are medical emergencies, and patients with these diseases require immediate resuscitation.
- In patients with sepsis without shock physiology, there should be a rapid assessment to determine the likelihood of an infectious etiology.
- Cultures should be obtained before the initiation of antibiotics if there are not significant delays (<45 minutes) in starting the appropriate antimicrobial therapy.
- With unconfirmed infection, there should be a continuous reevaluation of the patient in search of the infection source or alternative diagnosis. Empiric antibiotics should be discontinued if an alternative cause other than infection is demonstrated or suspected.
- Source control should be obtained as soon as possible.
- Patients at high risk of methicillin-resistant *Staphylococcus aureus* (MRSA) infections should be treated with appropriate antibiotic coverage.
- Antibiotic doses should be optimized based on their pharmacokinetic and pharmacodynamic properties.

- Intravascular access devices suspected of being the source of the infection should be removed as other intravascular access is obtained.
- Goals of care and prognosis should be discussed with the patients and their families as part of the resuscitation care. Aspects of palliative care should be integrated into the treatment plan as necessary.

The 2021 SSC guidelines also outline treatments based on existing evidence in the literature, characterized as strong and weak recommendations. Strong recommendations, with additional clarifications, include:

- The continued use of performance improvement programs for sepsis care with standardized treatment algorithms is recommended.
- Scoring tools, such as the quick Sequential Organ Failure Score (qSOFA), Sequential Organ Failure Score (SOFA), National Early Warning Score (NEWS), and Modified Early Warning Score (MEWS) should *not* be used as single-screening tools for sepsis or septic shock.
- Antibiotics should ideally be initiated within 1 hour of suspecting sepsis or septic shock.
- Crystalloids are recommended as the first-line treatment for fluid resuscitation.
- The initial mean arterial pressure (MAP) target for patients with septic shock requiring vasopressor should be ≥65 mmHg.
- Norepinephrine should be utilized as the first-line vasopressor.
- Starches or colloids should not be used in the resuscitation of these patients.
- In patients with sepsis-induced adult respiratory distress syndrome (ARDS):
  - Low tidal volume ventilation (6–8 mL/kg) should be utilized.
  - In general, the target plateau pressure should be ≤30 mmHg. As some patients with hypoxemic respiratory failure are responsive to higher levels of positive end-expiratory pressure (PEEP), individual PEEP titration to a driving pressure of <15 is recommended.
  - Incremental PEEP titration should not be utilized as a recruitment maneuver.

- Prone ventilation for >12 hours/day should be utilized in patients with moderate to severe ARDS, when feasible, and proning should be initiated as early as possible after ARDS is identified.
- Restrictive transfusion strategies should be utilized, transfusing to maintain hemoglobin levels >7 mg/dL.
- Unless contraindicated, venous thromboembolism prophylaxis should be utilized.
- Insulin therapy should be initiated in patients with glucose >180 mg/dL.

Other aspects of the resuscitation, including fluid administration, have been more controversial, with ongoing research to find the optimal recommendations.[14–16] Crystalloids are recommended as the first-line treatment for fluids resuscitation. Balanced crystalloid solution infusions are the preferred and suggested choice in the initial resuscitation of patients with sepsis and septic shock, as it is best to avoid some of the toxic effects, increased mortality, and high costs associated with colloids such as albumin. More recently, studies such as the SALT-ED[15] and SMART[16] trials have shown us that balanced crystalloids are associated with improved mortality and morbidity, as compared to normal saline solutions. The current guidelines suggest at least 30 mL/kg of body weight with crystalloid solutions during the initial 3 hours of the resuscitation. Ongoing research opens the opportunity for more personalization with fluid resuscitation both during and after the initial management, especially in patients with a predisposition to volume overload or significant third spacing (e.g., patients with congestive heart failure, end-stage renal failure, and decompensated liver failure).

The goal of the initial fluid resuscitation should be the restoration of adequate perfusion pressures to reverse and prevent further end-organ damage. As this might not be possible with a crystalloid resuscitation alone, SSC recommends the early initiation of vasopressors after an adequate initial fluid resuscitation. Norepinephrine infusion is the first-choice vasopressor in patients with septic shock, with a target MAP goal of ≥ 65mmHg or adequate end-organ perfusion. With increasing norepinephrine requirements, a second vasopressor could be added, such as vasopressin, to reach the target MAP and/or to decrease the norepinephrine requirement. In patients with a poor cardiac output, inotropes such as dobutamine can also be added to meet the targets of resuscitation.[17,18]

Just as with fluids and vasopressors, there has been much controversy and research over the past few decades about the appropriateness and timing of corticosteroids in the management of patients with septic shock. Routine use is not recommended for all patients, but stress-dose hydrocortisone should be considered for patients with ongoing or increasing vasopressor (norepinephrine ≥0.25 mcg/kg/min for ≥4 hours), addition of a second vasopressor, and ongoing resuscitation requirements despite an adequate initial management as outlined above.

During the past 20 years there has been a significant transformation in the management of sepsis and septic shock. Earlier recognition and treatment of these disease processes has resulted in a significant reduction in mortality. Additionally, there has been standardization of the terms associated with these disease processes, ongoing evaluation of the optimal fluids and vasopressors for resuscitation, incorporation of algorithms in resuscitation bundles in most hospitals, and a standardization of the care delivered. While some components of the EGDT are not used routinely, this landmark trial transformed the management of sepsis and septic shock around the world and opened the opportunity for multiprofessional quality and process implementation science in sepsis care. Ongoing trials strive to identify better targets of resuscitation and end-organ perfusion, in hopes of creating a more individualized approach to care and a more tailored resuscitation with selective vasopressors. While great strides have been made in the past 20 years, these disease processes still carry a high mortality, especially with delayed diagnosis and inadequate treatment. Therefore, adherence to newer standards of care is paramount in the treatment of severe sepsis and septic shock to prevent mortality and end-organ damage.

KEY POINTS TO REMEMBER

- Shock is a disease state characterized by organ hypoperfusion. It can be mediated by different mechanisms, including low intravascular volume (hypovolemic/hemorrhagic), decreased cardiac output (cardiogenic) or pump failure (obstructive), or vasodilation (distributive).

- Distributive shock results from arterial or venous vasodilation, leading to an inadequate intravascular tissue perfusion. It can be due to anaphylaxis, neurologic injury, drug overdoses, or sepsis.
- Septic shock is a subset of sepsis and occurs with dysregulation of circulatory and cellular metabolism resulting in end-organ hypoperfusion.
- The resuscitation of patients with sepsis and septic shock was improved, and mortality was significantly reduced, as a result of algorithmic and standardized care of patients with these disease processes.

References

1. Rivers E, Nguyen B, Havstad S, et al. Early goal-directed therapy in the treatment of severe sepsis and septic shock. *N Engl J Med*. 2001;345:1368–1377.
2. Angus DC, Barnato AE, Bell D, et al. A systemic review and meta-analysis of early goal-directed therapy for septic shock: The ARISE, ProCESS, and ProMISe Investigators. *Intensive Care Med*. 2015;41:1549–1560.
3. Nguyen HB, Jaehne AK, Jayaprakash N, et al. Early goal-directed therapy in severe sepsis and septic shock: Insights and comparisons to ProCESS, ProMISe, and ARISE. *Crit Care*. 2016;20:160–176.
4. ProCESS Investigators, Yealy DM, Kellum JA et al. A randomized trial of protocol-based care for early septic shock. *N Engl J Med*. 2014;370:1683–1693.
5. Mouncey PR, Osborn TM, Power GS, et al. Protocolised Management in Sepsis (ProMISe): A multicentre randomised controlled trial of the clinical effectiveness and cost-effectiveness of early, goal-directed, protocolised resuscitation for emerging septic shock. *Health Technol Assess*. 2015;19:i–xxv.
6. ARISE Investigators; ANZICS Clinical Trials Group, Peake SL, et al. Goal-directed resuscitation for patients with early septic shock. *N Engl J Med*. 2014;371:1496–1506.
7. PRISM Investigators, Rowan KM, Angus DC, et al. Early, goal-directed therapy for septic shock—a patient-level meta-analysis. *N Engl J Med*. 2017;376:2223–2234.
8. Shankar-Hari M, Philips GS, Levy ML, et al. Developing a new definition and assessing new clinical criteria for septic shock. *JAMA*. 2016;315:775–787.
9. Singer M, Deutschman CS, Seymour CW, et al. The Third International Consensus Definitions for Sepsis and Septic Shock (Sepsis-3). *JAMA*. 2016;315:801–810.
10. Evans L, Rhodes A, Alhazani W, et al. Surviving Sepsis Campaign: International guidelines for the management of sepsis and septic shock 2021. *Crit Care*. 2021;49:e1063–e1143.

11. Levy MM, Evans LE, Rhodes A. The Surviving Sepsis Campaign Bundle: 2018 update. *Intensive Care Med*. 2018;44:925–928.

12. Rhodes A, Evans LE, Alhazzani W, et al. Surviving Sepsis Campaign: International guidelines for management of sepsis and septic shock 2016. *Crit Care Med*. 2017;45:486–552.

13. Dellinger AP, Schorr CA, Levy MM. A users' guide to the 2016 Surviving Sepsis Guidelines. *Crit Care Med*. 2017;45:381–385.

14. Marik PE, Weinmann M. Optimizing fluid therapy in shock. *Curr Opin Crit Care*. 2019;25:246–251.

15. Self WH, Semler MW, Wanderer JP, et al. Saline versus balanced crystalloids for intravenous fluid therapy in the emergency department: Study protocol for a cluster-randomized, multiple-crossover trial. *Trials*. 2017;13:178–185.

16. Brown RM, Wang L, Coston TD, et al. Balanced crystalloids versus saline in sepsis: A secondary analysis of the SMART clinical trial. *Am J Respir Crit Care Med*. 2019;200:1487–1495.

17. Russell JA. Vasopressor therapy in critically ill patients with shock. *Intensive Care Med*. 2019;45:1503–1517.

18. Annane D, Renault A, Brun-Buisson C, et al. Hydrocortisone plus fludrocortisone for adults with septic shock. *N Engl J Med*. 2018;378:809–818.

13 The engine isn't working: Cardiogenic shock states

Daniel J. Rowan

A 57-year-old man presents to the ED complaining of difficulty breathing, palpitations, dizziness, and decreased urinary output. His wife states that he normally walks for a block before feeling short of breath but is now experiencing dyspnea at rest. Past medical history includes congestive heart failure with reduced ejection fraction, hypertension, and previous alcohol use. Home medications include aspirin, carvedilol, valsartan, spironolactone, and furosemide, but his wife informs of poor adherence to his regimen. His examination is notable for atrial fibrillation with HR 133 bpm, temperature 98.2°F, BP 90/50 mmHg with mean arterial pressure (MAP) 63, RR 34 breaths/min, and oxygen saturation 87% on room air. He appears anxious, diaphoretic, and dyspneic, with conversational dyspnea and accessory muscle use. His extremities are cool to the touch, appear mottled with delayed capillary refill, and demonstrate peripheral edema. His EKG shows atrial fibrillation with rapid ventricular response and LV hypertrophy, without ST elevations or depressions. Chest x-ray demonstrates cardiomegaly, pleural effusions, and pulmonary vascular congestion without focal infiltrate. Labs are notable for acute kidney injury, transaminitis, elevated BNP and troponin, as well as lactic acidosis.

What do I do now?

Patients presenting to the ED with acute decompensated heart failure exacerbation manifest a spectrum of illness, including symptoms suggesting occult and overt cardiogenic shock. This case highlights the challenge encountered by the ED provider when caring for these patients, as optimal care requires timely identification and management. With the use of a thorough history and physical examination, reasoned interpretation of laboratory, EKG, and radiology results, as well as focused assessment with point-of-care ultrasound (POCUS), the diagnosis can be made expeditiously.

Cardiogenic shock is defined as systemic hypoperfusion with impairment in tissue oxygen delivery as a result of reduced cardiac output (CO) despite adequate LV filling pressures. Historically, the insertion of a pulmonary artery catheter (PAC) has been utilized to establish the diagnosis. The PAC measures invasive hemodynamic parameters, specifically the CO and pulmonary artery occlusion or "wedge" pressure, which in the appropriate context can be interpreted as a surrogate of the LV end-diastolic pressure (LVEDP). Given the invasive nature of the procedure, controversy surrounding its universal use, and nuances in interpretation of PAC data, its role in the ED setting is unclear.

Cardiogenic shock may complicate up to 5% of presentations of acute heart failure. Acute coronary syndrome (ACS) accounts for ~30% to 50% of cases of cardiogenic shock and carries a high mortality. Patients with progression of ischemic and non-ischemic cardiomyopathies represent 30% to 40% of cases, while those with tachydysrhythmias and severe valvular disease represent a smaller subset. Rarer causes include stress-induced cardiomyopathy, pregnancy-related cardiomyopathies, thyroid disorders, and acute myocarditis. Mortality remains high, ranging from 30% to 50% in the hospital and ~50% 1 year following discharge.

Regardless of the cause of cardiogenic shock, declining cardiac function manifests as a reduction in CO, with a subsequent decrease in BP, leading to impairment in cardiac and systemic oxygen delivery. The baroreceptors in the great vessels sense this BP drop and release endogenous catecholamines; this results in an increase in HR and systemic vascular resistance (SVR). This peripheral vasoconstriction causes recruitment of unstressed blood volume from the peripheral and splanchnic circulation to the central venous circulation in an effort to increase intravascular volume. While increasing

HR, systemic vascular tone, and preload will improve the blood pressure, this also increases the filling pressures and afterload, challenging the failing heart and potentially leading to further decline in cardiac function.

As this spiral continues, end-organ perfusion grows progressively compromised as the effect of a reduced CO in conjunction with elevated SVR leads to declining perfusion pressures and decreased oxygen delivery. Acute kidney failure, hepatopathy, bowel ischemia, and lactic acidosis may develop, resulting in progressive metabolic acidosis. With elevated LV filling pressures due to declining cardiac function, pulmonary edema occurs, causing hypoxemia and further impairing systemic oxygen delivery. If the oxygen supply continues to fall and fails to meet growing peripheral tissue demand, activation of the inflammatory cascade can arise. Consequently, patients develop a systemic inflammatory response syndrome (SIRS)-like response with transition to vasodilatory shock, worsening multisystem organ failure, and development of disseminated intravascular coagulation.

On presentation, patients may complain of chest pain, fatigue, progressive dyspnea, worsening peripheral edema, weight gain, decreased urinary output, dizziness/syncope, recent illness, and palpitations. Attention should be focused for symptoms suggestive of an infectious or bleeding nidus, with resultant volume loss and decreased cardiac filling, leading to progression of stable cardiomyopathy into cardiogenic shock. Past medical history may note congestive heart failure (CHF), coronary artery disease (CAD), prior cardiac arrest, hypertension, diabetes mellitus, valvular disorders, arrhythmias, drug use, pulmonary hypertension, and thyroid disorders. Review of prior cardiac imaging, including transthoracic echocardiography (TTE) and coronary angiography, can identify the presence of CHF, valvular disease, pulmonary hypertension, LV or RV dysfunction, as well as evidence of preexisting CAD.

Cardiogenic shock may present as hypotension, with a systolic BP <90 or a decrease in MAP >30 from baseline, with evidence of end-organ dysfunction. Importantly, some patients present with "normotensive" or occult cardiogenic shock, with a relatively preserved BP and evidence of peripheral hypoperfusion. Clinical manifestations include altered mental status, tachy- or brady-dysrhythmias, increased work of breathing, diaphoresis, mottling of the extremities, delayed capillary refill, poor pulse oximeter waveform with inconsistent registry of oxygen saturation, oliguria, peripheral edema, and jugular venous distention.

Initial workup should focus on ruling out ACS as the primary etiology of cardiogenic shock. An EKG is obtained to evaluate for the presence of dysrhythmias, atrioventricular nodal blocks, ST elevation myocardial infarction or its equivalent, ST depressions, as well as t-wave inversions. Chest x-ray can identify the presence of pulmonary vascular congestion, pleural effusions, and cardiomegaly. Laboratory assessment includes CBC, a basic metabolic panel with full electrolyte panel, liver function tests, troponin, BNP, and lactic acid. Elevated liver transaminases and nonspecific gastrointestinal symptoms (nausea, vomiting, abdominal pain and distention) can be clinical manifestations of cardiogenic shock.

Bedside evaluation should include a basic POCUS of the heart and lungs, specifically assessing for pericardial effusion, cardiac dysfunction, lung pathology, and volume status. LV systolic function can be assessed using TTE, with focused evaluation assessing for overt reduction in ejection fraction and regional wall-motion abnormalities in the apical four-chamber and parasternal short axes. Evaluation for marked RV dilation, indicating acute or chronic dysfunction, is performed in the apical four-chamber view, where the RV normally appears less than two-thirds the size of the LV. Assessment of the lungs can quickly identify pulmonary edema and pleural effusions, suggesting elevated LVEDP. Identification of multiple or confluent B-lines can be indicative of pulmonary edema. Pleural effusions are also visualized with the aid of ultrasound. While controversial, absolute diameter and respiratory variation of the inferior vena cava can provide insight into a patient's likelihood of volume responsiveness. Further discussion of advanced ultrasonography and TTE exceeds the scope of this chapter.

Patients in cardiogenic shock can present with respiratory distress and failure, due to the development of pulmonary edema, as well as increased metabolic demand leading to higher minute ventilation with subsequent respiratory muscle fatigue. Supplemental oxygen can be used to target oxygen saturation of >92%, but hyperoxia should be avoided. Early use of noninvasive ventilation can help decrease work of breathing, LVEDP, cardiac afterload, preload, and oxygen demand. Mechanical ventilation may be required for patients with significant respiratory distress, altered mental status, and shock with multisystem organ failure. Patients undergoing mechanical ventilation benefit from lung-protective ventilatory strategies, targeting a tidal volume of 6 cc/kg of ideal body weight.

Unfortunately, there is not a perfect vasopressor for use in hypotension associated with cardiogenic shock, as they all increase myocardial oxygen demand, cardiac afterload, and risk of arrhythmia. Pure alpha agonists, such as phenylephrine, should never be used. Dopamine carries an increased risk of arrhythmogenesis when compared to norepinephrine and has been associated with comparatively worse outcomes. Recent evidence suggests higher mortality with epinephrine use in cardiogenic shock compared to other vasopressor/inodilator regimens. Temporary low-dose norepinephrine may carry the lowest risk of harm, demonstrating predominantly alpha-1 agonism, inducing peripheral vasoconstriction with elevation to SVR and MAP, while having slight effect on beta-1 receptors and increasing inotropy. Vasopressin is a reasonable consideration, particularly in cardiogenic shock with discordant RV failure, due to its predominant effect on the peripheral vasculature resulting in increased MAP, and lack of elevation of the pulmonary vascular resistance (PVR).

Inodilator agents, such as milrinone and dobutamine, play a more important role in treating cardiogenic shock. Dobutamine is a beta-1 and beta-2 agonist that increases cardiac inotropy. At lower doses (2.5–5 ucg/kg/min), its effect is primarily on the beta-1 receptors, resulting in increased stroke volume and cardiac output, while higher doses stimulate greater beta-2 agonism, causing a decrease in SVR and PVR. Consequently, systemic hypotension and arrhythmias may occur with higher doses. Milrinone is a phosphodiesterase-3 inhibitor that inhibits breakdown of cAMP, indirectly resulting in increased intracellular calcium with subsequent increase in cardiac contractility, chronotropy, and a reduction in SVR and PVR. Drawbacks include the relatively frequent development of hypotension, as well as ventricular arrhythmias. It has a delayed onset of action and a prolonged half-life, remarkably longer in renal failure, making initiation in the ED difficult.

Initial treatment of hypotension should focus on integrating the history, exam features, and imaging findings. If concern is present for cardiogenic and/or multifactorial shock arising in the setting of concomitant illness leading to insensible losses, absent evidence of severe volume overload, a bolus of 250 to 500 cc IV crystalloid can be given. Ideally, clinical and ultrasonographic evaluation is undertaken while this is provided, focusing on work of breathing, hemodynamics, and systemic perfusion. Norepinephrine may be utilized initially for hypotension to maintain MAP >65, while ongoing assessment of the etiology of shock is undertaken. Inotropic therapy with low-dose dobutamine can be considered if concern is present for persistent global hypoperfusion, despite an improving hemodynamic profile, in the setting of clinical and ultrasonographic evidence of cardiogenic shock.

Direct therapy of the primary cause of cardiogenic shock is essential. Early revascularization for shock due to ACS is associated with improved outcomes, particularly when percutaneous coronary intervention focused on the culprit lesion is undertaken. If high suspicion is present that tachydysrhythmia-induced cardiomyopathy is causing cardiogenic shock, direct-current cardioversion along with administration of antiarrhythmic medications may be performed. Administration of diuretics for patients with progressive cardiomyopathy resulting in volume overload and hypoperfusion is essential to decrease cardiac preload and improve systemic oxygen delivery. Targeted treatment of infectious or bleeding etiologies resulting in decompensation of CHF into cardiogenic shock should be undertaken. Avoidance of common medications used in chronic heart failure, particularly beta-blockers, calcium channel blockers, mineralocorticoid antagonists, ACE inhibitors, and angiotensin receptor blockers is imperative until shock resolves.

For patients with refractory cardiogenic shock, specialist consultation should be made urgently to assess candidacy for mechanical circulatory support (MCS) devices such as veno-arterial extracorporeal membrane oxygenation (VA ECMO), an intra-aortic balloon pump, or a temporary percutaneous ventricular assist device (VAD) such as the Impella. Broadly speaking, the net effect of these devices is to decrease cardiac work and oxygen consumption while improving systemic perfusion, albeit by different mechanisms. Importantly, MCS devices should function as a bridge to recovery, heart transplantation, or VAD placement, with decision-making guided by a multidisciplinary shock/ECMO team.

Further reading

Chioncel O, Parissis J, Mebazaa A, et al. Epidemiology, pathophysiology and contemporary management of cardiogenic shock—a position statement from the Heart Failure Association of the European Society of Cardiology. *Eur J Heart Fail.* 2020;*22*(8):1315–1341.

Combes A, Price S, Slutsky AS, Brodie D. Temporary circulatory support for cardiogenic shock. *Lancet.* 2020;396(10245):199–212.

Blanco P, Aguiar FM, Blaivas M. Rapid ultrasound in shock (RUSH) velocity-time integral: A proposal to expand the RUSH protocol. *J Ultrasound Med.* 2015;34(9):1691–1700.

Berg DD, Bohula EA, van Diepen S, et al. Epidemiology of shock in contemporary cardiac intensive care units. *Circ Cardiovasc Qual Outcomes*. 2019;12:e005618.De Backer D, Biston P, Devriendt J, et al. Comparison of dopamine and norepinephrine in the treatment of shock. *N Engl J Med*. 2010;362(9):779–789.

Farkas J. Cardiogenic shock & severe CHF. 2016. https://emcrit.org/ibcc/chf/#top

Hochman JS, Buller CE, Sleeper LA, et al. Cardiogenic shock complicating acute myocardial infarction—etiologies, management and outcome: A report from the SHOCK Trial Registry. SHould we emergently revascularize Occluded Coronaries for cardiogenic shocK? *J Am Coll Cardiol*. 2000;36(3 Suppl A):1063–1070.

Karami M, Hemradj VV, Ouweneel DM, et al. Vasopressors and inotropes in acute myocardial infarction related cardiogenic shock: A systematic review and meta-analysis. *J Clin Med*. 2020;9(7):2051.

Kim JH, Sunkara A, Varnado S. Management of cardiogenic shock in a cardiac intensive care unit. *Methodist Debakey Cardiovasc J*. 2020;16(1):36–42.

Léopold V, Gayat E, Pirracchio R, et al. Epinephrine and short-term survival in cardiogenic shock: An individual data meta-analysis of 2583 patients. *Intensive Care Med*. 2018;44(6):847–856.

Muller L, Bobbia X, Toumi M, et al. Respiratory variations of inferior vena cava diameter to predict fluid responsiveness in spontaneously breathing patients with acute circulatory failure: Need for a cautious use. *Crit Care*. 2012;8;16(5):R188.

Rudski LG, Lai WW, Afilalo J, et al. Guidelines for the echocardiographic assessment of the right heart in adults: A report from the American Society of Echocardiography endorsed by the European Association of Echocardiography, a registered branch of the European Society of Cardiology, and the Canadian Society of Echocardiography. *J Am Soc Echocardiogr*. 2010;23(7):685–713.

Shah M, Patnaik S, Patel B, et al. Trends in mechanical circulatory support use and hospital mortality among patients with acute myocardial infarction and non-infarction related cardiogenic shock in the United States. *Clin Res Cardiol*. 2018;107:287–303.

Sionis A, Rivas-Lasarte M, Mebazaa A, et al. Current use and impact on 30-day mortality of pulmonary artery catheter in cardiogenic shock patients: Results from the CardShock Study. *J Intensive Care Med*. 2020;35(12):1426–1433.

Stub D, Smith, Bernard S, et al. Air versus oxygen in ST-segment-elevation myocardial infarction. *Circulation*. 2015;24:2143–2150.

Thiele H, Akin I, Sandri M, et al. CULPRIT-SHOCK Investigators: PCI strategies in patients with acute myocardial infarction and cardiogenic shock. *N Engl J Med*. 2017;377(25):2419–2432.

Vahdatpour C, Collins D, Goldberg S. Cardiogenic shock. *J Am Heart Assoc*. 2019;16;8(8):e011991.

van Diepen S, Hochman JS, Stebbins A, Alviar CL, Alexander JH, Lopes RD. Association between delays in mechanical ventilation initiation and mortality in patients with refractory cardiogenic shock. *JAMA Cardiol*. 2020;5(8):965–967.

van Diepen S, Katz JN, Albert NM, et al. Contemporary management of cardiogenic shock: A scientific statement from the American Heart Association. *Circulation.* 2017;136(16):e232–e268.

van Diepen S, Reynolds HR, Stebbins A, et al. Incidence and outcomes associated with early heart failure pharmacotherapy in patients with ongoing cardiogenic shock. *Crit Care Med.* 2014;42(2):281–288.

14 A pump replacement: The bleeding LVAD patient

Alexandra June Gordon and
Andrew W. Phillips

A 55-year-old male with a history of
hypertension, hyperlipidemia, and severe
left heart failure who is 1 year status post left
ventricular assist device (LVAD) placement
presents with 1 day of bright-red blood
per rectum. He complains of dizziness and
lightheadedness. He takes aspirin, metoprolol,
lisinopril, and coumadin. On exam he is alert
and oriented, but fatigued. You note a humming
sound over his chest; his abdomen is soft; and
the driveline site is clean, dry and intact. He is
afebrile with HR 110 bpm and RR 12 breath/min.
He is pulseless, and the automated BP cuff is
unable to take a measurement.

What do I do now?

In this case, you have an LVAD patient with a gastrointestinal (GI) bleed. LVADs are continuous-flow mechanical pumps that augment or replace LV function in patients with severe left heart failure. They consist of the pump itself, an inflow cannula from the left ventricle, an outflow cannula to the aorta, a percutaneous driveline, and external components (controller and two batteries). RVADs (for the right side of the heart) are very rare, as are total mechanical hearts, and are beyond the scope of this chapter.

LVAD patients are always anticoagulated with coumadin and often on antiplatelet therapy with aspirin as well (although antiplatelet therapy is trending out of favor with newer models) to minimize thrombotic and embolic risk, so this is not an uncommon presentation. Furthermore, LVAD patients are often coagulopathic from the device itself because of an acquired von Willebrand factor deficiency thought to be from LVAD shear stress and ADAMTS-13 excessively cleaving von Willebrand multimers as a result of continuous flow.[1-3] The nonpulsatile flow of the LVAD also predisposes patients to arteriovenous malformations and angiodysplasias of the GI tract for reasons that are still not entirely understood.[4] For all of these reasons, nonsurgical bleeding is the most common reason LVAD patients present to the ED.[5]

The assessment of an LVAD patient does not differ in order from your usual patient, but your initial assessment requires some data that are atypical. First the airway must be assessed, which this patient is currently protecting; moreover, he has normal bilateral breath sounds with no increased work of breathing. Next, circulation must be assessed. The patient is pulseless and has no BP, although he is alert and oriented. LVADs have constant flow, so there is often not a palpable pulse—anywhere. BP is measured via Doppler and a manual cuff at the brachial artery. The pressure when you hear flow is reported as the mean arterial pressure (MAP). If the patient does have some pulse pressure, the first pressure is technically the systolic, but it is still uniformly reported as the MAP for LVAD patients. You can also use ultrasound with color flow for this task. Once obtained, you can get a truer sense of whether your patient is unstable. Normal MAP for an LVAD patient (60–80 mmHg) is different from the general population because the pump is so afterload sensitive.[6,7] If all else fails, it is very reasonable to have a low threshold to place an arterial catheter, especially in an ill-appearing LVAD patient.

An additional part of the assessment of an LVAD patient beyond the ABCs is assessing the device itself, much like assessing a ventilator circuit. First, listen for a precordial or epigastric hum. The presence of this hum reassures you that the pump is running and has not malfunctioned. After auscultating, check the connections between the controller and all its parts (driveline from patient to controller; controller to two power sources). Inspect the driveline site, typically in the abdomen (sometimes behind the ear in Europe) for signs of infection. There is also important information to be gleaned from the controller of all LVAD models currently on the market. The controller displays the battery life, speed in RPMs of the pump, flow in L/min, and power usage in watts. Alarms are also displayed here and color-coded for severity (green, yellow, red; red = life-threatening). Heartmate LVADs also report a pulsatility index (PI), which is a proprietary calculation that suggests an overall sense of how well the LVAD is performing—grossly speaking. Because of variability between patients, the PI is less helpful as a surrogate for vital signs, but often more useful as indicating trends, and consultants will want to know the PI if it is available. Patients often know their baseline numbers, or they are commonly written on the back of the controller, so remove the controller from its pouch to see any notes. Each institution that implants LVADs has an LVAD coordinator and/or an LVAD team. If there is not one specific to your institution, your patient should have their information, or you can always call the device manufacturer, printed on the controller.

LVAD patients with GI bleeding need large-bore access just like any other patient with a GI bleed. Two 18 gauge or greater peripheral IVs in the antecubital fossa or above is always preferred. In any ED assessment of an LVAD patient, an EKG should be obtained, and serum labs should be sent. In addition to a typical complete blood count, complete chemistry, and lactic acid, LVAD patients should have coagulation studies, liver function panel, cardiac enzymes, brain natriuretic peptide (BNP) or NT-pro BNP, as well as lactate dehydrogenase (LDH) sent.[8] BNPs can assist in determining atrial stretch and therefore volume status, as they would in a typical patient. Elevated LDH can be a marker of hemolysis: a level two to three times the upper level of normal is suggestive of pump thrombosis. A chest x-ray can help evaluate the lungs and confirm appropriate placement of the LVAD in the chest, and a bedside echo can help assess for valve issues and investigate right heart function (to a limited degree).

Resuscitating LVAD patients is tricky in that they are preload-dependent but still advanced heart failure patients. In the case of the LVAD patient with GI bleeding, the GI bleed is managed similarly to any other bleeding patient, just more cautiously. You should resuscitate per usual standards of hemoglobin > 7–8 and MAP > 60. If able, it is prudent to transfuse crossmatched blood since these patients are often awaiting heart transplantation, and you do not want to give them antibodies to multiple blood donors. Given that their underlying cardiac function is depressed even after LVAD augmentation, a cautious volume resuscitation is advisable. Remember, too, that although the left heart has mechanical support, the right heart does not, so fluid overloading the right heart can be deadly. Then again, so can hypoperfusion secondary to hypovolemic shock. It is a fine line.

At this point it is prudent to stop anticoagulation and antiplatelet agents, but the decision on whether to reverse anticoagulation is not one to be taken lightly. Given the thrombotic risk of these patients, it is best to have a very high threshold to reverse them and to reserve this for cases of immediately life-threatening hemorrhage. Thrombosis of the pump is a very morbid complication, and the risk of recurrence after an initial thrombus is very high. These patients are also at risk of other thromboembolic events, which is why they are anticoagulated in the first place.[9] This decision should *always* be made in conjunction with your hospital's VAD or mechanical circulatory support (MCS) team. It may be advisable to give vitamin K (if the patient is on a vitamin K antagonist) and platelets (if the patient is on an antiplatelet agent) in consultation with the VAD team. If you and the team decide to reverse the patient's anticoagulation, the VAD team will likely have to change the device's settings to compensate. However, it cannot be overstated: Reversing anticoagulation in an LVAD patient is essentially a salvage maneuver only for when the patient is peri-arresting or actively arresting from hemorrhage. Even infusing blood with a rapid infuser (e.g., Level 1, Belmont) in these patients with heart failure is generally preferable to reversing anticoagulation.

LVAD patients with GI bleeding should undergo endoscopy like any other GI bleeding patient. You can treat with a proton pump inhibitor

(PPI) and consider octreotide and antibiotics if your patient has liver dysfunction. You can consider CT angiography if bleeding cannot be localized or treated by gastroenterology. There should be a low threshold to admit GI bleeding LVAD patients to the ICU.

KEY POINTS TO REMEMBER

- Assess an LVAD patient the way you would any other patient (ABCs), but remember you will need an ultrasound or Doppler to obtain a blood pressure; this pressure is the MAP.
- Nonsurgical bleeding is the most common reason LVAD patients present to the ED because they are both anticoagulated and coagulopathic.
- LVADs are both preload dependent and afterload sensitive.
- Don't be afraid of the device itself. Check all the connections and look for alarms.
- Make early and frequent contact with the LVAD coordinator and/ or LVAD/advanced heart failure team at your institution or the patient's primary institution.

References

1. Spanier T, Oz M, Levin H, et al. Activation of coagulation and fibrinolytic pathways in patients with left ventricular assist devices. *J Thorac Cardiovasc Surg.* 1996;112(4):1090–1097.

2. Nascimbene A, Neelamegham S, Frazier O, Moake J, Dong J. Acquired von Willebrand syndrome associated with left ventricular assist device. *Blood.* 2016;127(25):3133–3141. doi:10.1182/blood-2015-10-636480

3. Suarez J, Patel C, Felker G, Becker R, Hernandez A, Rogers J. Mechanisms of bleeding and approach to patients with axial-flow left ventricular assist devices. *Circ Heart Fail.* 2011;4(6):779–784. doi:10.1161/circheartfailure.111.962613

4. Crow S, John R, Boyle A, et al. Gastrointestinal bleeding rates in recipients of nonpulsatile and pulsatile left ventricular assist devices. *J Thorac Cardiovasc Surg.* 2009;137(1):208–215. doi:10.1016/j.jtcvs.2008.07.032

5. Givertz M, DeFilippis E, Colvin M, et al. HFSA/SAEM/ISHLT clinical expert consensus document on the emergency management of patients with ventricular assist devices. *J Card Fail.* 2019;25(7):494–515. doi:10.1016/j.cardfail.2019.01.012

6. Bennett MK, Adatya S. Blood pressure management in mechanical circulatory support. *J Thorac Dis.* 2015;7(12):2125–2128. doi:10.3978/j.issn.2072-1439.2015.11.05

7. Khan A, Sultanik E, Racherla M, et al. Time spent out of mean arterial blood pressure (MAP) goal correlates with adverse events in patients on left ventricular assist device. *J Heart Lung Transplant.* 2018;37(4):S60. doi:10.1016/j.healun.2018.01.133

8. Trinquero P, Pirotte A, Gallagher LP, Iwaki KM, Beach C, Wilcox JE. Left ventricular assist device management in the emergency department. *West J Emerg Med.* 2018;19(5):834–841. doi:10.5811/westjem.2018.5.37023

9. Upshaw J, Kiernan M, Morine K, Kapur N, DeNofrio D. Incidence, management, and outcome of suspected continuous-flow left ventricular assist device thrombosis. *ASAIO J.* 2016;62(1):33–39. doi:10.1097/mat.0000000000000294

15 The other heart failure: Pulmonary hypertension and right ventricular dysfunction

John C. Greenwood

A 38-year-old, previously healthy male presents to the ED with fever and shortness of breath. The patient's symptoms have progressed over the past 2 to 3 days, along with generalized arthralgias, myalgias, and a nonproductive cough. He appears ill, he has coarse, bilateral breath sounds, and his vital signs are temperature 39°C, HR 128 bpm and regular, BP 86/56 mmHg, RR 28 breaths/min, and SpO_2 84% on 100% FiO_2.

The patient receives an empiric IV crystalloid fluid bolus and is emergently intubated for hypoxemic respiratory failure. His post-intubation chest x-ray shows bilateral, patchy infiltrates consistent with acute respiratory distress syndrome (ARDS). Ten minutes after intubation, the nurse calls you to the bedside because the patient is now more tachycardic with a BP of 74/58 mmHg and notable jugular venous distention.

What do I do now?

This patient's diagnosis is pulmonary hypertension and right ventricular (RV) failure with cor pulmonale caused by ARDS. Post-intubation hypotension occurs in ~20% to 30% of critically ill patients and is associated with a significant increase in morbidity and mortality.[1] The patient's pre-intubation shock index (HR/systolic BP) was >0.9, indicating he is at high risk for cardiopulmonary compromise post-intubation unless promptly addressed.[2] Rapid differentiation to determine the type of shock and time-sensitive interventions must be completed. The initial differential diagnosis should include significant vasoplegic shock due to sepsis or rapid sequence induction (RSI) medications, pure hypovolemia, obstructive physiology due to acute pulmonary hypertension leading to RV failure, tension pneumothorax, or acute left ventricular (LV) failure due to a sepsis-induced cardiomyopathy.

A rapidly obtained point-of-care ultrasound is the best initial diagnostic test to examine the patient's cardiac function and would reveal the diagnosis (Figure 15.1). Qualitative assessment of this image reveals a significantly dilated RV, with a RV:LV end-diastolic diameter of ≥1 in the four-chamber view. Additional findings might include other signs of RV strain, including

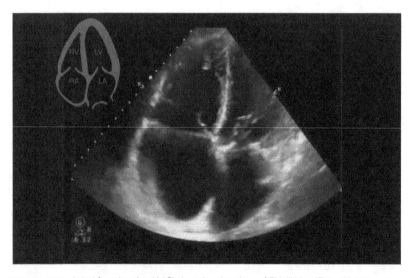

FIGURE 15.1   Apical four-chamber (A4C) view showing signs of RV dilation (RV > LV diameter) along with pathologic septal bowing during systole. An illustration of normal cardiac structures during an A4C view is indicated in the upper left-hand corner.

severe tricuspid regurgitation, septal wall flattening during diastole (commonly referred to as a D-sign), displacement of the septum toward the LV during systole, and a dilated inferior vena cava without respiratory variation. Quantitative assessment of RV function can also support the diagnosis by measuring the tricuspid annular plane systolic excursion (TAPSE) using the ultrasound's M-mode function.[3] A TAPSE of ≤1.0 cm indicates severely impaired RV function.

Routine laboratory testing will have likely been sent on this critically ill patient, but most tests will be nonspecific in the evaluation of acute pulmonary hypertension and RV failure. It is important to pay particular attention to elevations in troponin (indicating myocardial ischemia) or b-type natriuretic peptide, which are both associated with increased morbidity and mortality.[4] Elevated liver function tests, lactate, and coagulation panel can reflect liver congestion and are a poor prognostic finding.

Diagnostic testing confirms this patient has acute RV failure and signs of cor pulmonale. A comprehensive treatment strategy that includes guideline-recommended treatments for ARDS and interventions that address the pathophysiologic causes of RV failure should be initiated. In this patient, his acute pulmonary hypertension is most likely the result of significant hypoxic pulmonary vasoconstriction. Other reversible causes of increased pulmonary vascular resistance (PVR) include significant inspiration-associated hyperinflation of the lung with improper mechanical ventilation settings and worsening acidosis. The RV needs to be supported during the patient's initial resuscitation. The clinician should focus on improving RV function, increasing the patient's BP to ensure adequate coronary perfusion, and reducing the PVR and improving the RV afterload.

Improving systemic oxygenation and optimizing mechanical ventilation should be the first steps to reduce RV afterload and PVR. In general, consensus opinion is to provide supplemental oxygen to maintain an SpO_2 of >90%.[5] An arterial blood gas measurement should be drawn to ensure initial SpO_2 targets are correlating with an adequate PaO_2. Increases in PVR can quickly escalate with a PaO_2 of <60 mmHg. If the decision to initiate mechanical ventilation is made, as in this case, the patient should be prescribed ventilator settings that are protective of the RV. First, it is important to maintain low airway pressures to minimize the impact of positive-pressure ventilation on intrathoracic pressure. Lung-protective ventilation strategies can often be implemented, targeting a tidal volume of 6 to 8 cc/ kg of ideal body weight. In this patient with ARDS, lower tidal volumes may be needed to maintain a plateau pressure of ≤30 mmHg.[6] A strategy of "permissive hypercapnia" may need to be avoided, as significant acidosis may lead to worsening PVR and impair RV function further.[7] Positive end-expiratory pressure (PEEP) optimization to reduce driving pressure (P_{plat} − PEEP) to ≤15 mmHg may also be beneficial to minimize mechanical power delivery to lungs, improve oxygenation, and reduce any deleterious effects of pulmonary over- or under-inflation on PVR.[8,9]

In severe cases, RV afterload can also be reduced by initiating inhaled pulmonary vasodilator therapy. Inhaled epoprostenol or nitric oxide therapy causes local smooth muscle dilation leading to reduced pulmonary arterial pressures. Both of these medications can be delivered via facemask, high-flow nasal cannula, or endotracheal tube, and can improve patient hemodynamics.[10] Table 15.1 includes a summary of pharmacologic interventions that may be required in this patient.

TABLE 15.1 **Pharmacotherapy for pulmonary hypertension and RV failure**

Target	Drug, Dose[16]	Comments
RV systolic dysfunction	Dobutamine Dose: 2–20 mcg/kg/min	Beware of doses >10 mcg/kg/min due to higher risk of arrhythmias.
	Milrinone Dose: 0.125–0.75 mcg/kg/min	Higher doses will cause hypotension. Will also reduce PVR.
RCA malperfusion	Norepinephrine Dose: 0.05–0.5 mcg/kg/min	Avoid dopamine and phenylephrine.
	Vasopressin Dose: 0.01–0.06 units/min	
	Epinephrine Dose: 0.05–0.5 mcg/kg/min	
Increased RV afterload	Inhaled epoprostenol Dose: 50 ng/kg/min	Inhaled therapy limits vasodilatory effect to pulmonary circulation.
	Inhaled nitric oxide Dose: 20–80 ppm	

In this patient with hypotension, prompt initiation of vasoactive therapy should begin to achieve a mean arterial pressure of ≥65 mmHg. Hypotension is poorly tolerated, as the RV is particularly prone to ischemia due to limited right coronary artery (RCA) collateral blood flow. There are minimal evidence-based recommendations on which vasopressor would be best for this patient, but a norepinephrine infusion, starting at 0.05 mcg/kg/min, would be reasonable. Vasopressin has been found to improve systemic vascular resistance without increasing PVR,[11] while epinephrine infusion may also improve RV systolic function. Inodilator therapy to improve RV function and pharmacologically reduce RV afterload may be needed once a stable mean arterial pressure is achieved. Options include dobutamine (a beta-1/beta-2 agonist) or milrinone (a phosphodiesterase-3 inhibitor). Inodilator therapy can be effective to reduce PVR in addition to increasing RV stroke volume and improving systemic perfusion.

In general, it is preferred to avoid significant volume resuscitation in patients with ARDS and RV dysfunction as the cause for RV failure in this case is a significantly increased PVR. Excessive volume or crystalloid administration in this patient can lead to worsening RV dilation, septal displacement toward the LV, pulmonary edema, LV filling, and tissue perfusion. Increased RV dilation also increases free wall tension, resulting in increased oxygen demand and reduced RCA blood flow, reducing RV perfusion. Beware of false-positive measures of volume responsiveness, as this patient has RV failure, which invalidates most predictive tools.[12] These patients often need diuresis, not volume resuscitation.

Patients with ARDS or RV failure are critically ill and require ICU admission, as their anticipated recovery course is often days to weeks. Advanced interventions for patients with significant hypoxemia, such as prone position therapy, continuous paralytic treatment, and even extracorporeal membrane oxygenation, may be needed in the ICU.[13–15]

KEY POINTS TO REMEMBER

- Management goals for patients with pulmonary hypertension are to optimize preload and volume status, maintain RV function, prevent RCA malperfusion, reduce RV afterload, and reverse the underlying cause whenever possible.

- RV failure is a hallmark finding in patients with decompensated pulmonary hypertension.
- Point-of-care echocardiography is an invaluable tool when evaluating a patient with pulmonary hypertension and suspected right heart failure.
- Unmonitored, continuous fluid administration should be avoided in patients with pulmonary hypertension, because it often worsens pressure overload of the right heart.
- Mechanical ventilation settings should be prescribed to avoid excessive hypercapnia, achieve an $SpO_2 > 90\%$, and optimize recruitable lung volume to avoid excessive increases in intrathoracic pressure.

References

1. Heffner AC, Swords DS, Nussbaum ML, Kline JA, Jones AE. Predictors of the complication of postintubation hypotension during emergency airway management. *J Crit Care*. 2012;27(6):587–593. doi:10.1016/j.jcrc.2012.04.022

2. Trivedi S, Demirci O, Arteaga G, Kashyap R, Smischney NJ. Evaluation of preintubation shock index and modified shock index as predictors of postintubation hypotension and other short-term outcomes. *J Crit Care*. 2015;30(4):861. doi:10.1016/j.jcrc.2015.04.013

3. Rudski LG, Lai WW, Afilalo J, et al. Guidelines for the echocardiographic assessment of the right heart in adults: A report from the American Society of Echocardiography endorsed by the European Association of Echocardiography, a registered branch of the European Society of Cardiology, and the Canadian Society of Echocardiography. *J Am Soc Echocardiogr*. 2010;23(7):685–713; quiz 786–788. doi:10.1016/j.echo.2010.05.010

4. Warwick G, Thomas PS, Yates DH. Biomarkers in pulmonary hypertension. *Eur Respir J*. 2008;32(2):503–512. doi:10.1183/09031936.00160307

5. Hoeper MM, Granton J. Intensive care unit management of patients with severe pulmonary hypertension and right heart failure. *Am J Respir Crit Care Med*. 2011;184(10):1114–1124. doi:10.1164/rccm.201104-0662CI

6. Acute Respiratory Distress Syndrome Network, Brower RG, Matthay MA, et al. Ventilation with lower tidal volumes as compared with traditional tidal volumes for acute lung injury and the acute respiratory distress syndrome. *N Engl J Med*. 2000;342(18):1301–1308. doi:10.1056/NEJM200005043421801

7. Mekontso Dessap A, Charron C, Devaquet J, et al. Impact of acute hypercapnia and augmented positive end-expiratory pressure on right ventricle function in severe acute respiratory distress syndrome. *Intensive Care Med*. 2009;35(11):1850–1858. doi:10.1007/s00134-009-1569-2

8. Hakim TS, Michel RP, Chang HK. Effect of lung inflation on pulmonary vascular resistance by arterial and venous occlusion. *J Appl Physiol*. 1982;53(5):1110–1115. doi:10.1152/jappl.1982.53.5.1110

9. Amato MBP, Meade MO, Slutsky AS, et al. Driving pressure and survival in the acute respiratory distress syndrome. *N Engl J Med*. 2015;372(8):747–755. doi:10.1056/NEJMsa1410639

10. Buckley MS, Feldman JP. Inhaled epoprostenol for the treatment of pulmonary arterial hypertension in critically ill adults. *Pharmacotherapy*. 2010;30(7):728–740. doi:10.1592/phco.30.7.728

11. Sarkar J, Golden PJ, Kajiura LN, Murata L-AM, Uyehara CFT. Vasopressin decreases pulmonary-to-systemic vascular resistance ratio in a porcine model of severe hemorrhagic shock. *Shock*. 2015;43(5):475–482. doi:10.1097/SHK.0000000000000325

12. Monnet X, Marik PE, Teboul J-L. Prediction of fluid responsiveness: An update. *Ann Intensive Care*. 2016;6(1):111. doi:10.1186/s13613-016-0216-7

13. Guérin C, Reignier J, Richard J-C, et al. Prone positioning in severe acute respiratory distress syndrome. *N Engl J Med*. 2013;368(23):2159–2168. doi:10.1056/NEJMoa1214103

14. Vieillard-Baron A, Charron C, Caille V, Belliard G, Page B, Jardin F. Prone positioning unloads the right ventricle in severe ARDS. *Chest*. 2007;132(5):1440–1446. doi:10.1378/chest.07-1013

15. Papazian L, Forel J-M, Gacouin A, et al. Neuromuscular blockers in early acute respiratory distress syndrome. *N Engl J Med*. 2010;363(12):1107–1116. doi:10.1056/NEJMoa1005372

16. van Diepen S, Katz JN, Albert NM, et al. Contemporary management of cardiogenic shock: A scientific statement from the American Heart Association. *Circulation*. 2017;136(16):e232–e268. doi:10.1161/CIR.0000000000000525

16 Vasopressor cocktails (we all have drug shortages)

John C. Greenwood

A 28-year-old male with a history of IV drug abuse presents to the ED with a fever and shortness of breath. His symptoms have progressed over the past week, along with malaise, myalgias, and a worsening rash on his left arm. He appears ill and has clear bilateral breath sounds and a faint systolic murmur. Vital signs are temperature 38.5°C, HR 122 bpm, and regular, BP 98/32 mmHg (mean arterial pressure [MAP] 54), RR 26 breaths/min, and SpO_2 94% on 4 L of nasal cannula oxygen. On exam, you notice multiple injection sites on his left arm and a 4 × 4 cm, erythematous, indurated area over his left antecubital fossa. The patient receives a 1-L fluid bolus along with IV antibiotics. His chest x-ray shows bilateral, patchy infiltrates and his initial blood gas results are pH 7.15, pO2 86, pCO2 14, HCO_3 9, and lactate 6 mmol/dL. The patient remains hypotensive; his current BP is 96/38 mmHg.

What do I do now?

This acutely ill patient presents with what appears to be the clinical syndrome of septic shock, with multiple potential sources. While the initial source may be related to his injection-site cellulitis, it is likely he has additional, more challenging, infectious sources, including a perivascular abscess, bacteremia, endocarditis, osteomyelitis, or other sources leading to secondary hematogenous spread. Early, appropriate antibiotic therapy and source control are critical, followed by differentiation of this patient's shock and rapid resuscitation.

The hemodynamic phenotype can be readily determined with a point-of-care ultrasound that includes a focused transthoracic echocardiogram and an estimate of the central venous pressure by visualizing the inferior vena cava diameter and variability. A hyperdynamic left ventricle (LV) with a flat inferior vena cava would suggest a vasoplegic (low systemic vascular resistance [SVR]), and high cardiac output (CO) state. A more advanced, objective assessment that includes an LV outflow tract velocity time integral (LVOT-VTI) can quantify the patient's stroke volume. This can then be used to calculate CO, which is particularly useful in patients with an unclear or reduced ejection fraction.

Early resuscitation goals should start with achieving evidence-based macrocirculatory endpoints. Vasopressor (Table 16.1) and inotropic (Table 16.2) therapy will be critical to consider during this resuscitation. After achieving macrocirculatory targets, we will need to assess whether hemodynamic changes have translated into improved tissue perfusion.

Macrocirculatory targets can usually be measured rapidly at the bedside. This patient clearly has an inadequate MAP with a wide pulse pressure. The differential diagnosis begins with vasoplegia due to sepsis but should also include new aortic insufficiency from an aortic valve vegetation. Additional fluid resuscitation could be considered; however, early vasopressor initiation may be preferred in this case. The patient has a diastolic BP of <40 mmHg, indicating a critically low SVR, where fluid resuscitation is unlikely to result in an improved MAP.[1] The initial vasopressor of choice in this patient with sepsis is norepinephrine, as it will address the patient's vasoplegia (alpha agonist) and improve venous return and CO (beta effect).

Epinephrine,[2] phenylephrine,[3] or vasopressin[4] are not first-line recommendations for patients with septic shock but could be considered as

TABLE 16.1 **Vasopressor considerations in circulatory shock**

Goal: MAP ≥ 65 mmHg

Drug	Mechanism, effect, and dose[12]	Comments
Norepinephrine	**Mechanism** • α_1: ↑ SVR • β_1: ↑ HR, stroke volume, CO • β_2: ↑ vascular smooth muscle dilation in some organ beds **Dose:** 0.05–0.5 mcg/kg/min	• Per Surviving Sepsis Campaign: first-line vasopressor[8] • Consider early initiation if diastolic BP is <40 mmHg. • Greater α than β effect
Epinephrine	**Mechanism** • Targets α_1, β_1, β_2 **Dose:** 0.05–0.5 mcg/kg/min	• Per Surviving Sepsis Campaign: second-line vasopressor[8] • Consider in patients with impaired cardiac index (CI) • Equivalent α and β effect
Vasopressin	**Mechanism** • V_1: ↑ vascular smooth muscle tone • V_2: Renal antidiuretic effect **Dose:** Fixed at 0.03 units/min • Titratable: 0.02–0.04 units/min	• Per Surviving Sepsis Campaign: second-line vasopressor at fixed dose[8] • No effect on CO or HR
Phenylephrine	**Mechanism** • α_1: ↑ SVR **Dose:** 0.1–10 mcg/kg/min	• No *direct* effect on CO or HR; may cause *secondary* decrease in CO and HR due to increased afterload
Angiotensin II	**Mechanism** • AT II: ↑ SVR, renal antidiuretic effect **Dose:** 5–40 ng/kg/min	• Novel treatment for catecholamine-refractory vasoplegia • Too early to recommend routine use

Note: These are general dosing recommendations.

TABLE 16.2 **Inotropic considerations in circulatory shock**

Goal: Cardiac index > 2.2 L/min/m²

Drug	Mechanism, effect, and dose[12]	Comments
Epinephrine	**Mechanism** · Targets α_1, β_1, β_2 **Dose:** 0.01–0.5 mcg/kg/min	· Provides CO support without significant reduction in SVR
Dobutamine	**Mechanism** · β_1: ↑ HR, stroke volume, CO · β_2: ↑ vascular smooth muscle dilation; ↓ SVR **Dose:** 2–20 mcg/kg/min	· Can cause tachydysrhythmias at higher doses · Can cause hypotension due to ↓ SVR
Milrinone	**Mechanism** · Phosphodiesterase-3 inhibition: ↑ stroke volume/CO · Vascular smooth muscle: ↓ SVR **Dose:** 0.125–0.75 mcg/kg/min	· Will cause hypotension due to ↓ SVR

Note: These are general dosing recommendations.

both will increase the patient's SVR.[5] Phenylephrine may be a useful alternative to norepinephrine if the patient develops a tachydysrhythmia with a hyperdynamic LV, as phenylephrine does not have any beta-agonist effects. Vasopressin can also be considered as a secondary vasopressor to improve MAP, if norepinephrine requirements are rapidly escalating. Angiotensin II (AT II) has become recently available and has been studied clinically in catecholamine-refractory vasoplegic shock.[6] If available, AT II could be considered as an adjunct to norepinephrine therapy. Dopamine is no longer recommended.[7,8]

Sepsis-induced cardiac dysfunction is a well-described phenomenon that leads to a reduction in LV stroke volume and impaired myocardial performance. Myocardial depression is estimated to occur in up to 60% of patients with septic shock.[9] CO in patients with septic shock can be assessed using several minimally invasive and noninvasive methods, including commercially available pulse-wave-contour analysis devices, or focused echocardiography, where cardiac output and index can be quantified using the pulsed-wave Doppler function.[10]

If a patient continues to have low CO (cardiac index of <2.2 L/min/m²) with evidence of poor perfusion, it is reasonable to add inotropic therapy. Dobutamine is recommended as the first-line inotropic infusion in sepsis, at a starting dose of 2.5 mcg/kg/min in patients with adequate ventricular filling and MAP.[8] Alternatively, epinephrine may provide adequate inotropic support if given at lower infusion doses (up to 0.1 mcg/kg/min) without the vasodilatory effects caused by dobutamine's beta-2 activity.[11] If you choose epinephrine, it is important to remember that the ability to monitor lactate clearance may be impaired due to increased aerobic glycolysis causing lactate generation.

After initiating norepinephrine therapy, re-evaluation found improved signs of tissue perfusion, including lactate normalization and normal capillary refill. A comprehensive echocardiogram was performed later in the day and showed that the patient had a moderate aortic root abscess with trace aortic insufficiency. It is worth discussing additional interventions that may be required, as aortic root abscesses may progress to fulminant heart failure, aortic insufficiency, conduction abnormalities, fistula formation, and often require surgical correction. Conduction abnormalities can be temporized with an epinephrine infusion, utilizing its significant beta-1 activity while preparing to insert an emergent transvenous pacemaker.

Severe or worsening mitral or aortic valvular insufficiency can present with challenging clinical symptoms. Worsening cardiogenic pulmonary edema can often masquerade as pneumonia or acute respiratory distress syndrome. Severe tricuspid regurgitation can present as acute liver failure due to a congestive hepatopathy. Acute valvular insufficiency, usually diagnosed by echocardiogram, often requires the clinician to modify traditional interventions for vasoplegic shock in exchange for combined vasopressor and inodilator therapy to minimize the patient's regurgitant fraction to optimize CO (see Table 16.2).

Finally, current guidelines have been written to provide clinicians with general recommendations for a simplified approach to patients with a specific shock state. While patients often begin with one primary form of macrocirculatory shock (hypovolemic/hemorrhagic, obstructive, cardiogenic, neurogenic, or vasoplegic), over time, prolonged tissue malperfusion will lead to multiorgan dysfunction and mixed shock states. In patients with mixed shock, careful attention to hemodynamics with invasive monitoring should be performed to choose vasoactive medications that will address multiple competing pathophysiologies appropriately. Balanced, multimodal vasoactive therapy may be required to reverse multiple shock states.

Unfortunately, there are no current guidelines for vasopressor management in patients with mixed shock states. It is up to the clinician to choose a combination of vasoactive therapies that are specific for the individual patient. For example, in patients with both vasoplegia (low SVR) and low CO output (cardiac index <2.2 L/min/m^2), initiation of both vasopressor (norepinephrine or phenylephrine) and inotropic (epinephrine or dobutamine) support may be necessary. Patients with systolic heart disease can present with a traumatic injury and hemorrhagic shock. While performing source control and balanced blood volume resuscitation, temporary inotropic support with dobutamine may be required to improve stroke volume and prevent cardiogenic pulmonary edema. Understanding the side effects of each vasoactive is also critical. It would be expected for dobutamine to decrease SVR in this hemorrhaging patient, which is clearly not ideal. A low-dose alpha-agonist such as phenylephrine may offset this undesired effect.

Understanding the primary effects of each vasoactive, in addition to the anticipated side effects, is critical for all resuscitation physicians. In 2011 the United States experienced a critical norepinephrine shortage that was associated with a 4% mortality increase in patients with septic shock. Clinicians often substituted phenylephrine or vasopressin to achieve MAP goals at that time, but it is possible that the rise in mortality was due to a subtle decrease in cardiac support that norepinephrine provides through beta-receptor stimulation. Multimodal vasoactive therapy can often address therapeutic gaps that may be present with the use of alternative strategies during periods of critical drug shortages.

KEY POINTS TO REMEMBER

· **Norepinephrine is generally recommended as the first-line vasopressor for patients with vasoplegic circulatory shock caused by sepsis.**

- Individual patient physiology should be taken into account when choosing vasopressor and inotropic therapy, as shock is often multifactorial.
- Vasopressor and inotropic therapy should be used to target macrocirculatory endpoints, but should be titrated to achieve improved tissue perfusion as evidenced by normalized lactate, capillary refill, and other markers of perfusion.
- Point-of-care echocardiography is a valuable tool for early recognition of cardiovascular complications of sepsis.
- Common vasopressors include norepinephrine, epinephrine, phenylephrine, and vasopressin—all of which have a slightly different clinical effect that the clinician must be prepared to manage.

References

1. Monnet X, Jabot J, Maizel J, Richard C, Teboul J-L. Norepinephrine increases cardiac preload and reduces preload dependency assessed by passive leg raising in septic shock patients. *Crit Care Med*. 2011;39(4):689–694. doi:10.1097/CCM.0b013e318206d2a3

2. Myburgh JA, Higgins A, Jovanovska A, et al. A comparison of epinephrine and norepinephrine in critically ill patients. *Intensive Care Med*. 2008;34(12):2226–2234. doi:10.1007/s00134-008-1219-0

3. Morelli A, Ertmer C, Rehberg S, et al. Phenylephrine versus norepinephrine for initial hemodynamic support of patients with septic shock: A randomized, controlled trial. *Crit Care*. 2008;12(6):R143. doi:10.1186/cc7121

4. Russell JA, Walley KR, Singer J, et al. Vasopressin versus norepinephrine infusion in patients with septic shock. *N Engl J Med*. 2008;358(9):877–887. doi:10.1056/NEJMoa067373

5. Hamzaoui O, Georger J-F, Monnet X, et al. Early administration of norepinephrine increases cardiac preload and cardiac output in septic patients with life-threatening hypotension. *Crit Care*. 2010;14(4):R142. doi:10.1186/cc9207

6. Khanna A, English SW, Wang XS, et al. Angiotensin II for the treatment of vasodilatory shock. *N Engl J Med*. 2017;377(5):419–430. doi:10.1056/NEJMoa1704154

7. De Backer D, Biston P, Devriendt J, et al. Comparison of dopamine and norepinephrine in the treatment of shock. *N Engl J Med*. 2010;362(9):779–789. doi:10.1056/NEJMoa0907118

8. Rhodes A, Evans LE, Alhazzani W, et al. Surviving Sepsis Campaign: International guidelines for management of sepsis and septic shock: 2016. *Intensive Care Med*. 2017;43(3):304–377. doi:10.1007/s00134-017-4683-6

9. Vieillard-Baron A, Caille V, Charron C, Belliard G, Page B, Jardin F. Actual incidence of global left ventricular hypokinesia in adult septic shock: *Crit Care Med.* 2008;36(6):1701–1706. doi:10.1097/CCM.0b013e318174db05

10. Mercado P, Maizel J, Beyls C, et al. Transthoracic echocardiography: An accurate and precise method for estimating cardiac output in the critically ill patient. *Crit Care.* 2017;21(1):136. doi:10.1186/s13054-017-1737-7

11. Le Tulzo Y, Seguin P, Gacouin A, et al. Effects of epinephrine on right ventricular function in patients with severe septic shock and right ventricular failure: A preliminary descriptive study. *Intensive Care Med.* 1997;23(6):664–670.

12. van Diepen S, Katz JN, Albert NM, et al. Contemporary management of cardiogenic shock: A scientific statement from the American Heart Association. *Circulation.* 2017;136(16):d232–e268. doi:10.1161/CIR.0000000000000525

17 Cardiac arrest and ED ECLS/ECPR

Katrina Augustin and Torben Becker

A 55-year-old male presents to the ED in cardiac arrest. EMS reports they were called for a complaint of chest pain. On arrival, they found the patient diaphoretic, complaining of midsternal chest pain radiating to his jaw that started while he was moving furniture into his daughter's college dorm room. The patient was initially hypotensive with BP 88/56 mmHg and HR 90 bpm but subsequently complained of worsening chest pressure before becoming unresponsive. EMS noted ventricular fibrillation (VF) on the monitor and commenced with standard ACLS protocol including defibrillation, epinephrine, and continuous CPR. The patient was intubated during transport. EMS transport time was 12 minutes with total time of CPR estimated to be approximately 20 minutes since arrest. On arrival the patient was noted to still be in VF and was treated with additional defibrillation, epinephrine, and amiodarone according to ACLS protocol with no return of spontaneous circulation (ROSC). The patient's wife arrived and reported that the patient has a history of hypertension and hyperlipidemia but was otherwise healthy and working full time as an engineer. At this time the code has been in process for ~25 minutes since arrest with no ROSC.

What do I do now?

This case represents a classic conundrum that most emergency physicians will be faced with not infrequently during their careers. In refractory cardiac arrest where conventional ACLS therapies prove inadequate, extracorporeal life support (ECLS) can lead to early stabilization, allowing time for diagnosis and potentially life-saving interventions in patients who may otherwise not survive. ECLS is an emerging therapeutic treatment that, with additional training and expertise, falls within emergency physicians' scope of practice.

ECLS is able to temporarily replace heart and lung function by providing circulatory support and/or gas exchange, thus providing a bridge to recovery or more definitive long-term treatments. Primary modes of ECLS are veno-arterial (VA), veno-venous (VV), and veno-arterial-venous (VAV). VA ECLS provides cardiac support as well as combined cardiopulmonary support in patients with cardiopulmonary failure. VV ECLS provides gas exchange in patients with severe hypoxemia who have adequate cardiac function. The hybrid VAV ECLS provides an additional option for combined cardiopulmonary support in select patients. Terminology can be confusing, with terms such as extracorporeal membrane oxygenation (ECMO) and extracorporeal life support (ECLS) used interchangeably as they refer to the same process. Extracorporeal cardiopulmonary resuscitation (ECPR) refers to ECLS being initiated in a patient with cardiac arrest.

One of the more challenging aspects of ECLS initiation for emergency physicians is determining who would benefit from ECLS. As these patients are critically ill and frequently have very little history known, it can be difficult to ascertain whether the patient is an appropriate candidate for ECLS/ECPR initiation. While still an evolving topic, commonly accepted indications include conditions that cause acute cardiac and/or respiratory failure and have expected reversible etiologies or etiologies that can be bridged to definitive therapy. Refractory cardiac arrest secondary to acute coronary occlusion is the classic indications for ECPR. In these patients, ECPR allows for early stabilization and time to perform cardiac catheterization with percutaneous coronary intervention, which can potentially be a life-saving intervention. Massive pulmonary embolus with circulatory arrest or refractory shock is another classic condition where ECPR can be life-saving. In these patients, ECPR can provide temporary stabilization for treatments such as thrombolysis, surgical thrombectomy, or even endogenous lysis of the clot over time. Other potential indications for VA ECLS include cardiogenic shock, cardiodepressant drug overdose, electrolyte disturbances, rewarming in hypothermia with hemodynamic instability, stabilization for damage-control surgery secondary to trauma, and aortic dissection causing AV disruption and pericardial tamponade. Conditions causing severe hypoxemia such as status asthmaticus, near-drowning, severe pulmonary contusions secondary to trauma, acute respiratory distress syndrome (ARDS), anaphylaxis with failure to ventilate, foreign body obstruction, and fat/air/amniotic fluid embolism are all indications that may benefit from VV ECLS.

While there are few absolute contraindications, conditions that are associated with limited benefit from ECLS/ECPR include unwitnessed cardiac arrest (unknown no-flow duration), increased length of no-flow time with little chance of intact neurologic survival, such as seen with prolonged time without CPR, conditions incompatible with life, patients with end-stage heart or lung disease who are not candidates for transplant/long-term mechanical support, and patients with advanced malignancy with limited life expectancy. Other factors that may pose relative contraindications but need to be assessed on an individual basis include advanced age, previous intracranial hemorrhage or hemorrhage at other noncompressible sites, as well as anatomic constraints secondary to vascular anomalies or previous surgical intervention that could prevent successful cannulation. As ECPR becomes more advanced, inclusion criteria have broadened, with subsequent studies showing no increased risk of complications despite inclusion of patients who were previously thought to be less-than-ideal candidates. Additionally, while patients with shockable rhythms were shown to have better neurologically intact survival, pulseless electrical activity (PEA) and asystole are no longer considered absolute contraindications to ECPR. Patients with an initial rhythm of asystole have the lowest chance of intact neurologic survival when compared to initial shockable rhythms or even PEA.

As ECLS/ECPR continues to evolve, more centers are developing ED ECMO programs. Program development requires a multidisciplinary approach with collaboration among specialties such as cardiothoracic surgery, cardiology, pulmonary medicine, emergency medicine, pharmacy, and perfusion. While historically the majority of ECLS/ECPR cannulations have been performed by cardiothoracic surgeons, emergency physicians can acquire the required skills through additional training. As ECLS does require a multidisciplinary team with expertise and extensive resources, it may not be feasible at all facilities, especially nonacademic or rural facilities. Thus, transfer to an ECLS-capable facility or having an outside ECLS team come to these facilities may be indicated in a select group of patients who meet inclusion criteria.

Cannulation during ongoing CPR is perhaps the most challenging aspect of ECPR initiation in the ED. Cannulation can be achieved through several different routes, including percutaneous insertion, surgical cutdown, and a hybrid combining these two techniques. Currently, percutaneous cannulation has become the preferred method at most institutions—bleeding risks are lower, it allows better distal limb perfusion (as it avoids vessel ligation), and it has a decreased risk of infection when compared to the cutdown technique. This technique does have an increased risk of vessel injury when compared to surgical cutdown; however, the risk can be mitigated by using dynamic ultrasound guidance, allowing for visualization of vessel size and location and any vessel anomalies. ECLS cannulation sites vary and depend on the type of ECLS being performed. The femoral vessels are commonly cannulated in both VA and VV ECLS, while the right internal jugular vein is another frequently utilized site for cannulation in VV and VAV ECLS. ECLS cannulation can also be performed centrally in contrast to the peripheral techniques described in this chapter; however, this technique requires a surgeon's expertise and is outside the scope of practice for emergency physicians.

Blood flow through the circuit in VA ECMO is provided retrograde through the arterial circulation to the aortic arch, thus delivering oxygenated blood to not only the lower body but also the upper extremities and head. This becomes slightly more nuanced in patients with residual native cardiac function, as their upper extremities and head are often perfused by blood circulating antegrade through their native heart and lungs. This blood flowing antegrade then mixes more distally in the aorta with the oxygenated blood flowing retrograde from the ECLS circuit. In this situation, the ECLS circuit is only perfusing the lower part of the body, which may be adequate in patients who have good pulmonary function. However, in patients with pulmonary failure, blood flowing antegrade through the heart/lungs is often not adequately oxygenated, thus requiring an additional venous return (VAV) to provide oxygenated blood from the ECLS circuit to the head and upper extremities by way of the right atrium. In VV ECLS performed for refractory hypoxia, deoxygenated blood is commonly drained from the inferior vena cava by way of a femoral vein. Oxygenated blood is then returned to the body by way of the contralateral femoral vein (return cannula situated higher in the inferior vena cava than the access cannula) or the right internal jugular vein. VV ECLS can also be done with insertion of right internal jugular dual-lumen transatrial bicaval catheter, but this is best done with the aid of concurrent imaging such as fluoroscopic guidance to aid in correct placement (Figure 17.1).

After successful cannulation, patients are connected to the extracorporeal circuit, which contains a centrifugal pump and a membrane oxygenator as well as internal heat exchangers. Following initiation of ECLS, management consists of anticoagulation, adjusting flow rates through the circuit to meet oxygen demands and hemodynamic stability, and maintenance of normocapnia through manipulation of oxygenator sweep gas. Anticoagulation is important to prevent thrombus formation; however, newer circuits may be heparin-coated, decreasing the need for systemic anticoagulation. While heparin is the most common anticoagulant used, newer direct thrombin inhibitors such as argatroban or bivalirudin are increasingly used in ECLS and come with the advantage of eliminating heparin-induced thrombocytopenia from the differential diagnosis when evaluating drops in platelet count. Oxygenation can be maximized through the circuit by manipulating flow rate and to a lesser extent the FiO_2 of the sweep gas (gas passing through the oxygenation filter). In patients with primary lung pathology, care should be taken to perform lung-protective ventilation in order to prevent barotrauma and allow lung rest. In patients who are cannulated peripherally, an arterial line is ideally placed in the right upper extremity as it allows for the closest approximation of upper body and cerebral blood flow oxygenation. Arterial line placement is also useful to measure continuous mean arterial pressure and left ventricular (LV) pulsatility, which can provide insight into LV function. Increased pulsatility can indicate improving LV function; conversely, decreased pulsatility can indicate worsening LV function and increased risk of blood stasis and LV thrombus.

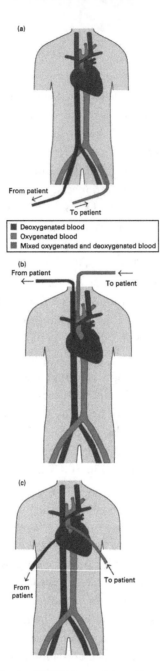

FIGURE 17.1 Illustrations of various VA-ECMO cannulations. Diagram (a) femoral vein-femoral artery peripheral cannulation. Retrograde flow from a femoral arterial cannula competes with anterograde cardiac output ejected from the left ventricle. Poor lung function results in the ejection of deoxygenated blood from the left ventricle, which mixes with oxygenated blood from the ECMO circuit. Mixing of oxygenated and deoxygenated blood will vary depending on the patient's heart function and ECMO flow. Poor lung function and good heart function in femoral-femoral ECMO cannulation may result in upper body hypoxemia. Diagram (b) internal jugular-carotid artery peripheral cannulation. Diagram (c) right atrium-ascending aorta central cannulation.

From Chung M, Shiloh AL, Carlese A. Monitoring of the adult patient on venoarterial extracorporeal membrane oxygenation. Scientific World Journal. 2014;2014:393258; open access article distributed under the Creative Commons Attribution License [https://creativecommons.org/licenses/by/3.0/legalcode]

Despite its life-saving potential, ECLS can be associated with many complications. Cannulation can lead to injury of major blood vessels, cardiac injury, and hemorrhage. To minimize these complications, ultrasound can be used to help determine the appropriate cannula size based on vessel size as well as to direct cannula placement. In addition, fluoroscopic imaging can guide wire and cannula positioning. Additional complications of ECLS include hemorrhage secondary to anticoagulation, systemic fibrinolysis and coagulopathy, thromboembolism, air embolism, cannula clotting, hemolysis, distal limb ischemia, LV distention, pulmonary edema, infection, and equipment malfunction. Distal limb ischemia can be mitigated by placement of a distal perfusion catheter either at the time of cannulation or when clinical signs of impaired blood flow to the distal extremity occur. The risk of hemorrhage secondary to anticoagulation can be minimized either by targeting lower therapeutic levels of systemic anticoagulation in high-risk patients or by using circuits that are heparin-bonded in the absence of systemic anticoagulation. Both methods, though, come at the expense of an increased risk of circuit thrombosis. VA ECLS can cause LV distention and pulmonary edema, especially in patients with poor native cardiac function, leading to elevated pulmonary pressures, LV stasis of blood, and impaired myocardial recovery. If inotropes and diuresis are unsuccessful in these patients, they may require additional support to allow for LV decompression, such as with an intra-aortic balloon bump, temporary LV assist device, or atrial septostomy to allow for blood to be redirected through the venous outflow cannula.

Outcome studies of ECPR/ECLS are promising. Studies analyzing patients with in-hospital cardiac arrest and refractory VF treated with ECPR, as compared to conventional CPR, show increased neurologically intact survival. Initial studies showed these outcomes are most significant in patients with in-hospital cardiac arrest and those presenting with refractory VF. Two initial randomized controlled trials (RCT) studying patients with out-of-hospital cardiac arrest, ARREST and Prague OHCA, support improved neurologically intact survival with ECPR compared to standard ACLS/conventional CPR. However, a subsequent RCT, INCEPTION, did not show a significant difference. While the ARREST trial was performed in a single highly experienced center with a defined prehospital algorithm for potential patients, the INCEPTION trial was a multi-center study of hospitals without extensive experience with ECPR and without a definitive prehospital care pathway. Therefore, the current evidence suggests that ECPR is most effective if performed in experienced centers and as part of an organized care system. This continues to be an area of active research, with more hospital systems creating ECPR programs.

While multiple scoring systems have been developed to predict survival after cardiac arrest in patients undergoing ECLS, the SAVE score or modified SAVE score (SAVE score + plasma lactate) has been found to be a useful tool in predicting in-hospital survival in patients undergoing VA ECLS in the ED.

In patients presenting in cardiac arrest meeting specific criteria, emergent ECLS is an increasingly important treatment modality. This therapeutic intervention may allow for intact neurologic survival in patients who likely would not survive otherwise, as it provides early stabilization, allowing for diagnosis and critical interventions. Emergency physicians play an increasingly important role in this therapy.

KEY POINTS TO REMEMBER

- In patients with refractory cardiac arrest, ECPR/ECLS can lead to early stabilization, allowing time for diagnosis and potentially life-saving interventions in patients who may otherwise not survive.
- Commonly accepted indications for ECLS include conditions that cause acute cardiac and/or respiratory failure with expected reversible etiologies, such as acute occlusive coronary disease requiring percutaneous coronary intervention or massive pulmonary embolus requiring thrombolysis.
- With additional training, emergency physicians can acquire the skills needed to perform ECLS cannulation.
- At facilities without the resources to perform ECLS, transfer to an ECLS-capable facility may be indicated in a select group of patients who meet inclusion criteria.
- Outcomes are promising, with many studies showing increased neurologically intact survival in patients treated with ECPR when compared to conventional CPR.

Further reading

American Heart Association. Cardiac arrest statistics 2016. http://www.heart.org/
HEARTORG/General/Cardiac-Arrest- Statistics_UCM_448311_Article.jsp

Belohlavek J, Kucera K, Jarkovsky J, et al. Hyperinvasive approach to out-of-hospital
cardiac arrest using mechanical chest compression device, prehospital intraarrest
cooling, extracorporeal life support and early invasive assessment compared
to standard of care: A randomized parallel groups comparative study proposal,
"Prague OHCA study." J Transl Med. 2012;10:163. https://doi.org/10.1186/
1479-5876-10-163

Belohlavek J, Smalcova J, Rob D, et al. Prague OHCA Study Group. Effect of intraarrest transport, extracorporeal cardiopulmonary resuscitation, and immediate
invasive assessment and treatment on functional neurologic outcome in
refractory out-of-hospital cardiac arrest: A Randomized Clinical Trial. JAMA.
2022;327(8):737–747.

Brogan TV, Lequier L, Lorusso R, MacLaren G, Peek G. Extracorporeal Life
Support: The ELSO Red Book. ELSO; 2017.

Chen WC, Huang, KY, Yao CW, et al. The modified SAVE score: Predicting survival
using urgent veno-arterial extracorporeal membrane oxygenation within 24
hours of arrival at the emergency department. Critical Care. 2016;20:336.

Choi DS, Kim T, Ro YS, et al. Extracorporeal life support and survival after out-of-
hospital cardiac arrest in a nationwide registry: A propensity score-matched
analysis. Resuscitation. 2016;99:26–32.

Haas NL, Coute RA, Cranford JA, Neumar RW. Descriptive analysis of extracorporeal
cardiopulmonary resuscitation following out-of-hospital cardiac arrest: An ELSO
registry study. Resuscitation. 2017;119:56–62.

Keebler ME, Haddad EV, Choi CW, et al. Venoarterial extracorporeal membrane
oxygenation in cardiogenic shock. JACC Heart Fail. 2018;6:503–516.

Lamhaut L, Hutin A, Puymirat E, et al. A pre-hospital extracorporeal cardiopulmonary
resuscitation (ECPR) strategy for treatment of refractory out-of-hospital
cardiac arrest: An observational study and propensity analysis. Resuscitation.
2017;117:109–117.

Lamhaut L, Tea V, Raphalen JH, et al. Coronary lesions in refractory out-of-hospital
cardiac arrest (OHCA) treated by extracorporeal pulmonary resuscitation (ECPR).
Resuscitation. 2018;126:154–159.

Richardson AC, Schmidt M, Bailey M, Pellegrino VA, Rycus PT, Pilcher DV. ECMO
cardiopulmonary resuscitation (ECPR), trends in survival from an international
multicentre cohort study over 12 years. Resuscitation. 2017;112:34–40.

Siao FY, Chiu CC, Chen YC, et al. Managing cardiac arrest with refractory ventricular
fibrillation in the emergency department: Conventional cardiopulmonary
resuscitation versus extracorporeal cardiopulmonary resuscitation.
Resuscitation. 2015;92:70–76.

Suverein M, Delnoij R, Lorusso R, et al. Early Extracorporeal CPR for refractory out-of-hospital cardiac arrest. *N Engl J Med.* 2023;*388*(4):299–309.

Swol J, Belohavek J, Brodie D, et al. Extracorporeal life support in the emergency department: A narrative review for the emergency medicine physician. *Resuscitation.* 2018;133:108–117.

Tisherman SA, Menaker J, Kon Z. Are we ready to take ECPR on the road? Maybe. *Resuscitation.* 2017;117:A1–A2.

Tonna JE, Johnson NJ, Greenwood J, et al. Practice characteristics of emergency department extracorporeal cardiopulmonary resuscitation (ECPR) programs in the United States: The current state of the art of emergency department extracorporeal membrane oxygenation (ED ECMO). *Resuscitation.* 2016;107:38–46.

Wang CH, Chou NK, Becker LB, et al. Improved outcomes of extracorporeal cardipulmonary resuscitation for out-of-hospital cardiac arrest: A comparison with that for extracorporeal rescue for in-hospital cardiac arrest. *Resuscitation.* 2014;85:1219–1224.

Yannopoulos D, Bartos J, Raveendran G, et al. Advanced reperfusion strategies for patients with out-of-hospital cardiac arrest and refractory ventricular fibrillation (ARREST): A phase 2, single centre, open-label, randomised controlled trial. *Lancet.* 2020;*396*(10265):1807–1816.

18 Too slow to go: Symptomatic bradycardia

Tyler VanDyck and Scott Simpson

A 58-year-old male with past medical history of hypertension, hyperlipidemia, and coronary artery disease presents to the ED with lightheadedness that started 1 week ago. His symptoms are worse with mild exertion and relieved with rest. Your physical exam findings when he arrives at the ED are benign, and he appears well perfused. His vital signs are BP 146/67 mmHg, HR 39 bpm, temperature 37.5°C, RR 18 breaths/min, and SpO$_2$ 97% on room air. An EKG shows third-degree heart block. Laboratory evaluation is significant for a normal troponin level. Chest x-ray is unremarkable. You consult the cardiology department and the patient is ready for admission when the nurse notifies you that the patient feels lightheaded again. You reassess the patient and notice that he is pale, cold, and clammy on exam. His HR is now 24 and his BP is 79/42.

What do I do now?

Bradycardia can be life-threatening and technically challenging to treat. Expedient decision-making and interventions are necessary in the symptomatic patient to prevent progression to cardiac arrest. In this chapter, we will cover when bradycardia should be treated, which medications can be helpful, when to consider and how to perform transcutaneous or transvenous pacing, and appropriate settings for a temporary pacemaker.

In the initial assessment of the bradycardic patient, the provider must identify whether the current rhythm is stable or unstable, based on the adequacy of perfusion. This can be assessed objectively by BP and clinical examination (capillary refill, skin temperature, and presence of mottling) as well as subjectively by symptoms such as chest pain, shortness of breath, and altered mental status. In the case of unstable bradycardia, immediate action must be taken to avoid further deterioration in the patient. For cases of stable bradycardia, the provider may elect to seek expert consultation but should be prepared for subsequent action in case of sudden hemodynamic collapse.

The initial medication for treatment of symptomatic bradycardia is atropine (0.5 mg IV push). It is readily available in most cardiac arrest carts. Atropine increases the heart rate via anticholinergic effects at the AV node. It may not be effective in all cases, particularly those arising from infranodal/complete AV block. Atropine frequently needs to be re-dosed every 3 to 5 minutes (to a maximum of 3 mg). Inotropes can be used as second-line agents. These include epinephrine (0.02–0.2 mcg/kg/min IV) and dopamine (5–10 mcg/kg/min IV), both titrated upward until satisfactory HR and BP are achieved. However, these infusions take time to prepare, are temporizing, and may similarly lack efficacy. In an unstable patient who does not respond to atropine, treatment should proceed immediately to pacing modalities, which include transcutaneous and transvenous approaches.

Most modern defibrillators include transcutaneous pacing functionality. Providers should familiarize themselves with the equipment in use in their facilities and the manufacturer's specific instructions regarding pad placement and the specifics of pacing function. Some models require placement of a separate set of EKG electrodes connected to the device to provide detection of intrinsic rhythm ("sensing"), whereas others provide this functionality integral to the pads. After activating the pacemaker mode of the device, the provider must select a pacing rate and output. Reasonable initial settings include a pacing rate of 80 to 100 ppm with a supplied current of 10 mA. The patient should be monitored for electrical and mechanical capture while quickly increasing the pacemaker output by intervals of 10 mA. Electrical capture occurs when pacing spikes on EKG are followed by a wide-complex QRS complex signifying electrical conduction. This must be correlated to mechanical capture, which is defined as a perfusing pulse corresponding to each paced beat. It is important not to confuse stimulated muscle contraction with electrical or mechanical capture. Mechanical capture can be verified manually by palpating for a pulse, or by correlation to a pulse oximeter or arterial BP waveform. The threshold (the minimum current required to produce capture) can vary based on body habitus and pad position but typically occurs between 40 and 80 mA. The current should be set ~5 to 10 mA above the threshold to avoid inadvertent loss of capture. Persistent lack of mechanical capture despite electrical capture, known as electromechanical dissociation or pulseless electrical activity, should immediately prompt consideration for non-electrical etiologies as per standard life support guidelines. Transcutaneous pacing should be expected to be painful in the conscious patient and should prompt use of analgesic and/or sedative medications as tolerated by the patient's hemodynamics.

Transcutaneous pacing provides only a temporary bridge in a resuscitation scenario until a more definitive pacemaker can be placed. If the underlying rhythm disturbance is expected to be ongoing, a transvenous pacemaker should be inserted as a more reliable option until a durable permanent pacemaker can be placed. Placing a transvenous catheter involves placement of a small introducer (usually 6 French, but variable by manufacturer) in a central vein followed by the insertion ("floating") of a subsequent pacing electrode. The preferred access site is the right internal jugular vein, followed by the left subclavian vein, based on the anatomy that facilitates easy pacing electrode entry into the right ventricle. The placement of the initial introducer should proceed in the standard Seldinger fashion of central venous catheterization.

After the introducer catheter is placed, the pacing catheter can be prepared. Pacing catheters typically include a 1.5-mL balloon on the catheter tip to facilitate insertion. The integrity of this balloon must be checked prior to insertion by inflating with the included syringe. The catheter sheath must also be placed on the catheter prior to insertion to maintain sterility of a portion of the external catheter, should it need to be advanced after the sterile field has been taken down. The non-sterile end of the catheter (containing the balloon inflation port and the electrical connections) may be handed off to a non-sterile assistant, who will connect the catheter to the generator box and inflate/deflate the balloon upon direction of the primary proceduralist. The pacemaker catheter should be placed through the introducer to a depth of 15 cm and the assistant should be instructed to turn on the generator and program the pacemaker.

In emergency circumstances, the pacemaker mode should be set to DOO/VOO or VVI. DOO and VOO are asynchronous modes that provide pacemaker functionality regardless of native cardiac activity. VVI is a demand pacing mode, whereby the pacemaker senses native cardiac activity and only paces when the set pacemaker rate exceeds the native rate. Demand pacing is advantageous to asynchronous pacing to avoid the theoretical risk of R-on-T phenomenon and ventricular fibrillation if the pacemaker applies current during native ventricular repolarization. The use of VVI, while safer, requires understanding of pacemaker sensing and sensitivity. The pacemaker detects native cardiac activity as voltage at the electrode. The native cardiac voltage must exceed the voltage sensitivity setting on the pacemaker to be sensed as a beat. If the sensitivity is set too high (i.e., a low mV setting), low voltage artifact may be misinterpreted as native cardiac activity and the pacemaker will be suppressed, a phenomenon known as "over-sensing." The opposite can also occur if the sensitivity is too low (i.e., a high mV setting) such that the pacemaker will not recognize the native activity and pace regardless, a phenomenon known as "under-sensing." An under-sensing VVI pacemaker is functionally similar to asynchronous pacing. Additional initial settings include an output of 5 to 20 mA (higher outputs may allow for earlier capture but with suboptimal electrode placement), ventricular sensitivity of 3 mV, and a rate of 80 to 100 ppm. The proceduralist should be familiar with specific manufacturer's instructions for the equipment they are using and should follow manufacturer's guidance where it differs from the guidelines provided here.

After the catheter is inserted to 15 cm and the generator is turned on and programmed, the proceduralist should observe for pacemaker spikes on the EKG monitor. If spikes are not seen, the EKG monitor may need to be programmed to allow pacemaker detection, or the current may need to be increased. After visualization of pacemaker spikes, the balloon should be inflated, and the catheter should be advanced while monitoring the patient's EKG monitor for signs of electrical capture. This will manifest as wide-complex QRS complexes following each pacemaker spike. The ideal location for the tip of the catheter is the apex of the right ventricle. If the pacemaker is too shallow and some degree of native conduction is preserved, atrial pacing can occur, which will manifest as narrow-complex QRS complexes following the pacemaker spikes. If the catheter needs to be withdrawn at any point and at the completion of the procedure, the balloon must be deflated to avoid potential damage to valvular apparatus. As with transcutaneous pacing, electrical capture must be correlated with mechanical capture. After capture is achieved, the pacemaker output should be decreased until capture is lost, to determine the threshold. The pacemaker output should be set at 2.5 times the threshold to avoid inadvertent loss of capture that can occur with movement of the electrode. Ideal threshold is <1 mA with optimal placement. High thresholds should prompt expert consultation and/or repositioning. Chest x-ray should be obtained to verify correct position in the right ventricle. If asynchronous (DOO/VOO) mode was used during flotation, consideration should be made to reprogramming to a demand mode (VVI), to avoid the risks of R-on-T phenomenon as discussed earlier. The pacing wire should be looped and taped securely externally to avoid dislodging.

As an alternative to the blind advancement technique, real-time echocardiographic guidance can be used from the subxiphoid position to visualize the catheter tip during flotation and confirm appropriate position. Another method involves intracavitary EKG monitoring facilitated by attachment of the pacing electrode to a precordial lead of the EKG monitor to allow interpretation of the differing native QRS morphology as the electrode moves through the native beating heart (see the "Further reading" list at the end of the chapter). This requires disabling the pacemaker during flotation such that interpretation of the native QRS complex can guide location. The pacemaker is then enabled when satisfactory position has been achieved. Common troubleshooting of emergent transvenous pacing is summarized in Table 18.1.

TABLE 18.1 **Troubleshooting common pacing challenges**

Common challenge	Possible causes	Actions to try
Failure to pace	• No pacing spikes seen on EKG when intrinsic rate is less than pacemaker rate • Oversensing	• Check connections • Decrease sensitivity (turn mV up to make it harder to sense)
Failure to capture	Pacing spike seen but no widened QRS follows (in V-paced modes) or no P wave (in A-V sequential dual-chamber modes)	Increase output (turn up mA) energy
Failure to sense	• Pacer does not detect intrinsic myocardial activity • Regular pacing spikes unrelated to intrinsic rhythm, with or without capture • Beware: can cause torsades due to R-on-T phenomenon	Increase the sensitivity (turn mV down to make easier to sense)
Inappropriate/ over-sensing	• Skeletal muscle activity misinterpreted or P or T waves misinterpreted as QRS complex • Bradycardia persists	• Decrease sensitivity (turn mV up to make it harder to sense)

For all situations

- Check connections from patient to the pacemaker box.
- Check battery of the pacemaker box.
- Check lead connections.
- Check duration of time epicardial leads have been in place (the longer time post-operatively causes greater fibrosis at lead insertion in myocardium).
- Check chest x-ray for tip/balloon position in right ventricular myocardium.
- Check for electrolyte disturbances.

After successful pacemaker placement and patient stabilization, the provider should continue standard diagnostic evaluation, to include consideration of overdose, cardiac ischemia, and severe electrolyte abnormalities such as hyperkalemia. Antidotal therapy can be effective in cases of beta-blocker, calcium channel blocker, and digitalis toxicity. A cardiologist and/or electrophysiologist should be consulted to provide ongoing management of the pacemaker.

KEY POINTS TO REMEMBER

- In patients with bradycardia, assessment of the stability of the rhythm differentiates patients who need immediate resuscitation from those who may be observed.
- The right internal jugular vein is the preferred site for transvenous pacemaker placement.
- The balloon on the pacemaker catheter must always be deflated before withdrawing the catheter and reattempting placement.
- Electrical capture of a pacemaker must be correlated with mechanical capture to verify successful pacing.
- Common etiologies for bradycardia include medication overdose, acute coronary ischemia, and electrolyte abnormalities such as hyperkalemia.

Further reading

Bing O, McDowell J, Hantman J, Messer J. Pacemaker placement by electrocardiographic monitoring. *N Engl J Med*. 1972;287:651.

Blanco P. Temporary transvenous pacing guided by the combined use of ultrasound and intracavitary electrocardiography: A feasible and safe technique. *Ultrasound J*. 2019;11:8.

Fitzpatrick A, Sutton R. A guide to temporary pacing. *BMJ*. 1992;304:365–369.

Liu M, Han X. Bedside temporary transvenous cardiac pacemaker placement. *Am J Emerg Med*. 2020;38(4):819–822.

19 Choked off: Tamponade

Josh Krieger and Ashika Jain

A 76-year-old man with a known history of right upper lobe adenocarcinoma of the lung who is currently undergoing palliative chemotherapy presents to the ED with 2 days of worsening shortness of breath. He has chronic dyspnea, but he noticed it has become significantly worse over the last 2 days and he now feels short of breath with any movement. His vital signs are HR 106 bpm, BP 85/68 mmHg, RR 28 breaths/min, and oxygen saturation 92% on ambient air. He is afebrile. Lung exam demonstrates diminished breath sounds in the right anterior lung field, and the remaining lung fields are clear to auscultation. When seated and reclined to 30 degrees, he has jugular venous distention to the angle of the mandible. Unfortunately, the ultrasound machine is being used by a colleague at this moment. A chest radiograph demonstrates a stable mass-like opacity in his right upper lobe with an enlarged cardiac silhouette, new from prior studies, with no evidence of pneumothorax or mediastinal shift.

What do I do now?

This elderly gentleman with known non-small cell lung cancer is presenting with acute-on-chronic dyspnea. He is also hypotensive, tachycardic, and tachypneic with jugular venous distention and a normal lung exam, aside from the expected diminished breath sounds in the location of his mass. Radiographic imaging reveals a newly enlarged cardiac silhouette.

The differential diagnosis for dyspnea in this patient could include progression of malignancy, pulmonary embolism, pneumothorax, pulmonary toxicity from chemotherapy, new heart failure, acute anemia, pulmonary infection, and cardiac tamponade. If available, his immediate workup should include a bedside ultrasound of his heart to evaluate for an effusion (Figure 19.1) and evidence of tamponade physiology as well as chest CT with contrast enhancement of the pulmonary arteries to evaluate his lung parenchyma and to assess for pulmonary embolism. His chest radiograph does not demonstrate findings convincing for pneumothorax, but this could be further investigated by looking for lung sliding on ultrasound.

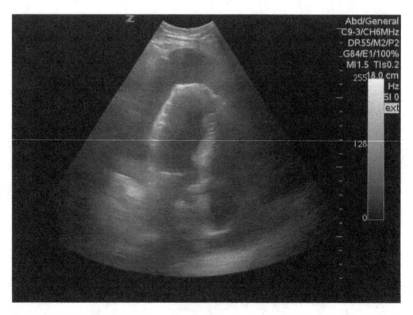

FIGURE 19.1 Large pericardial effusion on apical four-chamber (A4C) view on cardiac ultrasound

His newly enlarged cardiac silhouette should raise concern for a pericardial effusion, and bedside echocardiography demonstrates a large pericardial effusion with diastolic collapse of the right ventricle, concerning for cardiac tamponade. A CT demonstrates no pulmonary embolism with a stable mass in the right upper lobe and slightly enlarged metastases in multiple lung fields.

Cardiac tamponade can happen acutely as a result of penetrating injuries to the thorax or abdomen with hemopericardium, aortic dissection involving the aortic root, right atrial injury as a result of central venous catheter placement, or a slow-growing chronic effusion. Chronic effusions can be caused by malignancy, rheumatologic conditions, volume overload, uremia, or infections, among others. Tamponade is a form of obstructive shock wherein the right ventricle is unable to fill during diastole, causing blood to back up into the venous circulation. This backup of blood is manifested by jugular venous distention, and the absence of left ventricular preload causes hypotension. Clear lung sounds demonstrate that left ventricular forward flow is preserved. The muffled heart tones that complete Beck's classic triad are caused by fluid overlying the heart within the pericardium.

Pericardial involvement is found on autopsy in up to 20% of patients with malignancy. Effusions can result from direct or metastatic involvement of the pericardium, or as a complication of chemotherapy or radiation therapy. Lung cancer is the most common malignancy with pericardial involvement. A variety of older chemotherapy agents, as well as tyrosine kinase inhibitors and the newer class of agents known as immune checkpoint inhibitors, have been known to cause effusions and tamponade.

After establishing a diagnosis of pericardial effusion in a medical patient, workup should include inflammatory markers such as a C-reactive protein and erythrocyte sedimentation rate (ESR). An ECG may show sinus tachycardia, low-voltage QRS complexes in all leads, PQ-segment depression, or electrical alternans, which is beat-to-beat variation in QRS amplitude reflecting a swinging heart inside a large effusion. A chest radiograph may show an enlarged cardiac silhouette. Exam would be expected to show signs consistent with low right ventricular stroke volume and, in a chronic effusion, signs of elevated central venous pressure. These findings include cool and potentially edematous extremities with no pulmonary edema.

Transthoracic echocardiography should be the first-line imaging study to confirm the presence of an effusion and to evaluate the hemodynamic impact. The earliest sign of tamponade on echocardiography will be systolic right atrial collapse, as the right atrium is the lowest-pressure chamber in the heart. A longer duration of right atrial collapse throughout the cardiac cycle demonstrates more severe tamponade. The right ventricle collapses during diastole as intrapericardial pressures rise, and in early tamponade this may be seen only during expiration. The subxiphoid view is the best to visualize the right ventricle, followed by the parasternal long axis if the subxiphoid view is difficult. In an acute hemorrhagic effusion, a relatively effusion can rapidly lead to cardiogenic shock as there is no compensatory increase in the systemic venous pressure and there is a rapid rise in intrapericardial pressure. Chronic effusions will usually be larger before they cause tamponade, as the body raises its systemic venous pressure over time to maintain the venous/atrial pressure gradient.

Cardiac tamponade should be thought of as a continuum from mild to severe, depending on its impact on right heart filling and right ventricular stroke volume. As volume accumulates inside the pericardium, the intrapericardial pressure rises. As it nears and then surpasses the central venous pressure, the right atrial filling is limited, thus limiting right ventricular preload and stroke volume. Severity can be judged by tachycardia, tachypnea, and an elevated jugular venous pressure with pulsus paradoxus (a decrease in the systolic blood pressure of >10 mmHg during inspiration).

Treatment of cardiac tamponade from medical causes, once suspected, involves urgent consultation with an interventional cardiologist and an urgent formal echocardiogram. Temporizing measures prior to drainage of the effusion should include administration of volume to increase central venous pressure above right atrial pressure. Mitral and tricuspid valve inflow velocities and hepatic vein pulsed-wave Doppler variation with respiration should be assessed, and, in some cases, bedside echo-guided drainage will be performed. Other cases are more appropriate for drainage in the cardiac catheterization laboratory or for surgical drainage. Treatment of cardiac tamponade in the trauma setting is often best done with open thoracotomy and pericardiotomy. In facilities without access to immediate surgical management, the bedside provider may need to perform bedside pericardiocentesis as a last resort but should recognize that this is only a temporizing measure.

The classic blind subcostal approach to pericardiocentesis carries a substantial risk and is no longer a required procedure in the advanced trauma life support curriculum.

KEY POINTS TO REMEMBER

- One must suspect cardiac tamponade in order to look for it.
- Tamponade is manifested by tachycardia, tachypnea, and elevated central venous pressure.
- Pericardial effusions are best assessed with echocardiography, and the earliest evidence of tamponade is right atrial collapse.

Further reading

Alerhand S, Carter JM. What echocardiographic findings suggest a pericardial effusion is causing tamponade? *Am J Emerg Med*. 2019;37(2):321–326. doi:10.1016/j.ajem.2018.11.004

American College of Surgeons. *ATLS: Advanced Trauma Life Support for Doctors (Student Course Manual)*. 10th ed. American College of Surgeons; 2018.

Appleton C, Gillam L, Koulogiannis K. Cardiac tamponade. *Cardiol Clin*. 2017;35(4):525–537. doi:10.1016/j.ccl.2017.07.006

Imazio M, Colopi M, De Ferrari GM. Pericardial diseases in patients with cancer: Contemporary prevalence, management and outcomes. *Heart*. 2020;106(8):569–574. doi:10.1136/heartjnl-2019-315852

Klein AL, Abbara S, Agler DA, et al. American Society of Echocardiography clinical recommendations for multimodality cardiovascular imaging of patients with pericardial disease: Endorsed by the Society for Cardiovascular Magnetic Resonance and Society of Cardiovascular Computed Tomography. *J Am Soc Echocardiogr*. 2013;26:965–1012.

Maisch B, Ristić AD, Pankuweit S, Seferovic P. Percutaneous therapy in pericardial diseases. *Cardiol Clin*. 2017;35(4):567–588. doi:10.1016/j.ccl.2017.07.010

PART 4

Organ specific

20 Brain on fire: Status epilepticus

Michael Bux and Matthew T. Niehaus

A 28-year-old woman is brought by paramedics to the ED after a witnessed collapse and shaking spell at a grocery store. Bystanders estimate she was shaking for ~4 minutes before the ambulance arrived. When paramedics arrived on scene, she was only groaning to painful stimuli. En route to the ED, she again had whole-body stiffening followed by four-extremity rhythmic shaking. On arrival, you note continued rhythmic myoclonic activity despite 4 mg of lorazepam. She is not responsive to verbal or painful stimuli. Family is not present to provide additional history. Vitals signs are HR 82 bpm, BP 112/60 mmHg, RR 10 breaths/min, and oxygen saturation of 96% on room air. A brief physical exam shows an otherwise normally developed adult female with fixed left eye deviation whose pupils measure 3 mm bilaterally and symmetric myoclonus of the upper and lower extremities.

What do I do now?

MAKING THE DIAGNOSIS

The 2016 American Epilepsy Society Guidelines defined status epilepticus (SE) as either seizure activity (convulsive or nonconvulsive) lasting >30 minutes or two or more seizures in which full recovery of consciousness is not achieved between episodes. More recently, however, experts have proposed a simplified definition to define SE as any seizure lasting >5 minutes or multiple episodes within a 5-minute time period without return to pre-convulsive neurologic baseline.[1] This new definition seeks to cast a wide net in order to prevent a delay in providing expeditious care. Once a seizure continues despite adequate treatment with both first- and second-line medical therapies, it is considered refractory status epilepticus (RSE).[2]

Performing a thorough history and physical exam is essential to make the diagnosis of SE. While a history of epilepsy is helpful, providers must realize that most cases of SE present without any prior seizure history and are not due to a primary seizure disorder.[3] Secondary causes of SE are listed in Box 20.1, and the emergency provider needs to evaluate each patient with SE rapidly for these etiologies to provide adequate treatment and care.

Clues that should raise suspicion for the presence of SE are sudden and unexplained loss of consciousness without awakening,

---

BOX 20.1 **Secondary causes of SE**

Medication noncompliance

Acute alcohol withdrawal

Drug toxicity

Primary CNS disease (tumor, stroke, meningitis, encephalitis)

Trauma

Anoxic brain injury

Hypoglycemia

Primary seizure disorder (rare)

Psychogenic non-epileptiform seizures (formerly "pseudoseizures")

---

repetitive body movements, and loss of bladder continence. Physical exam findings that may be present include tongue biting, fever with meningismus, fixed eye deviation, and episodes of rigidity followed by flaccidity.

Clinicians must have a high index of suspicion for SE as the presentation can be variable. SE can be divided into three categories: convulsive, nonconvulsive, and partial. Convulsive SE is persistent or repeated generalized tonic-clonic seizures with a persistent postictal phase between repeated episodes. Nonconvulsive SE is a continuous or fluctuating suppression in level of consciousness. Partial SE likewise is a pattern of continuous or repeating fluctuations in motor signs, sensory symptoms, or impairment of function (speech) without changes in consciousness.[4]

TREATMENT

Pharmacotherapy for seizures should begin immediately when the diagnosis of SE is made. It has been demonstrated that seizures will become increasingly refractory to treatment the longer they continue.[5] Therefore, rapid identification, initiation of treatment, and movement through a management algorithm is essential in the treatment of SE. The American Epilepsy Society categorizes management into phases based on duration of seizure (Box 20.2). If the seizure breaks at any point along the algorithm, stop and continue with supportive care.

The algorithm in Table 20.1 has been adapted from the American Epilepsy Society.[4]

BOX 20.2   **Phases of SE management**

0–5 minutes	Stabilization phase
5–20 minutes	Initial therapy phase
20–40 minutes	Second therapy phase
40–60 minutes	Third therapy phase

TABLE 20.1 **Treatment algorithm for SE**

Seizure duration	Phase of treatment	What to do
0–5 min	Stabilization	• Primary survey—ABCs (airway, breathing, circulation, disability, exposure) • Monitor oxygenation and provide supplemental oxygenation as needed. • Gain IV access, attach patient to monitors, and begin timing the seizure. • Intubate as necessary for airway protection. • Labs: capillary blood glucose, electrolytes, complete blood count, toxicology screen, antiepileptic drug levels (if applicable) • Correct blood glucose if <60 mg/dL.

5–20 min	Initial therapy	• Give initial medication: a benzodiazepine.
		  • Choose ONE of the following:
		    • IV therapy
		      • Lorazepam: 0.1 mg/kg/dose (max 4 mg/dose)
		        • Preferred in pregnancy*
		      • Diazepam: 0.15–0.20 mg/kg/dose (max 10 mg/dose)
		    • If no IV access, give intramuscular midazolam: 10 mg if >40 kg or 5 mg for 13–40 kg
		  • If lorazepam or diazepam was given, one repeat dose may be given if seizure persists. Do not give a repeat dose of midazolam.
		  • If none of the three options is available, alternative therapy includes:
		    • IV phenobarbital: 15 mg/kg/dose
		    • Rectal diazepam: 0.2–0.5 mg/kg (max 20 mg/dose)

TABLE 20.1 **Continued**

Seizure duration	Phase of treatment	What to do

20–40 min	Second-tier therapy	• Give single dose of ONE of the following:
		  • IV fosphenytoin: 20 mg/kg (max 1,500 mg/dose)
		    • Patient should have cardiac monitoring due to risk of QT prolongation and arrhythmia.*
		    • Preferred control therapy in pregnancy*
		  • IV valproic acid: 40 mg/kg (max 3,000 mg/dose)
		    • Avoid in pediatric patients age <2 yr due to risk of hepatotoxicity.*
		  • IV levitiracepam: 60 mg/kg (max 4,500 mg/dose)
		    • Preferred second-line agent in pregnancy.
		• If none of the three options is available, alternative therapy includes IV phenobarbital: 15 mg/kg/dose (only if not previously given during initial therapy phase).

40–60 min	Third-tier therapy	• Choose one of the following:
		  • Repeat second-line therapy.
		  • Propofol: loading dose 1–2 mg/kg; initial maintenance 20 mcg/kg/min titrate to 30–200 mcg/kg/min based on EEG
		    • Pediatric patients: avoid doses >65 mcg/kg/min; contraindicated in young children
		  • Pentobarbital: loading dose 5–15 mg/kg; maintenance 0.5–5 mg/kg/hr
		  • Thiopental: loading dose 2–7 mg/kg at rate of <50 mg/min; maintenance 0.5–5 mg/kg/hr
		  • Midazolam: loading dose 0.2 mg/kg at rate of 2 mg/min; maintenance 0.05–2 mg/kg/hr
		• Intubate if not previously performed.
		• Begin continuous EEG monitoring.

*Reference: Brophy et al., 2012 (reference 2).

SPECIAL POPULATIONS

Pregnancy

Pregnant patients require special consideration when choosing medication and dose. The increased circulating blood volume (i.e., volume of distribution) and increased drug clearance may necessitate dosing adjustments. Lorazepam, fosphenytoin, and levetiracetam should be used for pregnant patients if available. Treat pregnant patients as aggressively as non-pregnant patients since fetal outcome depends upon rapid seizure control in the mother. Late pregnancy also adds eclampsia to the differential diagnosis, for which a bolus of 6 mg magnesium sulfate should be given and an obstetrics consult should be placed for potential emergent delivery of the fetus. When sending blood tests in a pregnant patient, consider sending a vitamin B6 (pyridoxine) level, as pyridoxine deficiency can lead to seizure just as in patients experiencing isoniazid toxicity.[2]

Pediatrics

The listed therapy algorithm can be used for patients of any age. The first-line therapies have all been shown to be efficacious in pediatric populations. Unfortunately, there are insufficient data on the use of second- and third-line medications in children.[4] In addition to the antiepileptic drugs in the therapy algorithm, all young children should be given IV pyridoxine.[4]

PROGNOSIS

The morbidity and mortality rates of SE are high relative to patients presenting with brief seizures. Overall prognosis is influenced by the etiology of seizure, duration of SE, and patient age. It is estimated that the mortality in adults can be up to 30%. Fortunately, mortality in pediatric populations is significantly lower, typically considered to be <3%.[4] Rapid recognition, stabilization, and initiation of antiepileptic medications can reduce the risk of morbidity and mortality.

· SE is a seizure lasting >5 minutes.

· SE can consist of convulsive, nonconvulsive, or partial seizures.

· First 5 minutes: Stabilize the patient via ABCs, oxygen, and airway protection as needed. Get patient on monitors. Obtain IV access. Check blood glucose and send labs.

· After 5 minutes: Initiate medication. Start with benzodiazepines. May repeat dose of lorazepam or diazepam.

· At 20 minutes: Give second-line therapy.

· At 40 minutes: Initiate third-line therapy.

· Use recommended weight-based doses for all medications

· All intubated patients need to be admitted to an ICU with continuous EEG capabilities.

References

1. Al-Mufti F, Claassen J. Neurocritical care: Status epilepticus review. *Crit Care Clin*. 2014;30(4):751–764.

2. Brophy GM, Bell R, Claassen J, et al. Guidelines for the evaluation and management of status epilepticus. *Neurocrit Care*. 2012;17(1):3–23.

3. Shorvon S. The management of status epilepticus. *J Neurol Neurosurg Psychiatry*. 2001;70(suppl 2):ii22–ii27.

4. Glauser T, Shinnar S, Gloss D, et al. Evidence-based guideline: Treatment of convulsive status epilepticus in children and adults: Report of the Guideline Committee of the American Epilepsy Society. *Epilepsy Curr*. 2016;16(1):48–61.

5. Zaccara G, Giannasi G, Oggioni R, et al. Challenges in the treatment of convulsive status epilepticus. *Seizure*. 2017;47:17–24.

21 The pressure is too much: Traumatic brain injuries and intracranial hypertension

Jesse Shriki and Wan-Tsu Wendy Chang

A 28-year-old male was brought to the ED via EMS after being found down by friends. Per report, the patient went outside to smoke. After a short but unknown amount of time, his friends heard a "thud" and went to investigate. They found the patient unresponsive, supine on the ground. As the friends were unsure whether pulses were present, one round of CPR was performed. Upon EMS arrival, spontaneous pulses were noted. The patient's initial Glasgow Coma Scale score (GCS) was 5 (E1V1M3); thus, EMS intubated him using ketamine, placed a cervical collar, and brought him into the ED. On evaluation, the patient was afebrile, HR 82 bpm, BP 91/70 mmHg, and oxygen saturation 82% on maximal ventilator settings. His GCS was 3T and pupils were 8 mm equal and minimally reactive bilaterally. The only sign of trauma was an occipital hematoma, and a non-contrast CT scan was read as diffuse axonal injury. He had coarse breath sounds with rhonchi bilaterally.

What do I do now?

Traumatic brain injury (TBI) can be classified by the mechanism of injury, pattern of brain injury, and clinical severity. Severe traumatic brain injury (sTBI) is defined as a GCS of 3 to 8.[1] TBI causes significant morbidity and mortality, necessitating 2.5 million ED visits in the United States in 2014 alone.[2] Overall, TBI-related deaths represent 2.2% of all deaths in the United States, especially those with a GCS of ≤6.[3] The most severely brain-injured patients with a GCS of 3 have up to 76% mortality.[4] For these reasons, the emergency physician should have a thorough understanding of the early management of the sTBI patient.

While the clinician cannot undo the primary insult to the brain, prevention of further (secondary) injury to the at-risk brain is a key focus in the early management of TBI. The deadly duo of hypotension and hypoxia should be avoided. BP control is important in brain injury as cerebral autoregulation may be impaired. Normally, the brain is able to maintain a constant cerebral blood flow for a range of mean arterial pressure (MAP) between 50 and 150 mmHg. sTBI can narrow or completely disrupt this cerebral autoregulation mechanism, thereby increasing the risk of cerebral ischemia and hyperemia, both of which can worsen cerebral edema. In addition, hypocapnia can be detrimental, despite its use as rescue therapy for cerebral herniation, given that alkalosis is a potent trigger for cerebral vasoconstriction.

Intracranial pressure (ICP) is the result of a rigid calvarium only able to accommodate a fixed volume of brain tissue, blood, and CSF. When that volume is increased by mass lesions such as hemorrhage or edema, ICP increases. Intracranial hypertension is a significant cause of secondary injury given that elevated ICP can decrease cerebral perfusion, as cerebral perfusion pressure (CPP) is the difference between MAP and ICP. However, it is not the magnitude of the ICP alone that is detrimental; the duration of the raised pressure or the "ICP dose" is similarly alarming.[5] Guidelines recommend maintaining ICP at <22 mmHg and CPP at >60 mmHg, though many hospitals still use an ICP of 20 mmHg as a threshold. Physical exam findings of elevated ICP include a decrease in motor GCS of >2, loss of pupillary reactivity, pupillary asymmetry of >2 mm, new focal motor deficit, or herniation syndrome. The classic Cushing's triad of hypertension, bradycardia, and irregular respirations is a late finding. These signs should prompt empiric treatment of raised ICP and repeat neuroimaging even if there is no ICP monitor in place.[6,7]

Indications for ICP monitoring per guidelines are necessarily broad. ICP should be monitored in all salvageable patients with sTBI and an abnormal head CT that appears causal for the presenting clinical exam findings.[1] An abnormal head CT includes findings such as hematomas, contusions, edema, compressed basal cistern, or herniation. In a normal head CT such as that seen in diffuse axonal injury, ICP monitoring is indicated if there is posturing or systolic blood pressure (SBP) of <90 mmHg.[1] As emergency physicians, we should also be mindful of other conditions that may cause a confounding neurologic exam. Drug overdose, especially with baclofen and other sedative-hypnotics, sepsis, seizures, and stroke may all masquerade as sTBI.

In order to optimize care of the brain-injured patient, consensus guidelines describe a tiered approach to the management of intracranial hypertension and herniation (Figure 21.1).[1,8,9] The tier system is graded from tier 0 (in which fundamental care for TBI is recommended) all the way to tier 4 (in which the most aggressive treatment of TBI is recommended). As most sTBI patients do not present to level 1 trauma centers, it is important

Tiers of ICP Treatment

TIER 0

• ICU Admit	• Avoid Fever	• Sedation to Prevent agitation	• Hgb >7
• Manage Airway	• Avoid IJ Acces	• O₂>94%	• Avoid hyponatremia
• HOB 30–45°C	• Place arterial line	• ETCo₂ Monitoring	• Serial Neurologic Exams
• Analgesia	• Prevent Seizures	• Keep Head Midline	

TIER 1

• CPP goal 60–70	• PaCO₂ 35–38	• EVD placement
• Increase analgesia	• Mannitol bolus (0.5–1g/kg)	• Drain CSF
• Increase sedation	• 3% Hypertonic Saline	• EEG monitoring

TIER 2

• PaCO₂ 32–35
• Paralysis
• Vasopressors, or bolus to raise CPP and lower ICP

TIER 3

• Barbital coma titrated to ICP
• Decompressive craniectomy
• Mild hypothermia (35–36°C)

FIGURE 21.1 Tiers of ICP treatment

to know the capabilities and limitations of the system so that appropriate care may be rapidly delivered. In some instances, a crucial intervention may be to transfer a patient to a tertiary-care center to expedite surgical interventions for these critically ill patients.

The tiered system begins at tier 0 and describes care that should be fundamental to all sTBI patients at any institution or level of care. Tier 0 treatments for intracranial hypertension and herniation include general clinical management. These are basic interventions such as elevating the head of bed to >30 degrees, keeping the head midline to facilitate cerebral venous drainage, and preventing fever. Seizure prophylaxis is recommended in patients with a GCS of <10, cortical contusion, depressed skull fracture, subdural hematoma, epidural hematoma, intracerebral hematoma, penetrating head wound, and seizure within 24 hours of injury.[10] While phenytoin has been the most studied, levetiracetam is an increasingly acceptable alternative given the ease of dosing and the absence of therapeutic drug monitoring.[11] Other tier 0 fundamentals include maintaining CPP at >60 mmHg in patients with ICP monitoring, hemoglobin >7 g/dL, and SpO$_2$ >94%. To avoid hypoxia, hypercapnia, or elevated ICP with multiple laryngoscopy attempts, the most experienced operator should intubate these patients.[4] Additionally, since hypotension, even in short episodes of <10 minutes, can result in increased mortality, guidelines recommend maintaining MAP at >80 mmHg and SBP at >100 mmHg, while not allowing the SBP to decrease to <90 mmHg in those 15 to 69 years old and 110 mmHg in patients >70 years.[1,4]

If the ICP is still elevated despite general clinical care and optimal physiologic parameters, tier 1 principles can be applied. Hyperosmolar therapy with either mannitol (0.5–1 g/kg) or hypertonic saline (2.5–5 mL/kg of 3% solution) can be given as an IV bolus via reliable peripheral lines. Hypertonic saline (HTS) concentrations >3% should be given via central or intraosseous access. Neither mannitol nor HTS has been shown to be superior; thus, the clinician should guide drug choice based on the patient's volume status, sodium concentration, and renal function. In addition, analgesia and sedation should be optimized. If an external ventricular drain (EVD) has been placed for ICP monitoring, CSF drainage can be considered. Hyperventilation to a PaCO$_2$ of 30 to 35 mmHg can be used as a temporary measure while definitive treatment is provided. However, prolonged hyperventilation of <25 mmHg is not recommended due to the risk of ischemia from cerebral vasoconstriction.

When ICP remains elevated after tier 1 interventions, tier 2 treatments can be initiated. Additional hyperosmolar therapies can be given, though a therapeutic ceiling is reached at a serum osmolarity of 320 mOsm/kg or an osmolar gap of 15 to 20 mOsm/kg for mannitol, and serum sodium of 155 mmol/L for HTS. Sedation with propofol can be increased to reduce cerebral metabolic demand and thereby lower ICP. Care must be taken to maintain CPP at >60 mmHg, which may require IV fluid boluses, vasopressors, or inotropes depending on the patient's underlying cardiac function. Neuromuscular paralysis may also be considered in a patient who is adequately sedated.

Finally, if ICP continues to remain elevated, surgical decompression may be considered. Decompressive craniectomy (DC) is the temporary removal of a large portion of the calvarium to allow expansion of the injured and edematous brain. Two major clinical trials on DC for the treatment of refractory intracranial hypertension, DECRA and RESCUEicp, found that DC after failed tier 2 interventions reduced 6-month mortality compared to medical management alone.[12,13] However, early or prophylactic DC is not recommended. Moderate hypothermia to 32°C to 34°C and barbiturate coma are additional tier 3 interventions. Whereas smaller EDs may not be comfortable using barbiturates or have access to neurosurgeons, most should feel comfortable with hypothermia. Cooling is an easy and high-yield intervention that can be done in the most rural of care centers. It should be emphasized that barbiturate coma should only be used concurrent with continuous EEG monitoring at centers with experience in this treatment. This last tier of treatment offers effective rescue therapies, but they are associated with a significant risk of adverse effects.

Corticosteroids are no longer recommended in initial management of TBI due to the increased risk of death demonstrated by the CRASH trial.[14] The application of cervical collars, while nearly universal in the management of trauma, should be done with caution in the sTBI patient. Rigid cervical collars, especially when poorly fitted, can obstruct cerebral venous outflow and cause an increase in ICP.[15] Fluid resuscitation should also be performed judiciously. Normal saline is the IV fluid of choice in sTBI patients given its isotonicity. HTS may be used both for volume resuscitation and treatment of intracranial hypertension. Albumin should not be used in the resuscitation of sTBI patients as it was associated with higher mortality than the use of normal saline.[16]

As exemplified in the case presented, sTBI can be associated with systemic complications. Acute respiratory distress syndrome (ARDS) occurs in up to 30% of sTBI cases.[17] This may be due to aspiration, catecholamine surge, or systemic inflammation. ARDS significantly complicates the management of sTBI patients since permissive hypercapnia and a lower PaO_2 target may not be tolerated. While an in-depth discussion of ventilator management in sTBI is beyond the scope of this chapter, a balance between brain and lung protection is important to maintain. Strategies such as low-tidal-volume ventilation with 6 to 8 mL/kg and the use of positive end-expiratory pressure should be applied cautiously while monitoring ICP and CPP to observe the effects of $PaCO_2$ and intrathoracic pressure on cerebral physiology.[18] If advanced neuromonitoring such as brain tissue oxygenation is available, this allows direct monitoring for cerebral hypoxia. In cases where traditional ventilation strategies fail, extracorporeal membrane oxygenation (ECMO) can be considered. The tradeoff in improved oxygenation and ventilation with ECMO comes at the cost of potential bleeding associated with the use of anticoagulation with cannulation and maintenance of the circuit as well as platelet dysfunction and depletion. Patient selection for this treatment strategy is vital for the success of its implementation.

Concluding the case, the patient was found to have a non-displaced basilar skull fracture and diffuse cerebral edema with effacement of the ventricles on head CT. No other traumatic injuries were found in his evaluation. Given his sTBI with radiographic evidence of intracranial hypertension, the head of the patient's bed was elevated, he was loaded with levetiracetam for seizure prophylaxis, and his oxygenation was optimized. Neurosurgery was consulted and an EVD was placed for ICP monitoring. While waiting for admission to the ICU, the patient developed worsening hypoxia with bilateral infiltrates on chest x-ray. Despite appropriate ventilator management including low tidal volumes, PEEP optimization, and FiO_2 of 100%, the patient had desaturations to SpO_2 <70% for prolonged periods. The decision was made to cannulate the patient for ECMO emergently. The patient also had severely elevated ICP, which was managed with tiered medical treatments, but he did not require DC. Ultimately, he was decannulated, liberated from the ICU, and discharged to a neurorehabilitation facility awake and interactive.

KEY POINTS TO REMEMBER

- A key focus in the management of sTBI is the prevention of secondary injuries.
- Hypotension, hypoxia, and hypocapnia can all worsen outcomes after sTBI due to impaired cerebral autoregulation and the effect of PaO_2 and $PaCO_2$ on cerebral blood flow.
- Cushing's triad of hypertension, bradycardia, and irregular respirations is a late finding in intracranial hypertension and cerebral herniation.
- Management of intracranial hypertension and herniation should follow a tiered approach, starting with basic interventions such as elevating the head of the bed and keeping the head midline to facilitate cerebral venous drainage.
- Treatment of raised ICP includes optimizing physiologic parameters, hyperosmolar agents, CSF drainage, analgesia, sedation, and surgical decompression.
- Hyperventilation, while an effective treatment of elevated ICP, should only be used as a temporary measure until definitive treatment can be given due to the risk of cerebral ischemia.
- Early transfer to a higher level of care with neurosurgical capability is critical to patient outcome.

References

1. Carney N, Totten AM, O'Reilly C, et al. Guidelines for the management of severe traumatic brain injury, fourth edition. *Neurosurgery*. 2017;80(1):6–15.
2. Centers for Disease Control and Prevention. TBI data and statistics. Updated March 29, 2019. Accessed February 1, 2021. https://www.cdc.gov/traumaticbrai njury/data/
3. Daugherty J, Waltzman D, Sarmiento K, Xu L. Traumatic brain injury-related deaths by race/ethnicity, sex, intent, and mechanism of injury—United States, 2000–2017. *MMWR Morb Mortal Wkly Rep*. 2019;68:1050–1056.
4. Shriki J, Galvagno SM. Sedation for rapid sequence induction and intubation of neurologically injured patients. *Emerg Med Clin North Am*. 2021;39(1):203–216.

5. Vik A, Nag T, Fredriksli OA, et al. Relationship of "dose" of intracranial hypertension to outcome in severe traumatic brain injury. *J Neurosurg.* 2008;109(4):678–684.

6. Chesnut RM, Temkin N, Carney N, et al. A trial of intracranial-pressure monitoring in traumatic brain injury. *N Engl J Med.* 2012;367(26):2471–2481.

7. Chesnut RM, Temkin N, Dikmen S, et al. A method of managing severe traumatic brain injury in the absence of intracranial pressure monitoring: The imaging and clinical examination protocol. *J Neurotrauma.* 2018;35(1):54–63.

8. Hawryluk GWJ, Aguilera S, Buki A, et al. A management algorithm for patients with intracranial pressure monitoring: The Seattle International Severe Traumatic Brain Injury Consensus Conference (SIBICC). *Intensive Care Med.* 2019;45(12):1783–1794.

9. Cadena R, Shoykhet M, Ratcliff JJ. Emergency neurological life support: Intracranial hypertension and herniation. *Neurocrit Care.* 2017;27(Suppl 1):82–88.

10. Brain Trauma Foundation, American Association of Neurological Surgeons, Congress of Neurological Surgeons. Guidelines for the management of severe traumatic brain injury. *J Neurotrauma.* 2007;24(Suppl 1):S1–S106.

11. Khan NR, VanLandingham MA, Fierst TM, et al. Should levetiracetam or phenytoin be used for posttraumatic seizure prophylaxis? A systematic review of the literature and meta-analysis. *Neurosurgery.* 2016;79(6):775–782.

12. Cooper DJ, Rosenfeld JV, Murray L, et al. Decompressive craniectomy in diffuse traumatic brain injury. *N Engl J Med.* 2011;364(16):1493–1502.

13. Hutchinson PJ, Kolias AG, Timofeev IS, et al. Trial of decompressive craniectomy for traumatic intracranial hypertension. *N Engl J Med.* 2016;375(12):1119–1130.

14. Roberts I, Yates D, Sandercock P, et al. Effect of intravenous corticosteroids on death within 14 days in 10008 adults with clinically significant head injury (MRC CRASH Trial): Randomised placebo-controlled trial. *Lancet.* 2004;364(9442):1321–1328.

15. Núñez-Patiño RA, Rubiano AM, Godoy DA. Impact of cervical collars on intracranial pressure values in traumatic brain injury: A systematic review and meta-analysis of prospective studies. *Neurocrit Care.* 2020;32(2):469–477.

16. SAFE Study Investigators, Australian and New Zealand Intensive Care Society Clinical Trials Group, Australian Red Cross Blood Service, et al. Saline or albumin for fluid resuscitation in patients with traumatic brain injury. *N Engl J Med.* 2007;357(9):874–884.

17. Hendrickson CM, Howard BM, Kornblith LZ, et al. The acute respiratory distress syndrome following isolated severe traumatic brain injury. *J Trauma Acute Care Surg.* 2016;80(6):989–997.

18. Boone MD, Jinadasa SP, Mueller A, et al. The effect of positive end-expiratory pressure on intracranial pressure and cerebral hemodynamics. *Neurocrit Care.* 2017;26(2):174–181.

Further reading

Cadena R, Shoykhet M, Ratcliff JJ. Emergency neurological life support: Intracranial hypertension and herniation. *Neurocrit Care*. 2017;27(Suppl 1):82–88.

Carney N, Totten AM, O'Reilly C, et al. Guidelines for the management of severe traumatic brain injury, fourth edition. *Neurosurgery*. 2017;80(1):6–15.

Garvin R, Mangat HS. Emergency neurological life support: Traumatic brain injury. *Neurocrit Care*. 2017;27(Suppl 1):159–169.

Hawryluk GWJ, Aguilera S, Buki A, et al. A management algorithm for patients with intracranial pressure monitoring: The Seattle International Severe Traumatic Brain Injury Consensus Conference (SIBICC). *Intensive Care Med*. 2019;45(12):1783–1794.

Shriki J, Galvagno SM. Sedation for rapid sequence induction and intubation of neurologically injured patients. *Emerg Med Clin North Am*. 2021;39(1):203–216.

22 Brain plumbing problems: Ischemic versus hemorrhagic strokes

Skyler Lentz and Evie Marcolini

EMS calls in with this report: "We are coming in with a 45-year-old male patient who was working out at the gym and suddenly had right-sided weakness and slurred speech. He currently has a FAST-ED score of 3 (1 for facial palsy, 1 for arm drift, and 1 for slurred speech). His blood pressure is 200/110 mmHg, heart rate is 60 per minute, SaO_2 98% on room air. He takes no medication and has no medical history."

What do I do now?

This young patient presents with symptoms of stroke, but the differential is broad, including toxicologic syndrome, seizure, stroke mimics, etc. If the cause is a stroke, the differential still includes ischemic versus hemorrhagic and anterior versus posterior circulation.

The emergency clinician must rapidly intervene for the best possible outcomes (Figure 22.1). The first step in evaluation and management is to obtain an accurate history, neurologic exam, serum glucose level, and a non-contrast head CT to rule out a hemorrhagic stroke. Once diagnosed, potential management options for an ischemic stroke include systemic thrombolysis (e.g., tissue plasminogen activator [tPA], tenecteplase) or referral for neuro-interventional thrombectomy. The patient with a hemorrhagic stroke requires reversal of anticoagulants, BP management, and consideration of neurosurgical intervention. Given lack of bed availability and the challenges of rural health, emergency clinicians must also be familiar with the care of ischemic and hemorrhagic stroke patients beyond the first few hours in care if there are delays in transfer.

INITIAL EVALUATION, PRESENTATION, AND MANAGEMENT

During the initial evaluation the emergency physician must determine the time the patient was last seen to be at his or her baseline (i.e., last known well), obtain vital signs, perform a neurologic exam, and obtain a point-of-care blood glucose measurement. This patient's National Institutes of Health Stroke Scale (NIHSS) score is 7 (2 for facial palsy, 1 for right upper extremity drift, 1 for right lower extremity drift, 1 for right lower extremity ataxia, 1 for aphasia, and 1 for dysarthria). The NIHSS (Table 22.1) serves as a useful tool in determining severity and management options and allows consistency in communicating exam findings with the consulting neurology team.[1] However, it should be noted that this tool will not necessarily help in diagnosing a stroke in the posterior circulation.

A non-contrast head CT is the first step to determine whether the patient has evidence of hemorrhage. This patient's non-contrast CT had no evidence of hemorrhage, so we are left with (anterior or posterior) ischemic stroke or a stroke mimic. Ischemic stroke mimics (e.g., complex migraine, conversion disorder, Todd's paralysis) are common and may represent as many as one third of cases. Factors associated with a mimic include a young

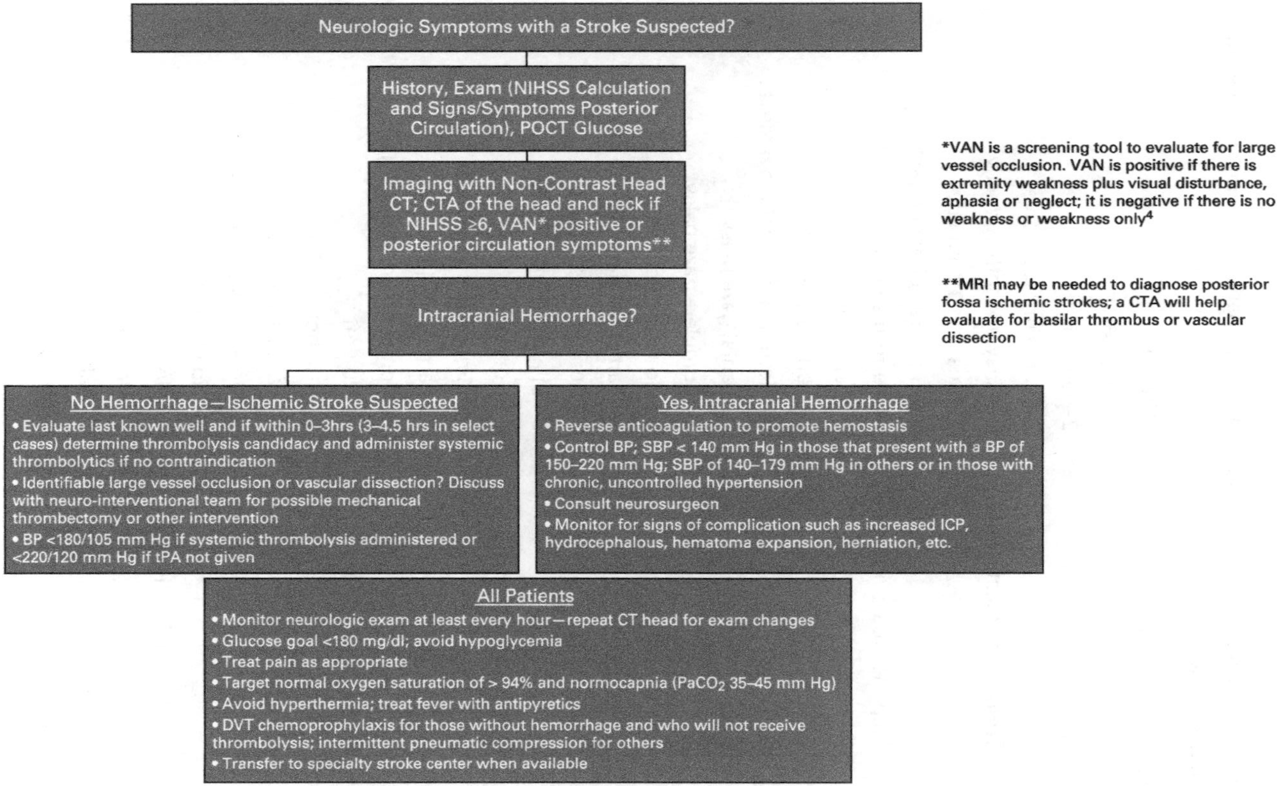

Neurologic Symptoms with a Stroke Suspected?

History, Exam (NIHSS Calculation and Signs/Symptoms Posterior Circulation), POCT Glucose

Imaging with Non-Contrast Head CT; CTA of the head and neck if NIHSS ≥6, VAN* positive or posterior circulation symptoms**

Intracranial Hemorrhage?

Yes: Intracranial Hemorrhage
- Reverse anticoagulation to promote hemostasis
- Control BP; SBP < 140 mm Hg in those that present with a BP of 150–220 mm Hg; SBP of 140–179 mm Hg in others or in those with chronic, uncontrolled hypertension
- Consult neurosurgeon
- Monitor for signs of complication such as increased ICP, hydrocephalous, hematoma expansion, herniation, etc.

<u>No Hemorrhage—Ischemic Stroke Suspected</u>
- Evaluate last known well and if within 0–3hrs (3–4.5 hrs in select cases) determine thrombolysis candidacy and administer systemic thrombolytics if no contraindication
- Identifiable large vessel occlusion or vascular dissection? Discuss with neuro-interventional team for possible mechanical thrombectomy or other intervention
- BP <180/105 mm Hg if systemic thrombolysis administered or <220/120 mm Hg if tPA not given

<u>All Patients</u>
- Monitor neurologic exam at least every hour—repeat CT head for exam changes
- Glucose goal <180 mg/dl; avoid hypoglycemia
- Treat pain as appropriate
- Target normal oxygen saturation of > 94% and normocapnia (PaCO₂ 35–45 mm Hg)
- Avoid hyperthermia; treat fever with antipyretics
- DVT chemoprophylaxis for those without hemorrhage and who will not receive thrombolysis; intermittent pneumatic compression for others
- Transfer to specialty stroke center when available

*VAN is a screening tool to evaluate for large vessel occlusion. VAN is positive if there is extremity weakness plus visual disturbance, aphasia or neglect; it is negative if there is no weakness or weakness only[4]

**MRI may be needed to diagnose posterior fossa ischemic strokes; a CTA will help evaluate for basilar thrombus or vascular dissection

FIGURE 22.1 The recommended approach to a patient with neurologic symptoms and a possible stroke

TABLE 22.1 **National Institutes of Health Stroke Scale (NIHSS)**

This is the recommended neurologic exam for patients having a suspected ischemic stroke.[1]

1A	Level of consciousness	0—Alert
		1—Drowsy
		2—Obtunded
		3—Coma/unresponsive
1B	Orientation questions (2)	0—Answers both correctly
		1—Answers 1 correctly
		2—Answers neither correctly
1C	Response to commands (2)	0—Performs both tasks correctly
		1—Performs 1 task correctly
		2—Performs neither
2	Gaze	0—Normal horizontal movements
		1—Partial gaze palsy
		2—Complete gaze palsy
3	Visual fields	0—No visual field defect
		1—Partial hemianopia
		2—Complete hemianopia
		3—Bilateral hemianopia
4	Facial movement	0—Normal
		1—Minor facial weakness
		2—Partial facial weakness
		3—Complete unilateral palsy
5	Motor function (arm)	0—No drift
	a. Left	1—Drift before 10 s
	b. Right	2—Falls before 10 s
		3—No effort against gravity
		4—No movement
6	Motor function (leg)	0—No drift
	a. Left	1—Drift before 5 s
	b. Right	2—Falls before 5 s
		3—No effort against gravity
		4—No movement

TABLE 22.1 **Continued**

7	Limb ataxia	0—No ataxia
		1—Ataxia in 1 limb
		2—Ataxia in 2 limbs
8	Sensory	0—No sensory loss
		1—Mild sensory loss
		2—Severe sensory loss
9	Language	0—Normal
		1—Mild aphasia
		2—Severe aphasia
		3—Mute or global aphasia
10	Articulation	0—Normal
		1—Mild dysarthria
		2—Severe dysarthria
11	Extinction or inattention	0—Absent
		1—Mild loss (1 sensory modality lost)
		2—Severe loss (2 modalities lost)

age, mild symptoms, and lack of cardiovascular risk factors.[2] Our patient's labs return, showing no evidence of toxicologic or metabolic abnormality, and the remainder of his labs are equally reassuring. The fingerstick glucose is 110; sodium and all other electrolytes are normal. If there is no alternative diagnosis found by history and exam, hemorrhage has been ruled out by imaging, and hypoglycemia has been ruled out by a point-of-care glucose (glucose is the only lab test required prior to thrombolytics), then an ischemic stroke is clinically suspected. Systemic thrombolysis is recommended if the onset of symptoms is confirmed within 3 to 4.5 hours and there is no contraindication. Further candidacy and contraindication questions for thrombolytics (Box 22.1) should be elicited—a checklist for contraindications is recommended. Common absolute contraindications include active hemorrhage, known bleeding diathesis, acute or prior intracranial hemorrhage, and uncontrolled hypertension (>180 mmHg SBP/>110 mmHg DBP). In specific select cases (i.e., those ≤80 years old, NIHSS score ≤25, without imaging findings of more than one-third middle cerebral artery (MCA) territory ischemia, and without a history of both

Most common absolute and relative contraindications to IV thrombolytics

Absolute thrombolytic contraindications

Onset of symptoms outside the recommended time window of 3–4.5 hours

Acute intracranial hemorrhage or prior intracranial hemorrhage

CT findings of extensive hypoattenuation suggesting widespread ischemic injury

Ischemic stroke within 3 months

Severe head trauma within 3 months

Acute head trauma

Intracranial intra-axial neoplasm

Intracranial or intraspinal surgery within 3 months

Subarachnoid hemorrhage or suggestive symptoms

GI bleeding within 21 days or known GI malignancy

Coagulopathy (platelets <100,000/mm^3; INR >1.7; aPTT >40 s; PT >15 s; treatment dose low-molecular-weight heparin within 24 hours; direct thrombin inhibitor or direct factor Xa inhibitor use within prior 48 hours)

Suspected infective endocarditis or septic emboli

Confirmed or suspected aortic dissection

BP uncontrolled >185/110 mmHg

Relative thrombolytic contraindications

Preexisting disability, dementia, or systemic malignancy with poor prognosis should be considered in individual cases.

Lumbar puncture within 7 days

Seizure at onset (unless deficits felt to be from ischemic stroke rather than the postictal state)

Arterial puncture within 7 days

Major trauma or major surgery within the last 14 days

Menstruation with a history of menorrhagia

Small intracranial aneurysm (<10 mm)

Intracranial arterial dissection

Intracranial vascular malformations

Extra-axial intra cranial neoplasm (e.g., meningioma)

Pregnancy

Acute pericarditis with only mild disability from ischemic stroke

The treatment decision should be made on an individual basis if relative contraindications are present.[1]

diabetes and prior stroke), the thrombolysis window can be extended to 4.5 hours.[1] Those beyond the thrombolysis time window may still be considered for mechanical thrombectomy.

Posterior circulation stroke may present with nonspecific signs and symptoms, including depressed global mental status or somnolence. It is important to look for evidence of a basilar artery hyperdensity on the non-contrast head CT while keeping in mind that the posterior circulation territory is not adequately viewed with this imaging modality.[3] History and exam findings may help guide further imaging. If the patient has posterior signs or symptoms of dizziness or vertigo, unilateral limb weakness, dysarthria, headache, fluctuating neurologic symptoms, ataxia, dysarthria, nystagmus, oculomotor abnormalities, tetraparesis, decreased level of consciousness, etc., then it is prudent to image appropriately. One rule of thumb is that if the neurologic exam does not match the imaging, we need to go a step further to evaluate—this will be with a CT angiogram (CTA) or MRI, if available, to evaluate for a basilar artery thrombosis or posterior circulation infarct.

Vascular imaging can evaluate for a large vessel occlusion (LVO), vascular dissection, or severe carotid stenosis. One method of determining whether to obtain an immediate CTA (at the time of the non-contrast CT) is the Vision, Aphasia, Neglect (VAN) stroke assessment tool (Table 22.2).[4] An NIHSS score of ≥6 is also associated with an LVO with 87% sensitivity and 52% specificity, but the VAN tool is more specific.[5] The FAST-ED score (Facial Palsy, Arm Weakness, Speech Changes, Time, Eye Deviation, and Denial/Neglect) can be used to triage the risk of LVO in the field; those with higher scores are more likely to have an LVO.[6] These assessment tools or the NIHSS will determine the likelihood of an LVO and guide more efficient management by obtaining vascular imaging, neuro-interventional resources, and transfer of the patient sooner.

In general, mechanical thrombectomy should be considered if the patient had a near-normal functional status preceding the event, an occlusion of the internal carotid or proximal M1 segment of the MCA, an NIHSS score of ≥6, an ASPECTS (Alberta Stroke Program Early CT Score) of ≥6, and age >18 years, and a thrombectomy can be performed within 6 hours of symptom onset.[1] ASPECTS scoring utilizes non-contrast head CT imaging to determine the likelihood of early MCA territory ischemic

TABLE 22.2 **The VAN stroke assessment tool and the FAST-ED score**

VAN	Finding	FAST-ED Score	Points
Weakness: Raise both arms?	**No weakness** (VAN screen negative) **Mild** (minor drift) **Moderate** (severe drift, touches or nearly touches the ground **Severe** (flaccid)	**Facial Palsy** Normal or minor paralysis Partial or complete paralysis	0 1
Visual Disturbance	**Field Cut** (test 4 quadrants) **Double Vision** (evaluate for uneven or abnormal extraocular movements) **New Blindness None**	**Arm Weakness** No drift Drift or some effort against gravity No effort against gravity or no movement	0 1 2
Aphasia	**Expressive** (unable to speak or unable to repeat or name two objects) **Receptive** (not understanding or not following commands) **Mixed None**	**Speech Changes** Absent Mild to moderate Severe, global aphasia or mute	0 1 2
Neglect	**Forced gaze or inability to track one side** **Unable to feel both sides at the same time or unable to identify own arm Ignoring one side None**	**Eye Deviation** Absent Partial Forced deviation	0 1 2

TABLE 22.2 **Continued**

VAN	Finding	FAST-ED Score	Points
		Denial/Neglect	
		Absent	0
		Extinction to bilateral, simultaneous sensory stimulation	1
		Does not recognize own hand or orients only to one side of the body	2

These tools can be used to assess the likelihood of an LVO and the need for initial vascular imaging or triage of neuro-interventional resources.

VAN is positive if there is weakness plus either a visual disturbance, aphasia, or neglect. Screening has been found to be 100% sensitive and 90% specific for LVO.[4] Patients who are VAN negative with posterior circulation symptoms may still require CTA to evaluate for a basilar thrombus.

FAST-ED shows a higher likelihood of LVO with an increasing score: 0 or 1, <15%; 2 or 3, 30%, and ≥4, 60% or higher likelihood of LVO.[6]

From references 4 and 6.

changes—a lower score predicts a poorer functional outcome (http://www.aspectsinstroke.com/).[7] The 6-hour thrombectomy window may be extended to 24 hours depending on local protocols and patient characteristics.[8] The thrombectomy window is also extended for those with a basilar artery occlusion due to the poor prognosis—every single case of a basilar artery occlusion should be discussed urgently with the consulting stroke and neuro-interventional team.

Per the VAN stroke assessment, our patient has drift and aphasia, so he gets a CTA at the same time of his non-contrast CT. It shows evidence of a left, MCA proximal M1 segment occlusion.

FIRST HOURS OF MANAGEMENT

Ischemic stroke

We are at a small ED and our patient has an acute ischemic stroke of the left MCA territory with an occlusion of the proximal M1 segment (proximal horizontal branch of the MCA). He has no contraindication to thrombolysis, which is recommended since his last known well time is within 3 hrs. The proximal M1 occlusion also makes him a candidate for thrombectomy.[1] If he was outside the thrombolysis window (3 or 4.5 hours), he may still be a candidate for thrombectomy typically within 6 hours but potentially up to 24 hours in special circumstances.

Urgent transfer for neuro-interventional capabilities is the next step, but this resource may not be available to everyone. While awaiting transfer—or if a blizzard prevents transfer—we must be ready to manage this patient with an acute ischemic stroke beyond the acute presentation (Table 22.3). His BP is significantly elevated, especially for a young healthy man. This likely represents the brain's innate attempt to perfuse the ischemic penumbra by elevating pressure, thus encouraging collateral circulation. In this case, we have a fine balancing act. Understanding that perfusion is key to the ischemic component of this stroke, we will lower the pressure gently and by no more than 15% to 20%. The guidelines

TABLE 22.3 **Extended and initial care considerations**

Glucose	Goal <180 mg/dL Hyperglycemia and hypoglycemia are associated with worse outcomes after stroke.
BP	**Ischemic stroke** <180/105 mmHg if systemic thrombolysis given <220/120 mmHg if systemic thrombolysis not given **ICH** SBP <140 mmHg in those who present with a BP of 150–220 mmHg SBP target of 140–179 mmHg reasonable in those with >220 mmHg on arrival or preceding untreated hypertension
Repeat imaging	For any exam changes or severe symptoms and 24 hours after thrombolysis
Prophylaxis of deep venous thrombosis	Use intermittent pneumatic compression devices (if available). Hold chemoprophylaxis (e.g., heparin, enoxaparin) if a thrombolytic is given or if ICH. Chemoprophylaxis may be used in those with an ischemic stroke without hemorrhage who have not received a thrombolytic.

TABLE 22.3 **Continued**

Cerebral or cerebellar edema	A large MCA territory stroke may lead to malignant cerebral edema and herniation in the first 72 hours. Surgical decompressive craniectomy is an option in select cases. Osmotic therapy (mannitol or hypertonic saline) may be considered as a temporizing treatment. A large cerebellar infarct may cause edema, obstructive hydrocephalus, and herniation; possible interventions include ventriculostomy and/or craniectomy.
Neurologic checks	Should be performed every hour
Hyperthermia	Evaluate for source and control the temperature with antipyretic therapy.
Respiratory support	Patients unable to protect their airway should be intubated. Once intubated, the goal should be a normal oxygen saturation of >94% and normocapnia with a $PaCO_2$ of 35–45 mmHg.

From references 1 and 11.

recommend BP <180/105 mmHg in cases where thrombolysis is given. If thrombolysis is not given, then the BP is permitted to be higher for the first 24 hours, up to <220/120 mmHg.[1] The first consideration to reduce BP is to treat pain or anxiety. Analgesia is a gentle way of reducing BP, as well as a small dose of a benzodiazepine if needed. Using a directed antihypertensive agent may lower BP excessively (especially in a young, otherwise medication-naive patient) and may risk extension of the ischemic area or transformation to infarction. If the systolic pressure persists after analgesia/anxiolytic, then a titratable agent such as nicardipine, labetalol, or clevidipine is preferred. Avoiding vasodilating agents such as nitroprusside or nitroglycerin is recommended so as to not precipitate an increase in intracranial pressure (ICP).

The importance of repeat neurologic exams cannot be overstated in this patient. Because he has received thrombolysis, there is a risk of hemorrhagic conversion of the ischemic/infarcted parenchyma—greater if the ischemic territory is larger. Our neurologic exam is the best immediate method of following the patient; any exam change warrants a repeat non-contrast head CT. The progression of this patient's stroke may also have implications for his candidacy for mechanical thrombectomy once he is at the tertiary-care center with interventional capacity. Glucose levels should be followed closely, as glucose is the brain's most important nutrient in the acute phase. IV hydration will help mitigate hemodynamic lability.

A rarer cause of an ischemic stroke is a cerebrovascular dissection. Now consider if our patient had radiologic evidence of a cervical artery dissection (i.e., carotid or vertebral) as well as clinical evidence of an acute ischemic stroke. A dissection is a separation of the layers of the vessel wall, causing arterial lumen narrowing and potentially resulting in thrombotic occlusion and subsequent downstream embolization. The first priority for this type of stroke is to treat with heparin or an antiplatelet agent to prevent further propagation of thrombus and/or embolization with ischemic consequence.[1,9] The definitive treatment for this is dependent on many factors—complete versus partial occlusion, age of occlusion (determined roughly by timing of symptoms), severity of ischemic (or infarcted) area, and the patient's preexisting risk factors. Neuro-interventional consultation is key and will determine the next course of action, which may be stenting, ligation, or observation. In the meantime, heparinization or antiplatelet therapy is the accepted standard of care, although some will opt for initial thrombolysis if the patient is within the time window and there are no contraindications. BP management for a patient with vascular dissection is the same as for one with ischemic stroke; this entails a fine balancing act between allowing enough pressure to perfuse, but minimizing the risk of further dissection or hemorrhage.

Hemorrhagic stroke

Now consider now if our patient had a spontaneous intracerebral hemorrhage (ICH) on his initial head CT. An ICH portends a high risk of morbidity and mortality and presents very similarly to an ischemic stroke. The most common cause is uncontrolled hypertension; other causes include vascular malformations and cerebral amyloid angiopathy.[10] The brain injury is caused by the mass effect of the hemorrhage and the increase in ICP. In addition to airway and breathing assessment, a patient with spontaneous hemorrhage requires BP control, neurologic checks for deterioration, and reversal and avoidance of anticoagulant medications to promote hemostasis.

The ideal BP target is debatable, but the American Heart Association/ American Stroke Association guidelines suggest that acute lowering of the SBP to <140 mmHg is reasonable in patients who present with a BP of 150 to 220 mmHg.[11] It is less clear in those who present with an SBP of >220 mmHg, but a similar target of <140 is reasonable according to the guidelines. However, aggressive control risks cerebral ischemia, and a more liberal SBP target of 140 to 179 mmHg in those presenting with very high BP (i.e., >220 mmHg) or who have known preceding untreated hypertension should be considered.[12]

Correction of coagulopathy is important to aid in hemostasis. For those taking vitamin K antagonists (i.e., warfarin), four-factor prothrombin complex concentrate (PCC) is recommended along with 5 to 10 mg IV vitamin K.[11,13] Xa inhibitors (e.g., rivaroxaban, apixaban) should be treated with four- factor PCC or andexanet—the superiority of andexanet over four-factor PCC is unknown.[14,15] The direct thrombin inhibitor dabigatran has a specific reversal agent, idarucizumab.[13] Platelets should be considered in those with thrombocytopenia or those who will be undergoing a neurosurgical procedure such as ventriculostomy or craniotomy, but a platelet transfusion is not routinely recommended in those taking antiplatelet therapy.[16]

Patients with an ICH should have hourly neurologic checks with repeat imaging for neurologic changes. They are at risk for deterioration from hydrocephalus, increases in ICP, herniation, and hematoma expansion. Neurosurgical intervention with an external ventricular drain may be indicated for those with evidence of increased ICP, intraventricular hemorrhage, transtentorial herniation, a deteriorating neurologic exam, or hydrocephalus.[11] Those with a cerebellar hemorrhage are at high risk for deterioration from obstructive hydrocephalus and brainstem compression and should be considered for surgical decompression.[11] Surgical evacuation of a supratentorial cerebral hemorrhage is controversial and should be decided on a case-by-case basis with a neurosurgical consultation either in person (if available) or remotely. Those with signs of complication or cerebellar hemorrhage should be transferred urgently to a neurosurgical center. Mannitol or hypertonic saline may be considered as a temporizing agent for signs of edema, increased ICP, or herniation.

With ischemic and hemorrhagic strokes, the emergency clinician must rapidly intervene for the best possible patient outcomes. Given lack of bed availability and the challenges of rural health, emergency clinicians must also be familiar with "what's next" in the care of ischemic and hemorrhagic stroke patients beyond the first few hours in care. A recommended approach is shown in Figure 22.1 and considerations for extended care are listed in Table 22.3.

References

1. Powers WJ, Rabinstein AA, Ackerson T, et al. Guidelines for the early management of patients with acute ischemic stroke: 2019 update to the 2018 guidelines for the early management of acute ischemic stroke: A guideline for healthcare professionals from the American Heart Association/American Stroke Association. *Stroke.* 2019;50(12):e344–e418. doi:10.1161/STR.0000000000000211

2. Merino JG, Luby M, Benson RT, et al. Predictors of acute stroke mimics in 8187 patients referred to a stroke service. *J Stroke Cerebrovasc Dis.* 2013;22(8):e397–e403. doi:10.1016/j.jstrokecerebrovasdis.2013.04.018

3. Asimos AW, Sassano DR, Jackson SC, et al. Assessment of vessel density on non-contrast computed tomography to detect basilar artery occlusion. *West J Emerg Med.* 2020;21(3):694–702. doi:10.5811/westjem.2019.12.45247

4. Teleb MS, Ver Hage A, Carter J, Jayaraman MV, McTaggart RA. Stroke vision, aphasia, neglect (VAN) assessment—a novel emergent large vessel occlusion screening tool: Pilot study and comparison with current clinical severity indices. *J Neurointervent Surg.* 2017;9(2):122–126. doi:10.1136/neurintsurg-2015-012131

5. Smith EE, Kent DM, Bulsara KR, et al. Accuracy of prediction instruments for diagnosing large vessel occlusion in individuals with suspected stroke: A systematic review for the 2018 guidelines for the early management of patients with acute ischemic stroke. *Stroke.* 2018;49(3):e111–e122. doi:10.1161/STR.0000000000000160

6. Lima FO, Silva GS, Furie KL, et al. The Field Assessment Stroke Triage for Emergency Destination (FAST-ED): A simple and accurate pre-hospital scale to detect large vessel occlusion strokes. *Stroke.* 2016;47(8):1997–2002. doi:10.1161/STROKEAHA.116.013301

7. Pexman JHW, Barber PA, Hill MD, et al. Use of the Alberta Stroke Program Early CT Score (ASPECTS) for assessing CT scans in patients with acute stroke. *Am J Neuroradiol.* 2001;22(8):1534–1542.

8. Nogueira RG, Jadhav AP, Haussen DC, et al. Thrombectomy 6 to 24 hours after stroke with a mismatch between deficit and infarct. *N Engl J Med.* 2018;378(1):11–21. doi:10.1056/NEJMoa1706442

9. Markus HS, Levi C, King A, Madigan J, Norris J, Cervical Artery Dissection in Stroke Study (CADISS) investigators. Antiplatelet therapy vs anticoagulation therapy in cervical artery dissection: The Cervical Artery Dissection in Stroke Study (CADISS) randomized clinical trial final results. *JAMA Neurol.* 2019;76(6):657–664. doi:10.1001/jamaneurol.2019.0072

10. Morotti A, Goldstein JN. Diagnosis and management of acute intracerebral hemorrhage. *Emerg Med Clin North Am.* 2016;34(4):883–899. doi:10.1016/j.emc.2016.06.010

11. Hemphill JC, Greenberg SM, Anderson CS, et al. Guidelines for the management of spontaneous intracerebral hemorrhage: A guideline for healthcare professionals from the American Heart Association/American Stroke Association. *Stroke.* 2015;46(7):2032–2060. doi:10.1161/STR.0000000000000069

12. Qureshi AI, Huang W, Lobanova I, et al. Outcomes of intensive systolic blood pressure reduction in patients with intracerebral hemorrhage and excessively high initial systolic blood pressure: Post hoc analysis of a randomized clinical trial. *JAMA Neurology.* 2020;77(11):1355–1365. doi:10.1001/jamaneurol.2020.3075

13. Frontera JA, Lewin III JJ, Rabinstein AA, et al. Guideline for reversal of antithrombotics in intracranial hemorrhage. *Neurocrit Care.* 2016;24(1):6–46. doi:10.1007/s12028-015-0222-x

14. Panos NG, Cook AM, Sayona J, et al. Factor Xa inhibitor-related intracranial hemorrhage. *Circulation.* 2020;141(21):1681–1689. doi:10.1161/CIRCULATIONAHA.120.045769

15. Connolly SJ, Crowther M, Eikelboom JW, et al. Full study report of andexanet alfa for bleeding associated with factor Xa inhibitors. *N Engl J Med.* 2019;380(14):1326–1335. doi:10.1056/NEJMoa1814051

16. Baharoglu MI, Cordonnier C, Salman RA-S, et al. Platelet transfusion versus standard care after acute stroke due to spontaneous cerebral haemorrhage associated with antiplatelet therapy (PATCH): A randomised, open-label, phase 3 trial. *Lancet.* 2016;387(10038):2605–2613. doi:10.1016/S0140-6736(16)30392-0

23 The worst headache of my life: Subarachnoid hemorrhage

Roderick W. Fontenette and

Andrew J. Branting

A 54-year-old female with a past medical history significant for hypertension presents to the ED with a chief complaint of a headache that began 2 hours prior to arrival. She was sitting at her desk at work when she developed a severe, persistent 10/10 headache that reached its maximum intensity almost immediately. She reports previously having headaches but has never been diagnosed with migraine headaches nor has she had a headache this severe before. Nothing makes her headache better or worse. She denies recent trauma. Co-workers denied loss of consciousness or syncope. She endorses neck pain and stiffness with associated nausea and one episode of vomiting. She denies tobacco or illicit drug use. Her BP is 173/94 mmHg, HR is 83 bpm and regular, and she is afebrile. Her neurologic exam is negative for meningismus and cranial nerve or focal sensorimotor deficit. She ambulated to her room without focal gait abnormality, dizziness, or acute visual changes.

What do I do now?

Headache is a common complaint, accounting for 1% to 2% of annual ED visits. Of those suffering from acute headache, ~1% have a spontaneous subarachnoid hemorrhage (SAH), making it relatively rare. Notably, the most common cause of subarachnoid blood is blunt head trauma resulting in traumatic SAH rather than spontaneous aneurysmal SAH. The management of traumatic SAH focuses on avoidance of secondary injury and transfer to a regionalized trauma center—this is not the focus of this chapter.

Aneurysmal rupture is the most common cause of spontaneous SAH, accounting for 80% to 85% of cases, and these aneurysmal SAHs account for 3% to 5% of all strokes. It is estimated that 1 in 50 people in the general population have intracranial aneurysms. Of these individuals, 1 in 5 have more than one, and the annual rate of rupture is ~8 to 10 per 100,000 people.[1] Risk factors for aneurysmal rupture include size (with larger aneurysms being more likely to rupture), multiple aneurysms, aneurysms in the posterior circulation, history of prior aneurysm rupture, substance abuse (cocaine, tobacco, alcohol), hypertension, and family history of SAH; there is a female predominance.

The associated morbidity and mortality of aneurysmal SAH is high, with ~10% to 15% of patients dying prior to reaching the hospital. Of those who do reach the hospital, 50% will not survive to hospital discharge. Up to one-third of survivors remain functionally dependent and 20% have substantial neurocognitive impairment.[2–4] The diagnosis is missed in ~1 in 20 patients who present to the ED with acute SAH, leading to a delay in care that increases mortality to 80%.[5] The most common reason for missed diagnosis is failure to perform non-contrast head CT.[6] This highlights the importance of an appropriate clinical evaluation and a stepwise approach in the diagnosis and management of acute SAH. Providers can utilize the Hunt and Hess clinical grading scale to aid in the prognosis following aneurysm rupture (Table 23.1).

There are several causes of non-aneurysmal SAHs. Perimesencephalic SAH makes up ~5% of all SAHs and one-third of non-aneurysmal SAHs.[7] Additional causes of non-traumatic, non-aneurysmal SAH includes arteriovenous malformations, coagulopathy, intradural cerebral artery dissection,

TABLE 23.1 **Hunt and Hess grading scale**

Grade	Criteria	Index of perioperative mortality (%)
0	Aneurysm is not ruptured	0–5
I	Asymptomatic or with minimal headache and slight nuchal rigidity	0–5
II	Moderate to severe headache, nuchal rigidity, but no neurologic deficit other than cranial nerve palsy	2–10
III	Somnolence, confusion, medium focal deficits	10–15
IV	Stupor, hemiparesis medium or severe, possible early decerebrate rigidity, vegetative disturbances	60–70
V	Deep coma, decerebrate rigidity, moribund appearance	70–100

Reference: Crespo J. Anesthesia for the surgery of intracranial aneurysms: Part II. *Internet J Anesthesiol.* 1997;2(2).

cerebral vasculitis, pituitary apoplexy, sickle cell disease, cerebral amyloid angiopathy, and cocaine or stimulant abuse.

PRESENTATION

The patient's initial presentation often includes a complaint of a diffuse, sudden, severe "thunderclap" headache. This "classic" headache occurs in ~80% of patients, with the headache reaching maximum intensity within seconds to minutes in as many as 50% of patients. It has been reported that 20% to 50% of patients will have a sentinel headache they experience days prior to the severe persistent headache.[8,9] The onset of headache with exertion is another classic part of the history that should raise the suspicion of SAH, and one less common presentation to consider is the individual waking up from sleep with acute headache. Associated symptoms vary but can include nausea and vomiting, photophobia, cranial nerve palsies, meningismus, depressed mental status, confusion, and focal neurologic deficits. Roughly 5% of patients will experience a seizure at the time of aneurysm rupture, with 20% having a seizure prior to arrival and another 5% to 10% having a seizure after admission.[10–12]

DIAGNOSIS

The initial evaluation of patients at high risk for acute aneurysmal SAH begins with assessing ABCs to ensure that definitive airway management is not clinically indicated. Neuroimaging is the cornerstone of diagnosis and begins with a non-contrast head CT, on which an acute bleed will appear as a hyperintense signal (Figure 23.1). The localization of the blood collection can help distinguish the type of SAH (Figure 23.2): Traumatic SAH typically occurs in the peripheral cortex, most frequently in the sylvian fissure, while aneurysmal SAH typically occurs around the circle of Willis,

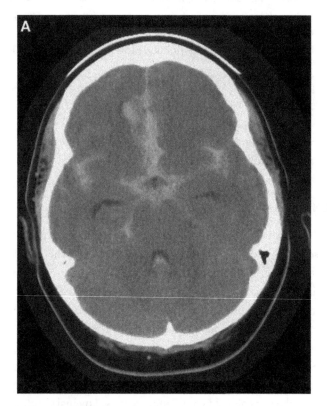

FIGURE 23.1 Aneurysmal SAH

With permission from Flemming, Kelly D., Tia Chakraborty, and Jennifer E. Fugate (ed.), 'Nontraumatic Subarachnoid Hemorrhage' in Kelly D. Flemming (ed.), *Mayo Clinic Neurology Board Review*, 2 edn (New York, 2021; online edn, Oxford Academic, 1 Nov. 2021), https://doi.org/10.1093/med/9780197512166.003.0058, accessed 16 Aug. 2022

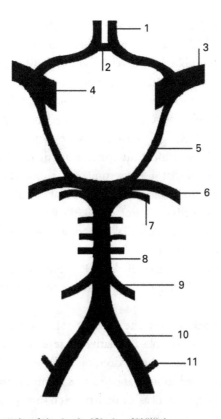

Arterial supply of the brain (Circle of Willis).
1: Anterior cerebral artery. 2: Anterior communicating artery.
3: Middle cerebral artery. 4: Internal carotid artery.
5: Posterior communicating artery. 6: Posterior cerebral artery.
7: Superior cerebellar artery. 8: Basilar artery.
9: Anterior inferior cerebellar artery. 10: Vertebral
artery. 11: Posterior inferior cerebellar artery.

FIGURE 23.2 Arterial anatomy of the brain

with aneurysms found at artery bifurcations. Perry et al. demonstrated that one can rule out acute SAH with 100% sensitivity if strict criteria are met, including a negative initial head CT that was obtained within 6 hours of symptom onset and a hematocrit of >30%.[13] If these criteria are not met and CT is done after 6 hours, lumbar puncture (LP) has been the typical next step in evaluation.

LP is performed to evaluate the CSF for the presence of blood and xanthochromia, which results from the breakdown of hemoglobin to oxyhemoglobin to bilirubin. The development of xanthochromia is time dependent, with 20% of samples positive in 6 hours and 100% at 12 hours. This is a critical point to recognize, as a "normal" sample prior to 12 hours could result in a false negative, leading the physician and patient to be inappropriately reassured. Roughly 30% of LPs are traumatic or "bloody" taps, rendering the results difficult to interpret. In another, retrospective analysis, the Perry group found that in the setting of a traumatic LP, the absence of xanthochromia and the presence of <2,000 × 10^6/L RBCs in the final tube holds a negative predictive value of 100% (95% CI 99.2–100%), allowing for the exclusion of SAH.[14] Potential complications of LP include postdural headache (occurring in up to 40% of patients) and infection and bleeding (occurring far less frequently). If the LP is nondiagnostic or the patient declines to consent, CT angiography (CTA) is another viable option to aid in diagnosis.

CTA is often used to detect the presence of intracerebral aneurysms and has been deemed a reasonable alternative by several societies when paired with adequately informed, shared decision-making.[15] CTA is not without fault: It has been noted to miss aneurysms ≤3 mm in size, which is problematic as aneurysms as small as 2 mm have been shown to cause significant complications. CTA also exposes the patient to additional radiation as well as IV contrast. MRI/MRA is another imaging modality available in the evaluation of aneurysmal SAH but is typically not used in the acute workup given the length of time to complete the study and the fact that it generally is a limited resource.

MANAGEMENT

Management of aneurysmal SAH prioritizes limiting secondary brain injury and preventing rebleeding. Rebleeding is reported to occur in 4% to 17% of patients, most commonly within the first 72 hours, and results in an increased morbidity and mortality, especially with a delay in diagnosis.[16] Broadly stated, management includes airway management, blood pressure and hemodynamic optimization, treatment and prevention of seizures, fever management, pain control/anxiolysis, monitoring for acute neurologic decline, and prevention of vasospasm.[17] Regardless of the practice environment, early neurosurgical consultation should take place with the goal of securing an aneurysm, if present, within 24 hours. Transfer to a high-volume, comprehensive stroke center should be strongly considered, with final disposition ultimately being an ICU.

The decision to place an advanced airway is dependent on a patient's mental status and ability to protect their airway—as always, this is a clinical judgment. The need for transfer should be considered in making this decision. Airway management goals should focus on maintaining eucapnia and avoiding hypoxemia. Utilizing the most skilled provider available as well as adjuncts to avoid stimulation and multiple attempts will avoid ICP spikes and diminish the risk of rebleeding.

Coagulopathy should be thoroughly investigated and treated. Patients who are taking vitamin K antagonists and are found to have an INR of >1[4] should be considered for IV vitamin K and prothrombin complex concentrates (PCC), with fresh frozen plasma (FFP) as a second-line alternative if PCC is unavailable.[18] For patient taking factor Xa and direct-thrombin inhibitors, please refer to your local reversal protocols. Patients taking oral antiplatelet agents are thought to be at a higher risk of more severe rebleeding events as well as neurosurgical procedure complications; thus, platelet transfusion is only recommended for those with a planned neurosurgical intervention.[18] Use of desmopressin (DDAVP) should be considered on an individual basis after weighing the risks and benefits. Patients with overall thrombocytopenia (platelets < 100,000) can be considered for transfusion. With regards to antifibrinolytic agents, we recommend discussing this with the treating neurosurgeon. The risk of rebleeding is greatest in the first 12 to 24 hours, and Hillman et al. found an 80% reduction in rebleeding before definitive treatment when tranexamic acid (TXA) was given within 24 hours; thus, short-term use of procoagulant drugs may be considered, but definitive treatment remains the priority.[19]

Recommendations for BP control in SAH are based on a low quality of evidence, but current major guidelines recommend the treatment of hypertension until the aneurysm is secured. The goal of management is to improve outcomes by reducing rebleeding risk, but this must be balanced with the risk of stroke and maintaining cerebral prefusion pressure. The goal BP is controversial and institution specific. Most recommend using a short-acting, easily titratable agent, such as clevidipine or nicardipine, with the goal of maintaining an SBP of ≤160 mmHg or an MAP of ≤100 mmHg.

In considering optimal BP management, one should adequately treat pain, anxiety, and nausea/vomiting. Thoughtful use of short-acting IV opioid analgesics for pain and small intermittent doses of benzodiazepines for anxiety may help control BP without the need for the aforementioned continuous infusions. NSAIDs and caffeine-containing medication combinations should be avoided in the acute period. Acetaminophen is a viable option in patients without preexisting liver disease or those with a known allergy. Aggressively treating nausea/vomiting minimizes rebleeding risk through limiting transient increases in ICP from gagging, retching, and straining. Oversedation should be avoided as it masks changes in neurologic status, but rapid reversal should not be performed as the risk of rebleeding is high with sudden agitation and potential precipitated seizures.

Seizures are not uncommon in aneurysmal SAH, and the treatment of active seizures should follow standard seizure treatment algorithms. Seizure prophylaxis is less clear, and standardized protocols are not in place, but many advocate for initiating a short course of prophylactic antiepileptic drugs, especially until the aneurysm is secured. The ultimate choice is left to the provider, but if antiepileptic drugs are desired, the use of phenytoin is strongly discouraged as it has been shown to worsen neurologic and cognitive outcomes following SAH.[20]

High-quality, vigilant nursing care is a must in these critically ill patients. Hourly neurologic checks—with special attention to level of consciousness, pupillary changes, gaze abnormalities, and focal deficits—are essential to follow the trajectory of the patient and identify early warning signs of deterioration from developing hydrocephalus or vasospasm. Nurses should maintain the head of the patient's bed elevated at 30 degrees and attempt to space care at intervals, with consideration of pretreating with medications to avoid ICP spikes. Nursing-driven protocols for electrolyte management can also be helpful in the prevention and treatment of hyponatremia, which has been associated with an increased incidence of vasospasm. Similar protocols can be used to monitor glucose control, with a goal of <200 mg/dL, while avoiding hypoglycemia, which could result in increased complications. Strict intake/output tracking aids in the goal of maintaining euvolemia and avoiding hypervolemia, which is associated with increased rebleeding in the acute, unsecured management period and an overall longer hospital stay. Finally, patients should be made NPO and this status should be maintained until proper swallow screens are performed.

Definitive management of intracranial aneurysm can be accomplished surgically with the placement of clips or through endovascular embolization with coils. The decision to choose one over another depends on several key factors and is institution dependent. Surgical management is typically chosen for large and complex aneurysms, aneurysms with wide bases, and aneurysms of the middle cerebral artery. Coils are placed for aneurysms in the posterior circulation and in patients deemed to be poor surgical candidates (e.g., patients with high-grade aneurysms, patients who are poor surgical candidates due to hemodynamic instability). The International Subarachnoid Trial (ISAT) found that, when appropriate, endovascular coiling was a safe alternative to clipping and should be considered when the patient is a candidate for either intervention.[21] Coiling has been endorsed by the American Heart Association/American Stroke Association.[22]

After being secured, vasospasm is the most feared complication of an aneurysmal SAH. Occurring in up to 70% of patients, it is thought to be due to an increase in intracellular calcium in the vascular smooth muscle of intracerebral arteries. Vasospasm typically presents between days 3 and 14 following rupture and is associated with delayed cerebral ischemia (DCI), with resultant functional neurologic impairment and increased mortality. DCI occurs in 20% to 30% of patients with aneurysmal SAH. Nimodipine is a dihydropyridine calcium channel blocker that, when administered early, ideally in the first 24 hours, has been shown to improve outcomes with reduced rates of delayed cerebral ischemia and functional impairment.[23] The true neuroprotective mechanism of nimodipine is unclear but is presumed to be at a cellular level as it does not improve angiographic evidence of vasospasm. Nimodipine is the agent of choice as this clinical benefit has not been found with the use of alternative calcium channel blockers. Angiographic vasospasm may require intra-arterial vasodilators, balloon angioplasty, or vasopressor therapy and should be treated in conjunction with neurosurgeons and/or endovascular neuro-interventionalists. The Modified Fisher Grading Scale is used to estimate the likelihood of clinically significant

TABLE 23.2 **Modified Fisher grading scale**

Grade	SAH	Intraventricular hemorrhage	Risk of vasospasm
I	No or minimal	–	24%
II	Minimal	+	33%
III	Diffuse focal or thick	–	33%
IV	Diffuse focal or thick	+	40%

Reference: Frontera JA, Claassen J, Schmidt JM, et al. Prediction of symptomatic vasospasms after subarachnoid hemorrhage: The Modified Fisher Scale. *Neurosurgery.* 2006;59(1):21–27.

vasospasm and DCI, with higher grades associated with an increased risk of vasospasm (Table 23.2).

Other complications following the rupture of an aneurysmal SAH include obstructive hydrocephalus, neurogenically mediated fevers, respiratory failure, and cardiac complications. Hydrocephalus results from obstructed flow of CSF between ventricles or impaired resorption via the arachnoid granulations and typically occurs 48 to 72 hours following rupture. Hydrocephalus, if symptomatic, requires CSF diversion via an external ventricular drain, which allows for both monitoring and treatment of elevated ICP. Fevers should be aggressively avoided with the goal of maintaining normothermia; aggressive cooling measures may be required and anti-shivering protocols should be in place if needed. While fevers of a neurologic origin are common, practitioners should be vigilant for infection, drug reactions, and other causes of fever, which should always be fully evaluated before reaching a diagnosis of neurogenic fever.

Neurogenic pulmonary edema and stress-induced cardiomyopathy are other well-known complications often requiring mechanical ventilatory support. Pneumonitis and pneumonia are potential complications secondary to acute and chronic aspirations, respectively. Finally, cardiac dysfunction resulting in hemodynamic instability has been documented in the literature, as well as EKG changes including T-wave inversions (neurogenic T-waves), QTc prolongation, and ST elevation. The pathophysiology is believed to be secondary to an increased catecholamine surge as a result of the acute intracranial bleed and not due to primary coronary artery occlusion from plaque rupture.

· Aneurysmal SAHs have a case fatality rate of 50%. This increases to 80% if diagnosis is delayed.

· Definitive management of the culprit aneurysm by clipping or coiling should be completed within 24 hours. Consider early transfer to a comprehensive stroke center with a high volume of aneurysm cases as this has been shown to improve outcomes. Specific BP target is institution specific, but most recommend an SBP of <160 mmHg.

· The sensitivity of modern non-contrast CT to rule out SAH nears 100% if performed within 6 hours if all qualifying criteria are met. The sensitivity falls to 90% on the first day, 60% to 85% on day 5, and 50% at 1 week.

· Following a negative non-contrast head CT, the decision to obtain an LP versus CTA is institution specific and should be made involving the patient using shared decision-making.

· Follow institution targets for SBP (or MAP), maximize PaO_2 and $PaCO_2$ goals, reverse coagulopathies, initiate seizure prophylaxis when appropriate, and treat pain/anxiety aggressively.

Common locations and frequencies of intracranial aneurysms

Location	Precent of Aneurysms Found
Pericallosal Artery (distal portion of Anterior Cerebral Artery)	4%
Anterior Communicating Artery	30%
Middle Cerebral Artery	20%
Internal Carotid Artery Bifurcation	7.5%
Posterior Communicating Artery	25%
Basilar Tip	7%
Posterior Inferior Cerebellar Artery	3%
Additional/Miscellaneous Locations	3.5%

Brisman JL, Song JK, Newell DW. Cerebral Aneurysms. *N Engl J Med.* August 31, 2006;355:9.

References

1. Brain Aneurysm Foundation. Statistics and facts. https://bafound.org/about-brain-aneurysms/brain-aneurysm-basics/brain-aneurysm-statistics-and-facts/

2. Hop JW, Rinkel GJ, Alga A, et al. Case-fatality rates and functional outcome after subarachnoid hemorrhage: A systematic review. *Stroke*. 1997;28(3):660–664.

3. Anderson SW, Todd MM, Hindman BJ, et al. Effect of intraoperative hypothermia on neuropsychological outcomes after intracranial aneurysm surgery. *Ann Neurol*. 2006;60(5):518–527.

4. Al-Khindi T, Macdonald RL, Schweizer TA. Cognitive and functional outcome after aneurysmal subarachnoid hemorrhage. *Stroke*. 2010;41:e519–e536.

5. Vermeulen MJ, Schull, MJ. Missed diagnosis of subarachnoid hemorrhage in the emergency department. *Stroke*. 2007;38:1216–1221.

6. Kowalski RG, Claassen J, Kreiter KT, et al. Initial misdiagnosis and outcome after subarachnoid hemorrhage. *JAMA*. 2004;291:866–869.

7. Flaherty ML, Haverbusch M, Kissela B, et al. Perimesencephalic subarachnoid hemorrhage: Incidence, risk factors, and outcome. *J Stroke Cerebrovasc Dis*. 2005;14(6): 267–271.

8. Suarez JI, Tarr RW, Selman WR. Aneurysmal subarachnoid hemorrhage. *N Engl J Med*. 2006;354(4):387–396.

9. Beck J, Raab A, Szelenyi A, et al. Sentinel headache and the risk of rebleeding after aneurysmal subarachnoid hemorrhage. *Stroke*. 2006;37(11):2733–2737.

10. Linn FH, Wijdicks EF, van der Graaf Y, et al. Prospective study of sentinel headache in aneurysmal subarachnoid haemorrhage. *Lancet*. 1994;344:590–593.

11. Rhoney DH, Tipps LB, Murry KR, et al. Anticonvulsant prophylaxis and timing of seizures after aneurysmal subarachnoid hemorrhage. *Neurology*. 2000;55:258–265.

12. Jaja BNR, Schweizer TA, Claassen J, et al. The SAFARI score to assess the risk of convulsive seizure during admission for aneurysmal subarachnoid hemorrhage. *Neurosurgery*. 2018;82:887–893.

13. Perry JJ, Stiell IG, Sivilotti LA, et al. Sensitivity of computed tomography performed within six hours of onset of headache for diagnosis of subarachnoid hemorrhage: Prospective cohort study. *BMJ*. 2011;343:d4277.

14. Perry JJ, Alyahya B, Sivilotti ML, et al. Differentiation between traumatic tap and aneurysmal subarachnoid hemorrhage: prospective cohort study. *BMJ*. 2015;350:h568.

15. Godwin SA, Cherkas, DS, Panagos PD, Shih RD, Byyny R, Wolf SJ. Clinical policy: Critical issues in the evaluation and management of adult patients presenting to the emergency department with acute headache. *Ann Emerg Med*. 2019;74(4):e41–e74

16. Starke RM, Connolly ES, Participants in the International Multi-Disciplinary Consensus Conference on the Critical Care Management of Subarachnoid

Hemorrhage. Rebleeding after aneurysmal subarachnoid hemorrhage. *Neurocrit Care*. 2011;15:241–246.

17. Diringer MN, Bleck TP, Hemphill JC III, et al. Critical care management of patients following aneurysmal subarachnoid hemorrhage: Recommendations from the Neurocritical Care Society's Multidisciplinary Consensus Conference. *Neurocrit Care*. 2011;15:211–240.

18. Frontera JA, Lewin JJ 3rd, Rabinstein AA, et al. Guideline for reversal of antithrombotics in intracranial hemorrhage: A statement for healthcare professionals from the Neurocritical Care Society and Society of Critical Care Medicine. *Neurocrit Care*. 2016;24:6–46.

19. Hillman J, Fridriksson S, Nilsson O, et al. Immediate administration of tranexamic acid and reduced incidence of early rebleeding after aneurysmal subarachnoid hemorrhage: A prospective randomized study. *J Neurosurg*. 2002;97:771–778.

20. Naidech AM, Kreiter KT, Janjua N, et al. Phenytoin exposure is associated with functional and cognitive disability after subarachnoid hemorrhage. *Stroke*. 2005 Mar;36(3):583–587.

21. Molyneux A, Kerr RS, Yu LM, et al. International Subarachnoid Aneurysm Trial (ISAT) of neurosurgical clipping versus endovascular coiling in 2143 patients with ruptured intracranial aneurysms: A randomized trial. *Lancet*. 2002;360(9342):1267–1274.

22. Connolly ES, Jr., Rabinstein AA, Carhuapoma JR, et al. Guidelines for the management of aneurysmal subarachnoid hemorrhage: A guideline for healthcare professionals from the American Heart Association/American Stroke Association. *Stroke*. 2012;43:1711–1737.

23. Allen GS, Ahn HS, Preziosi TJ, et al. Cerebral arterial spasm—a controlled trial of nimodipine in patients with subarachnoid hemorrhage. *N Engl J Med*. 1983;308:619–24.

24 I feel weak: Myasthenic or neuromuscular emergencies

Charles M. Andrews

A 36-year-old female presents to the ED with complaints that she feels weak. She states that she has been feeling more fatigued for several months now and believes her fatigue is worse, especially after working long days as a waitress. She even says that she can't keep her eyes open to watch television because it becomes difficult to see at night after working. She admits to a past medical history of type 2 diabetes and hypertension and thinks she may recently have had a "cold." Her vital signs are HR 92 bpm, BP 148/72 mmHg, temperature 37°C, RR 22 breaths/min, and O_2 95%. On examination you notice ptosis of the left eye with limited upgaze, and she is constantly trying to clear her throat and only talking in short sentences. The remainder of her cranial nerve exam is unremarkable, and she has reduced neck flexion but otherwise normal motor strength in her extremities.

What do I do now?

DIFFERENTIAL DIAGNOSIS AND PRESENTATION

Any patient presenting with symptoms of weakness should be assessed for focal weakness that may be consistent with acute ischemic stroke, given the timeframe for diagnosis, imaging, and benefit from potential treatments. If the weakness is more generalized or not in a cerebrovascular pattern, then further history and detailed neurologic examination is required for further differential and diagnosis of this patient. Although this patient has findings on her neurologic examination, none of these appear to be focal or consistent with stroke.

One should initially keep a broad differential when approaching a patient with nonspecific weakness as there are myriad causes and pathologies. Key initial clues include factors such as the abruptness of onset of weakness, presence or lack of fatigability, recent illnesses, and concurrent symptoms in additional to the neurologic findings. Patients with neuromuscular problems often present late in their disease process or present with no clear diagnosis, often requiring multiple repeated visits.

Myasthenia gravis (MG) and Lambert–Eaton myasthenic syndrome (LEMS) are the two primary diseases of the neuromuscular junction (NMJ). MG is caused by antibodies that interact with postsynaptic acetylcholine (Ach) receptors, while in LEMS, antibodies react with presynaptic voltage-gated calcium channels, leading to impairment in Ach release. More recently, additional antibodies causing MG have been found, including MuSK and LRP4 proteins that are involved in signaling at the NMJ. There are several subtypes of MG differentiated by antibody, early versus late onset, presence of thymoma, ocular, and even those that remain seronegative despite extensive testing. Despite different presentations and subtypes, these patients have a common feature: failure in transmission of signal from presynaptic neurons to muscle, ultimately causing weakness.

Weakness in MG almost always involves the eyes and causes diplopia as well as ptosis. This can be more pronounced on one side and is often asymmetric. Aside from the eyes, the weakness is typically symmetric and involves the proximal muscles of the upper body more than distal muscles. The classic symptom in MG is fatigability, or marked weakness after repeated muscle use or exercise, that is more noticeable throughout the day. Our patient clearly has ocular involvement and has worsening symptoms at night after work with visual complaints. Often MG patients will also have difficulty with dysphagia or managing secretions as their symptoms progress. In contrast, patients with LEMS typically present with distal weakness that progresses more proximally, their symptoms improve with exercise (more Ach release at the NMJ), and LEMS often is associated with malignancy.

Rare but treatable disorders of the NMJ include botulism and organophosphate toxicity. Both of these conditions typically present with weakness, although additional history of eating self-canned foods or working with insecticides and additional symptoms are often discovered. Botulism typically manifests with dilated pupils, ptosis, and diplopia and causes weakness cranial to caudal, with foodborne botulism causing nausea, vomiting, cramping, and diarrhea. Infantile botulism and wound botulism are additional subtypes. Organophosphate toxicity must also be considered, although most cases are related to interaction with pesticides today.

Guillain–Barré syndrome (GBS) presents with rapidly ascending weakness and, eventually, paralysis. This typically happens over weeks but can be much more rapid and occur in days. In addition to weakness, patients develop areflexia of the regions involved and may develop sensory changes. Autonomic dysfunction and back pain are frequently seen together with neurologic deficits. Often patients can detail a recent viral or bacterial illness, and *Campylobacter* has been repeatedly implicated in stimulation of the immune response through molecular mimicry causing autoimmune neurologic disease. Antibodies that cause axonal disease typically interact with gangliosides, causing demyelination, but can also interact directly with axonal proteins, which causes a more severe, longer-lasting disease course. GBS has many reported variants and can present with isolated motor disease, with motor and sensory symptoms, and with different presentations of weakness (cranial to caudal in Miller–Fisher GBS). Tick paralysis may be indistinguishable from GBS and may be only identified by finding and removing a tick, with improvement in symptoms. Tick paralysis occurs more often in children and individuals with a smaller body mass. It needs to be considered in the northwestern and southwestern United States as well as in Australia, where *Dermacentor/Ixodes* ticks are endemic.

Spinal cord ischemia and cord compression can also present with generalized weakness, although this is relatively rare. Most spinal infarcts occur from the anterior spinal artery and occur along with some vascular malformation. The presentation will depend on the region of involvement, but typically will also include pain along with motor loss at this level as well as loss of pain and temperature. Transverse myelitis, tumor-related spinal cord compression, spondylitis myelopathy, and even epidural abscess can present with a rapid onset of paralysis that is difficult to distinguish from GBS.

WORKUP

Given the wide and complex array of pathologies that can present with acute weakness, the approach to workup and diagnosis should be assessed with traditional ABCs with several caveats in mind. As pointed out, the description of the weakness is key to diagnosis. Is the weakness acute, subacute, rapidly progressive? Is it symmetric in presentation? Did this weakness begin in the lower extremities and advance cranially, or was it the opposite? Is this weakness consistently worsening, or does it change throughout the day (fatigability)? Are there any other historical findings, such as recent viral or bacterial illnesses? Is there any pain, or are associated symptoms other than weakness present?

One area an emergency provider should quickly be able to assess is breathing quality in patients with neuromuscular disease and weakness. As stated, many patients with neuromuscular illness may not be identified or may not present until their disease is advanced and leading to impending respiratory failure. Patients who cannot clear their secretions, cannot speak in full sentences, have a change in voice, or utilize abdominal breathing with use of accessory muscles are at clear risk for impending respiratory failure. If a patient has these findings, do not proceed with ABG analysis as normal results will not be reassuring, and hypercarbia and hypoxia are late findings given compensatory respiratory mechanisms. The 20/30/40 rule describes bedside pulmonary function tests and the thresholds to predict intubation in neuromuscular emergencies, although its use can be challenging in patients with impending need for intubation, as these tests heavily depend on patient effort and compliance. Bedside pulmonary assessment variables in the rule are <20 mL/kg vital capacity (full exhale after full inspiration), >$^-$30 cmH$_2$O maximum inspiratory pressure, and <40 cmH$_2$O maximum expiratory pressure. Any of these findings suggest the need for intubation.

The case described in the vignette is most consistent with an issue at the NMJ, likely MG. Botulism and organophosphate toxicity should be able to be ruled out easily with history and exam not demonstrating eating self-canned foods, work with insecticides, and lack of pupillary changes, gastrointestinal symptoms, and significant vital sign abnormalities. Laboratory workup for MG includes testing serum for Ach receptor antibodies as well as MuSK and LPR4 antibodies. If LEMS is considered, then serum may additionally be sent for voltage-gated calcium channel antibodies, and patients should be asked about and potentially screened for cancer. Ultimately a neurologist may be able to perform electromyography (EMG) to evaluate action potential transmission, but this is difficult to obtain in any hospitalized patients and is not practical to request in the ED. Given the limited availability of EMG and the fact that most laboratory tests will be sent out for analysis and will take days to return, treatment is typically initiated based on clinical symptoms and bedside diagnosis.

The diagnosis of GBS is clinical in nature and based on presentation and symptoms. Additional studies may be helpful in supporting this diagnosis, but there is no discrete serologic or CSF lab result that is confirmatory. CSF from lumbar puncture typically demonstrates no significant changes to cell counts but markedly elevated protein levels that peak ~4 to 6 weeks following onset of symptoms. For this reason, if the patient's course is rapidly progressive and lumbar puncture is completed early, marked protein elevation may not be present yet and CSF may essentially be normal. There are additionally several antiglycan antibodies that are associated with motor variants of GBS: GM1, GD1a, GalNAc-GD1a, and GM1b. GQ1b antibodies can also be sent as they are frequently positive in Miller–Fisher variants of GBS. EMG can also be used to demonstrate reduction in amplitude of muscle action potentials, but findings can be normal early in disease and, again, EMG is difficult to obtain in critically ill patients in the hospital. Given the number of spinal cord and compressive pathologies, MRI of the cervical spine should be undertaken to rule out any of these diseases.

TREATMENT

A specific approach to respiratory failure in patients with neuromuscular disease is essential. As the clinician may not know the true etiology of the neuromuscular weakness when it is determined that respiratory failure is imminent, there are some thoughts that one must consider. Negative-pressure ventilation (NPV) is often used in patients who are awake and alert but have increased work of breathing, either for treatment or for preoxygenation prior to intubation. MG patients may respond well, especially in milder cases, but if they are unable to clear their secretions from dysphagia, this will only make matters worse. In patients with GBS, NPV is contraindicated as patients who get to this point of weakness will need intubation and many times tracheostomy, given that the course of their disease is often much longer than with other neuromuscular causes. If MG patients require intubation, the dosage and type of paralytics will require specific attention. Depolarizing neuromuscular blockers (NMBs) such as succinylcholine require higher doses given the downregulation and decrease of functional ACh receptor. Patients taking anticholinesterase therapy will also have reduced metabolism of succinylcholine, leading to prolonged paralysis; for these reasons, it should be avoided. Using nondepolarizing NMBs such as rocuronium is preferred, but patients are very sensitive and require much less—usually one-quarter the typical dose. Rocuronium may also be reversed with sugammadex and is therefore the safest choice.

Medical treatment of MG is based largely on two types of drugs: anticholinesterases and immunosuppressants. Patients who present in myasthenic crisis with respiratory failure will also likely require plasma exchange (PLEX) or intravenous immune globulin (IVIG). Pyridostigmine is the most commonly used anticholinesterase and is typically given every 6 hours for symptom management. Patients who are receiving too much may present with the cholinergic crisis, which can present with muscle weakness and can also be accompanied by muscarinic effects (nausea, vomiting, diaphoresis, salivation, bronchorrhea, diarrhea, miosis, and bradycardia). Although much emphasis is placed on differentiating myasthenic from cholinergic crisis, the latter is extremely rare and the diagnosis is clear based on a history of large amounts of drug and concurrent symptoms. Corticosteroids are often used for worsening of MG symptoms; use is typically started at ~20 mg/day prednisone unless significant weakness and respiratory failure are present. When prednisone is started at higher doses (40–60 mg), worsening of weakness can occur, precipitating respiratory failure in some patients. Other immunosuppressive drugs used are azathioprine, mycophenolate, and rituximab, although these drugs would be expected to be started by a neurologist as an outpatient for chronic management therapy.

PLEX and IVIG have been shown to improve symptoms in severely affected patients. The efficacy of both treatments is similar in patients with generalized myasthenia and should be determined based on the patient's characteristics as well as the availability of each therapy. PLEX requires dialysis line access as well as availability of nephrologists (typically weekday, daytime hours) but has been more effective in MuSK Ab cases. IVIG appears less effective in ocular MG subtypes and milder cases and cannot be used in patients with renal failure. It would not be expected to initiate any of these treatments in the ED; rather, emergency physicians should identify the need and have patients admitted to ICUs capable of providing these treatments.

PLEX and IVIG are also the main treatments of GBS. After identification and diagnosis, the key to treatment is reaching the plateau phase, where symptoms no longer worsen and in fact slowly improve. IVIG may be used more often as first-line therapy given its availability and ease of administration, although no evidence has supported one treatment over the other. Unlike in MG, corticosteroids have not been shown to helpful and should not be used. Patients with GBS frequently have multiple medical problems, including dysautonomia, adynamic ileus, SIADH, and severe pain, that require critical care in ICUs that capable of and comfortable treating these patients. Given the increase in neurocritical care units, providers should consider transfer in severe cases.

KEY POINTS TO REMEMBER

- MG most often presents with asymmetric abnormalities in the cranial nerves (eye movements, ptosis) and symmetric weakness below the head.
- GBS classically presents with ascending lower extremity weakness, loss of reflexes, and sensory changes, but there are many variants to this presentation.
- Early recognition of neuromuscular disease is key, as undiagnosed neuromuscular disease can lead to respiratory failure and may be prevented with early diagnosis.

- Botulism toxicity may present similar to MG. Although rare, it is treatable and should be considered.
- Treatment for both MG and GBS typically involves immunosuppression with either IVIG or PLEX. Patients should be admitted to centers with these capabilities.
- Do not wait to intubate until PaO_2 or $PaCO_2$ changes occur. In fact, this means you have waited too long to intervene!

Further reading

Abel M, Eisenkraft JB. Anesthetic implications of myasthenia gravis. *Mt Sinai J Med.* 2002;69(1–2):31–37.

Ciafaloni E. Myasthenia gravis and congenital myasthenic syndromes. *Continuum.* 2019;25(6):1767–1784.

Gajdos P, Chevret S, Toyka KV. Intravenous immunoglobulin for myasthenia gravis. *Cochrane Database Syst Rev.* 2012;12:CD002277.

Gilhus NE. Myasthenia gravis. *N Engl J Med.* 2016;375(26):2570–2581.

Guidon AC. Lambert-Eaton myasthenic syndrome, botulism, and immune checkpoint inhibitor-related myasthenia gravis. *Continuum.* 2019;25(6):1785–1806.

Sanders DB, Wolfe GI, Benatar M, et al. International consensus guidance for management of myasthenia gravis: Executive summary. *Neurology.* 2016;87(4):419–425.

Sheikh KA. Guillain-Barre syndrome. *Continuum.* 2020;26(5):1184–1204.

25 Stop the bleed: Procedures for hemostatic control

Mark M. Ramzy

A 74-year-old male presents to your ED with epistaxis. His wife states that he was bleeding from both nostrils for 15 minutes before EMS arrived. Paramedics state that the patient has continued to bleed through multiple gauze pads despite direct pressure and leaning forward. He has a history of poorly controlled hypertension despite taking several medications. The patient is alert, awake, and oriented. He states this has happened multiple times in the past, all with spontaneous resolution and not requiring him to go to the ED. HR is 110 bpm, BP is 194/110 mmHg, and he is saturating well on room air. Physical exam is notable for an anxious male sitting upright and leaning forward while holding several blood-soaked gauzes. There are no signs of trauma. Further inspection of his oropharynx reveals a significant amount of clots and bleeding.

What do I do now?

Hemorrhage control is a fundamental skill that all emergency physicians need. From epistaxis to a bleeding dialysis fistula, proper control of bleeding will be required frequently throughout an emergency physician's career. Having a detailed treatment strategy with contingency plans is crucial in appropriately managing these patients and preventing further deterioration. All approaches should start with assessing the patient's airway and their ability to protect its patency. Establishing several large-bore IVs should take priority, followed by quickly identifying the bleeding source, applying direct pressure if able, correcting coagulopathies, and utilizing hemostatic chemical adjuncts or devices when appropriate.

In the case of our patient with significant bleeding from his oropharynx, his ability to talk, follow commands, and comply with treatment positions reassures us that his airway and mentation are patent. Given his prior episodes of self-resolving hemoptysis, he remains at a high risk for deterioration and requires immediate attention. This patient should have two 18G IVs placed right away in the event that he becomes hemodynamically unstable and requires immediate airway protection and volume resuscitation. Identifying the source of his bleeding is imperative as it will help guide the rest of his treatment and determine his disposition. Therefore, the use of a Frazier-tip suction catheter, often found in epistaxis kits, will assist in visual inspection of the nasopharynx.

First, have the patient blow their nose to expel any clots and allow for the application of topical vasoconstrictors such as oxymetazoline or phenylephrine. The patient should continue to lean forward and keep applying direct pressure for an additional 10 to 15 minutes. Should bleeding persist after this **and a bleeding vessel is visualized**, the use of chemical cauterization with silver nitrate is advised. In this patient, whose bleeding appears to be coming from both nostrils, the use of silver nitrate should not be attempted until his bleeding source is identified; more importantly, it should never be applied to both sides of the nasal septum, as this increases the risk of perforation.

Should bleeding continue, use of thrombogenic foams and gel may be considered if available. Oxidized cellulose or gelatin matrixes (known commercially as Gelfoam, Surgicel, or FloSeal) are biodegradable and bioabsorbable agents that provide effective hemostatic control when placed directly on bleeding mucus.[1] Another effective agent for bleeding control is injectable tranexamic acid (tXA).[2] Since there is no standardized approach in the application of tXA, several methods have been documented in the literature: 200 mg can be atomized and sprayed directly into the nasal cavity, or 500 mg can be soaked into a nasal tampon and packed into the affected nostril.[3,4]

If bleeding still continues, nasal tampons or sponges (such as the commercially available Merocel) can also be used. These compressed and dehydrated polyvinyl acetate sponges assist in the control of anterior or posterior nasal bleeding by expanding when irrigated with normal saline.[5] Lastly, in patients with known and uncontrolled anterior bleeding, use of an anterior epistaxis balloon (such as the RapidRhino) is highly encouraged. These devices, available in different lengths, are typically impregnated with cellulose to promote platelet aggregation. It is important to inflate them with the predetermined amount of air, stated on the package insert, and not saline to minimize any risk of balloon rupture or aspiration.

Persistent bleeding despite the use of direct pressure, topical vasoconstrictors, and nasal sponges or tampons should strongly suggest to the emergency physician that an uncontrolled bleeding source is present in the posterior nasopharynx, specifically from the sphenopalatine artery or one of its branches. In our patient, the lack of an obvious anterior source, the persistent bleeding despite continued direct pressure, and the patient's advanced age and elevated BP are all factors that point to the epistaxis coming from a posterior source. These patients require the placement of a specialized dual balloon that provides both anterior and posterior compression. Although varying in size, and various package inserts specify the exact volume to inflate, the anterior balloon typically holds 30 mL while the posterior holds 10 mL. If this specialized dual-balloon catheter is unavailable, a 14Fr Foley catheter with its tip cut off may also be utilized. The tip of the catheter is cut off because when left in place, it can sometimes stimulate the patient's gag reflex.

Upon hemorrhage control, patients with anterior packing should be closely monitored for complications and hemodynamic stability for ≥1 hour in the ED. Prior to discharge home, these patients should be given educational instructions for techniques on controlling repeat hemorrhage, with explicit return precautions to the ED and ENT follow-up within 48 to 72 hours. Patients with posterior packing should be admitted to the hospital for closer monitoring as complications such as bradycardia, pressure necrosis, hypoxia, and cardiac dysrhythmias may occur.[5]

Similar to epistaxis, bleeding that occurs in other areas of the body requires having a detailed treatment strategy that should also include a stepwise interventional plan. With this particular episode of hemoptysis, there's some concern in this patient that the bleeding may be coming from the esophagus or elsewhere in the upper GI tract. The airway should be promptly secured in patients with whom massive hemoptysis is suspected. Additionally, being familiar with placing the two-ballooned Sengstaken–Blakemore tube or the three-ballooned Minnesota tube is pivotal in controlling the bleeding source and preventing further hemodynamic compromise. Key steps in Minnesota tube placement are summarized in Box 25.1.

In patients with traumatic lacerations, the first step in intervention is to place direct pinpoint pressure over the area that is actively bleeding. This involves identifying the exact source of the bleeding and applying maximal pressure over that area alone. If bleeding continues despite direct pinpoint pressure, topical hemostatic agents can be deployed. These special gauzes are impregnated with kaolin, zeolite, or chitosan (often referred to as QuikClot, Combat Gauze, and ChitoGauze, respectively) and serve to accelerate the body's own coagulation cascade and platelet aggregation.[6] In settings of uncontrolled bleeding from traumatic injury, systemic use of 1 g tXA given in 100 mL normal saline over 10 minutes is recommended within 1 hour from the injury; it must be given within the first 3 hours.[7]

Windlass tourniquet use is becoming increasingly common for exsanguinating extremity injury in the prehospital setting.[8] When applied early and before the onset of hypovolemic shock, tourniquets have been shown to improve mortality up to 94%.[9] To properly use these devices, they should be placed 2 inches proximal to the wound and tightened to greater than arterial pressure, as noted by the disappearance of the patient's distal pulse. The application of a second tourniquet may be required. Although the safe time limit for tourniquet removal has yet to be determined, it should NOT be removed until the patient has reached definitive care in the operating room. The removal of a tourniquet after prolonged application may have detrimental effects due to the systemic release of potassium, lactate, and myoglobin from a severely acidotic limb.[7]

Procedural steps for Minnesota tube placement

1. Intubate and resuscitate the patient before placing any GI balloon tamponade device.
2. Ensure that all equipment is available at the bedside, including hemostats, manometers, and syringes for both suction and inflation ports, as well as sterile water for filling the balloons. Check the equipment for leaks by fully inflating and then completely deflating the balloons. If there is concern for air leak, place the balloons in water during inflation.
3. The esophageal and gastric balloons should be fully deflated and the inflation ports clamped with a tube clamp (hemostats), or plastic plugs inserted into the tube lumens.
4. Place the patient in the supine position with the head of the bed elevated to 45 degrees. Check the estimated length by measuring the tube from the bridge of the nose to the xiphoid process.
5. Lubricate the distal balloon and tube, which may facilitate passage.
6. Insert the balloon into the oral cavity followed by the esophagus using laryngoscopy and with the assistance of McGill forceps to the 50-cm mark.
7. Check with radiography prior to full inflation of the gastric balloon, as cases have been described of intrathoracic inflation of balloons; this pitfall also underscores the importance of intubation prior to balloon placement.
8. Inflate the gastric balloon with ~50 mL of fluid and then perform a chest radiograph to ensure that the balloon is located in the stomach and not in the esophagus.
9. After confirmation, fully inflate the gastric balloon in 50- to 10-mL increments, checking that the pressure does not exceed 15 mmHg on manometry after each 50- to 100-mL injection. A measurement of >15 mm Hg suggests that the gastric balloon may errantly be in the esophagus.
10. Once the gastric balloon is fully inflated, the inflation and pressure monitoring ports should be clamped. Bare metal hemostats are not recommended, as these will damage the tube; instead, place a piece of gauze between the hemostat and the tube to prevent any tube damage.
11. Slowly withdraw the tube until the operator encounters mild resistance, allowing the balloon to push against the gastric fundus. This will typically occur at 40 cm.
12. Secure the tube with traction applied, preferably with a securing device (i.e., endotracheal tube securing device). A 1-L bag of fluids can provide a similar effect with 1 to 2 pounds of traction.

13. Once traction has been applied, apply continuous aspiration. Consider aspiration of all gastric contents. Also decompress esophageal contents via the esophageal port. If the bleeding continues despite the gastric balloon inflation, increase tension by 1 to 2 pounds of traction by adding a second liter of fluids.
14. If the bleeding has not ceased (e.g., continued bleeding from the ports or oropharynx), inflate the esophageal or upper balloon to ~30 to 40 mmHg on manometry. The maximum pressure within the esophageal balloon should not exceed 45 mmHg. When the esophageal balloon has reached its end-inflation, it should be double clamped at the esophageal inflation port with two clamps. A repeat chest x-ray should be obtained after placement.

In the setting of non-compressible torso hemorrhage, surgically invasive procedures such as emergent thoracotomy and laparotomy have been historically used for definitive hemostatic control. Another tool that is being more commonly used is the resuscitative endovascular balloon occlusion of the aorta (REBOA). This procedure, performed by a previously trained professional who understands the indications, risks, benefits, and application of the technique, involves accessing the patient's common femoral artery in order to insert and inflate an endovascular balloon into the proximal aorta. Note that this temporizing measure is utilized until more definitive hemostasis can be achieved either surgically in the operating room or through interventional vascular means.

Hemorrhage control is a skill every emergency physician must master. The degree of complexity can vary based on the location and source of the bleeding. Whether it is uncontrolled bleeding from epistaxis or a traumatic laceration, having a stepwise and graded intervention plan ensures the greatest success for hemostatic control. These strategies may require a combination of direct pinpoint pressure, chemically infused gauze to accelerate coagulation cascade activation, or packing and balloon inflation.

KEY POINTS TO REMEMBER

- In patients with epistaxis, always assess their airway and breathing.

- Establish at least two large-bore IVs as soon as possible so they can be used in the event of clinical deterioration or hemodynamically instability.
- Direct pinpoint pressure to stop bleeding should be applied for ≥10 to 15 minutes.
- Patients with posterior nasal packing require hospital admission for close monitoring, given the high rate of associated complications.
- IV tXA should be given within 1 hour of traumatic injuries. The dose is 1 g given in 100 mL saline over 10 minutes. It must be given in the first 3 hours.
- Tourniquets should not be removed until the patient is in a setting where the bleeding can be properly controlled, such as the operating room.

References

1. Mathiasen RA, Cruz RM. Prospective, randomized, controlled clinical trial of a novel matrix hemostatic sealant in patients with acute anterior epistaxis. *Laryngoscope.* 2005;115(5):899–902. doi:10.1097/01.MLG.0000160528.50017.3C

2. Krulewitz NA, Fix ML. Epistaxis. *Emerg Med Clin North Am.* 2019;37(1):29–39. doi:10.1016/j.emc.2018.09.005

3. Heymer J, Schilling T, Räpple D. Use of a mucosal atomization device for local application of tranexamic acid in epistaxis. *Am J Emerg Med.* 2018;36(12):2327. doi:10.1016/j.ajem.2018.04.033

4. Birmingham AR, Mah ND, Ran R, Hansen M. Topical tranexamic acid for the treatment of acute epistaxis in the emergency department. *Am J Emerg Med.* 2018;36(7):1242–1245. doi:10.1016/j.ajem.2018.03.039

5. McGinnis HD. Nose and sinuses. In: Tintinalli JE, Ma O, Yealy DM, et al., eds. *Tintinalli's Emergency Medicine: A Comprehensive Study Guide, 9th ed.* McGraw-Hill; 2019:1572–1578.

6. Bennett BL, Littlejohn L. Review of new topical hemostatic dressings for combat casualty care. *Mil Med.* 2014;179(5):497–514. doi:10.7205/MILMED-D-13-00199

7. Baker DA, Keller AP IV, Knight RM, et al. Military medicine. In: Tintinalli JE, Ma O, Yealy DM, et al., eds. *Tintinalli's Emergency Medicine: A Comprehensive Study Guide, 9th ed.* McGraw-Hill; 2019:2007–2013.

8. Cameron PA, Knapp BJ, Teeter W. Trauma in adults. In: Tintinalli JE, Ma O, Yealy DM, et al., eds. *Tintinalli's Emergency Medicine: A Comprehensive Study Guide, 9th ed.* McGraw-Hill; 2019:1669–1676,

9. Kragh JF Jr, Littrel ML, Jones JA, et al. Battle casualty survival with emergency tourniquet use to stop limb bleeding. *J Emerg Med.* 2011;41(6):590–7. doi:10.1016/j.jemermed.2009.07.022

Further reading

Baker DA, Keller AP IV, Knight RM, et al. Military medicine. In: Tintinalli JE, Ma O, Yealy DM, et al., eds. *Tintinalli's Emergency Medicine: A Comprehensive Study Guide, 9th ed.* McGraw-Hill; 2019:2007–2013.

Kucik CJ, Clenney T. Management of epistaxis. *Am Fam Physician.* 2005;71(2):305–311.

Wyler B, Valenzuela RG. Epistaxis. https://www.emrap.org/corependium/chapter/reczzsotcDtSSQEgw/Epistaxis

26 I'm bleeding!: Hemorrhagic resuscitation

Samantha Strickler

Medical command reports that a 26-year-old male was involved in a motorcycle accident and has a right lower extremity deformity. He was combative and is now intubated. His vital signs are HR 126 bpm, BP 84/47 mmHg, RR 26 breaths/min, SpO_2 94% after intubation. Medical command tells you, "Level 1 trauma alert, ETA 10 minutes."

On arrival, the paramedic reports that the patient was struck by a car and then thrown about 20 feet. He was wearing a helmet. He remains hypotensive and the paramedic tells you that his most recent vital signs were HR 132 bpm, RR 32 breaths/min, manual BP 92/52 mmHg, and SpO_2 96%. Glucose was 102 mg/ dL. EMS started two 18G IVs in the upper extremities, administered 600 mL lactated Ringer's, and placed a cervical collar. The patient's medical history is unknown.

Repeat vital signs are manual BP 76/42 mmHg, RR 16 breaths/min, HR 142 bpm, and SpO_2 98%. Intubation is confirmed with end-tidal capnography, and bilateral breath sounds are present. Radial pulses are palpable in the upper extremities. Pulses are palpable in the left lower extremity and right lower extremity pulses are faint with palpation. The patient localizes to painful stimuli in all extremities.

What do I do now?

U pon the arrival of any patient who has suffered trauma, the initial
evaluation follows the stepwise ATLS approach of examining and
stabilizing airway, breathing, circulation, and disability.[1] For this young
man, airway and breathing were controlled in the field with intubation and
reassessed upon arrival as being intact. Rapid evaluation of his circulation,
however, reveals several concerning findings: persistent tachycardia and hypotension, as well as diminished pulses in his right lower extremity.

These initial findings of persistent hypotension and tachycardia raise
immediate concern for shock, which is defined as a hemodynamic state
with inadequate tissue perfusion and oxygenation. In the setting of trauma,
patients can develop various and concomitant types of shock. Shock may be
distributive (i.e., neurogenic shock from spinal cord injury, sepsis), cardiogenic (i.e., cardiac contusion causing arrhythmia), obstructive (i.e., tension
pneumothorax, cardiac tamponade), and/or hypovolemic (i.e., acute blood
loss). Among the various types of shock in trauma, hypovolemic shock secondary to bleeding is the most common.[1]

ATLS suggests four physiologic classifications of hemorrhagic shock:[1]

Class 1 corresponds with an estimated blood loss (EBL) of <15%
(–750 mL for the average adult), which typically has very little
physiologic effect on HR, BP, pulse pressure, RR, urine output, or
Glasgow Coma Scale (GCS) score.
Class II (mild) corresponds with an EBL of 15% to 30% (750–1,000 mL),
and the patient may have elevated HR and decreased pulse
pressure.
Class III (moderate) corresponds to 30% to 40% EBL
(1,500–2,000 mL).
Class IV corresponds to >41% EBL (>2,000 mL).

Class III and IV are characterized as having more physiologic derangements,
including elevated HR, decreased BP, decreased pulse pressure, increased
RR, and depressed GCS score. When considering a patient with hemorrhagic shock, it may not be feasible to definitively assign a specific hemorrhagic class as individual physiology may vary (i.e., pregnancy, advanced
age, medication effects) and clinical status can change quickly.

Due to the morbidity and mortality associated with hemorrhagic shock,
rapid recognition is imperative. A high degree of suspicion should be

maintained for any patient presenting with a high-energy mechanism of injury, as in this situation. Consider hemorrhagic shock in any patient who has signs or symptoms of chest, abdomen, pelvis, or long bone trauma. During the primary survey, the focus should be on damage control resuscitation to treat and prevent worsening of the acute coagulopathy of trauma. The principle of damage control resuscitation focuses on (1) balanced resuscitation, (2) early administration of blood products, and (3) prevention of hypothermia (e.g., use of warmers, blankets, increased room temperature), metabolic acidosis, and hypocalcemia.[1-5] Balanced resuscitation calls for limited use of crystalloids and permissive hypotension, which is thought to limit clot disruption. The optimal BP goal during damage control resuscitation has yet to be defined and requires ongoing evaluation. However, in clinical practice a goal SBP of 80 to 100 mmHg is suggested in patients without traumatic brain injury (TBI). For patients with TBI, a higher SBP (>120 mmHg) is suggested.[6]

During the primary survey, adequate IV access for resuscitation is needed; two short and large-bore IVs should be placed as close to central circulation as possible to facilitate optimal flow and delivery.[7] Under ideal settings, at least two 18G IVs are placed in the bilateral antecubital fossas. At times, this may not always be feasible due to a patient's trauma injury complex, body habitus, or comorbidities. If difficulties arise with establishing IV access, an intraosseous access (IO) device should be placed as soon as possible in the proximal humerus or tibia.[8] Central venous catheters can be considered, with preference for a dialysis catheter or introducer over a triple-lumen catheter due to higher flow rates. These catheters are, however, often more time-consuming to place and generally do not provide better flow when compared to a short and wide centrally placed IV.[7]

In this patient, transfusion of blood products should occur immediately upon recognition of shock due to hemorrhage or if there is concern for uncontrollable bleeding with impending shock. Uncrossed O Rh-negative blood or whole blood is typically reserved in hospital settings for these situations. In the past decade, there have been several military studies suggesting decreased mortality with the use of uncrossed whole blood rather than individual blood components; however, there are limited data in the civilian population.[9-12] If time permits, cross-matched blood should be used. This resource can take >60 minutes to obtain from the blood bank and therefore may be most appropriate for patients with Class I or II hemorrhage.

There is ongoing debate about the ideal transfusion ratios used to treat hemorrhagic shock. Current research suggests high ratios of plasma, platelets, and RBCs to improve patient outcomes. In patients with active hemorrhage, research supports administration of blood products in a ratio of 1:1:1 or 1:1:2 (plasma:platelets:packed RBCs [PRBCs]).[13-15] In a patient such as this, who may be anticipated to require massive transfusion (>10 units PRBCs in 24 hours or >4 units in 1 hour), a massive transfusion protocol should be initiated. Massive transfusion protocols have been shown to reduce mortality, incidence of trauma-induced coagulopathy, and use of blood products.[5,15,16]

Recently, there has been a growing body of literature supporting frequent monitoring and aggressive repletion of calcium with transfusion of blood products. During transfusion of blood products, the citrate preservative added to blood binds calcium, decreasing its bioavailability. As calcium is involved in numerous physiologic processes, including the coagulation cascade and platelet activation, hypocalcemia (ionized Ca <1.12 mmol/L) can be detrimental to an individual with hemorrhagic shock.[17] Studies have demonstrated that hypocalcemia in trauma is associated with worsened coagulopathy and increased mortality.[18] Studies have also demonstrated that as the number of blood products administered increases, as does the risk of severe hypocalcemia (ionized Ca <0.90 mmol/L).[19] To date there are no established guidelines to recommend frequency of monitoring or replacement strategies for hypocalcemia associated with massive transfusion of blood products. However, based upon the current literature, it may be reasonable to consider administering 1 to 3 g calcium chloride or gluconate following 2 units PRBCs and to frequently monitor ionized Ca levels during resuscitation.

Rapid infusers and warmed blood should be utilized in the delivery of blood to a patient with hypovolemic shock. If not immediately available in the ED, many operating rooms utilize rapid infusers, which can be brought to the ED. Blood products can also be placed inside an IV pressure bag to enhance administration.[7]

During the initial evaluation of this patient, basic laboratory tests should be sent to guide ongoing resuscitation. Specific tests include a complete blood cell count (CBC), complete metabolic panel (CMP), magnesium, phosphorus, ionized calcium, pregnancy test (serum hCG), venous blood gas (VBG), lactic acid, urinalysis, toxicology screening, blood type, Rh status, cross-match and coagulation tests, including prothrombin time (PT), activated partial thromboplastin time (APTT), international normalized ratio (INR), and fibrinogen. In pregnant patients, fibrin degradation products in conjunction with fibrinogen levels should be assessed to evaluate for signs of disseminated intravascular coagulation (DIC) and associated placental abruption.[20] The Kleihauer–Betke (KB) test should be pursued in Rh-negative pregnant patients if there is a concern for placental abruption. The KB test assists with determining additional dosing of anti-D immune globulin. Depending upon availability, point-of-care tests such as VBG and thromboelastography (e.g., TEG, ROTEM) should also be considered. Utilization of thromboelastography provides insight into clot development, firmness, and fibrinolysis and therefore provides guidance for ongoing resuscitation with blood products.[21]

Tranexamic acid, an anti-fibrinolytic agent, can also be utilized to assist in the management of hemorrhagic shock due to trauma. When bleeding occurs the coagulation cascade is activated to form clot and is simultaneously stimulated to break down clot (fibrinolysis). During trauma, this physiologic process may become pathologic and result in hyper-fibrinolysis. Tranexamic acid inhibits fibrinolysis by competitively binding to plasminogen, preventing the formation of plasmin. Early administration of tranexamic acid (within 3 hours) to individuals with, or at risk of, significant bleeding has been shown to reduce mortality due to hemorrhagic shock as well as all-cause mortality with no apparent increase in vascular occlusive events.[22] Aminocaproic acid is another anti-fibrinolytic agent with the same mechanism of action as tranexamic acid, but its use has only been validated in ocular trauma.[23]

During damage control resuscitation, efforts must simultaneously and continuously focus on response to resuscitation and definitive treatment of traumatic hemorrhagic shock. In individuals who show ongoing signs of hemorrhagic shock despite transfusion of blood products and correction of coagulopathies, immediate intervention needs to be pursued either in the operating room, with a focus on damage control surgery, or in the interventional radiology suite (i.e., angioembolization). Occasionally, patients stabilize with damage control resuscitation and do not require further intervention. This group of patients, however, must be cautiously watched for new or ongoing signs of hemorrhagic shock (e.g., tachycardia, hypotension, elevation of lactic acid, urine output, alteration of mental status). If an individual is considered to be at risk of ongoing bleeding, frequent monitoring of labs (i.e., hemoglobin, platelets, INR, fibrinogen, and lactic acid every 1–6 hours) and ongoing reevaluation (i.e., every 30 minutes) should be considered. In actively bleeding individuals, practitioners strive for hemoglobin >7 g, platelets >50,000, INR <1.8 to 2.0, fibrinogen >150 mg/dL, and lactic acid <2.0 mEq/L.

Depending upon local resource availability, individuals who have experienced significant trauma and/or have ongoing signs of hemorrhagic shock may require transfer to a trauma center for definitive treatment. Transfers should be initiated early during the initial resuscitation in order to optimize patient outcomes. While arrangements are made for transfer, damage control resuscitation should be aggressively continued in order to address ongoing physiologic derangements resulting from hemorrhagic shock.

KEY POINTS TO REMEMBER

- Rapid recognition of hemorrhagic shock is imperative. Two short and large-bore IVs should be placed as close to central circulation as possible for resuscitation of hemorrhagic shock.
- Damage control resuscitation includes (1) balanced resuscitation, (2) early administration of blood products, and (3) prevention of hypothermia, metabolic acidosis, and hypocalcemia.
- Current research suggests high ratios of plasma, platelets, and RBCs (1:1:1 or 1:1:2) in transfusions to improve patient mortality.
- Massive transfusion protocols have been shown to reduce mortality, incidence of trauma-induced coagulopathy, and use of blood products.
- Use of tranexamic acid can reduce mortality in patients with or at risk of significant hemorrhage when administered early in resuscitation (<3 hours from presentation).

- Definitive treatment of hemorrhagic shock may include going to the operating room for damage control surgery, going to the interventional radiology suite for angioembolization, or transfer to a trauma center for a higher level of care.

References

1. American College of Surgeons. *Advanced Trauma Life Support: Student Course Manual.* 10th ed. American College of Surgeons; 2018.

2. Holcomb JB, Jenkins D, Rhee P, et al. Damage control resuscitation: Directly addressing the early coagulopathy of trauma. *J Trauma.* 2007;62(2):307–310.

3. Duchesne JC, Mc Swain NE, Cotton BA, et al. Damage control resuscitation: The new face of damage control. *J Trauma.* 2010;69(4):976–990.

4. Shrestha B, Holcomb JB, Camp EA, et al. Damage-control resuscitation increases successful nonoperative management rates and survival after severe blunt liver injury. *J Trauma Acute Care Surg.* 2015;78(2):336–341.

5. Mizobata Y. Damage control resuscitation: A practical approach for severely hemorrhagic patients and its effects on trauma surgery. *J Intensive Care.* 2017;5(1):4.

6. Bouglé A, Harrois A, Duranteau J. Resuscitative strategies in traumatic hemorrhagic shock. *Ann Intensive Care.* 2013;3(1):1.

7. Reddick AD, Ronald J, Morrison WJ. Intravenous fluid resuscitation: Was Poiseuille right? *Emerg Med J.* 2011;28(3):201–202.

8. Ngo AS, Oh JJ, Chen Y, Yong D, Ong ME. Intraosseous vascular access in adults using the EZ-IO in an emergency department. *Int J Emerg Med.* 2009;2(3):155–160.

9. Spinella PC, Perkins JG, Grathwohl KW, Beekley AC, Holcomb JB. Warm fresh whole blood is independently associated with improved survival for patients with combat-related traumatic injuries. *J Trauma.* 2009;6(Suppl 4):S69–S76.

10. Perkins JG, Cap AP, Spinella PC, et al. Comparison of platelet transfusion as fresh whole blood versus apheresis platelets for massively transfused combat trauma patients. *Transfusion.* 2011;51(2):242–252.

11. Nessen SC, Eastridge BJ, Cronk D, et al. Fresh whole blood use by forward surgical teams in Afghanistan is associated with improved survival compared to component therapy without platelets. *Transfusion.* 2013;53:107S–113S.

12. Gallaher J, Robert J, Dixon A, et al. Large volume transfusion with whole blood is safe compared with component therapy. *J Trauma Acute Care Surg.* 2020;89(1):238–245.

13. Holcomb JB, Tilley BC, Baraniuk S, et al. Transfusion of plasma, platelets, and red blood cells in a 1:1:1 vs a 1:1:2 ratio and mortality in patients with severe trauma: The PROPPR randomized clinical trial. *JAMA.* 2015;313(5):471–482.

14. Holcomb JB, del Junco DJ, Fox EE, et al. The Prospective, Observational, Multicenter, Major Trauma Transfusion (PROMMTT) study: Comparative effectiveness of a time-varying treatment with competing risks. *JAMA Surg*. 2013;148(2):127–136.

15. Murphy CH, Hess JR. Massive transfusion: Red blood cell to plasma and platelet unit ratios for resuscitation of massive hemorrhage. *Curr Opin Hematol*. 2015;22(6):533–539.

16. Meneses E, Boneva D, McKenney M, Elkbuli A. Massive transfusion protocol in adult trauma population. *Am J Emerg Med*. 2020;38(12):2661–2666.

17. Lier H, Krep H, Schroeder S, Stuber F. Preconditions of hemostasis in trauma: A review. *J Trauma Injury Infect Crit Care*. 2008;65:951–960.

18. Giancarelli A, Birrer KL, Alban RF, et al. Hypocalcemia in trauma patients receiving massive transfusion. *J Surg Res*. 2016;202:182–187.

19. Hall C, Nagengast AK, Knapp C, et al. Massive transfusions and severe hypocalcemia: An opportunity for monitoring and supplementation guidelines. *Transfusion*. 2021;61:S188–S194.

20. Huls CK, Detlefs C. Trauma in pregnancy. *Semin Perinatol*. 2018;42(1):13–20.

21. Whiting D, DiNardo J. TEG and ROTEM: Technology and clinical applications. *Am J Hematol*. 2014;89:228–232.

22. CRASH-2 trial collaborators. Effects of tranexamic acid on death, vascular occlusive events, and blood transfusion in trauma patients with significant haemorrhage (CRASH-2): A randomised, placebo-controlled trial. *Lancet*. 2010;376(9734):23–32.

23. Crouch ER, Williams PB, Gray MK, Crouch ER, Chames M. Topical aminocaproic acid in the treatment of traumatic hyphema. *Arch Ophthalmol*. 1997;115(9):1106–1112.

Further reading

Huls CK, Detlefs C. Trauma in pregnancy. *Semin Perinatol*. 2018;42(1):13–20.

Mizobata Y. Damage control resuscitation: A practical approach for severely hemorrhagic patients and its effects on trauma surgery. *J Intensive Care*. 2017;5(1):4.

Whiting D, DiNardo J. TEG and ROTEM: Technology and clinical applications. *Am J Hematol*. 2014;89:228–232.

27 Reversal agents: Antidotes for anticoagulants

Jessica Downing, Meaghan Keville, and Daniel Haase

A 63-year-old female is brought to the ED by EMS after a fall. Arrival vital signs are BP 155/70 mmHg, temperature 37.1°C, HR 85 bpm and irregular, RR 14 breaths/min. Her husband reports they had "a couple of cocktails" this evening and she tripped and fell down "three or four stairs" and struck her head. She notes a past medical history of hysterectomy and "irregular heartbeat" for which she takes "a rhythm medicine" and "a blood thinner." On exam she is noted to have a large frontal cephalohematoma with overlying laceration that continues to ooze. She opens her eyes to verbal command and is confused, with slurred speech. She localizes to pain with bilateral upper extremities. CT scan demonstrates a large left subdural hematoma with 2 mm of midline shift. Your hospital has no neurosurgeon and the nearest hospital with neurosurgical capability is an hour away by ground transportation.

What do I do now?

E mergency management of the hemorrhaging patient with anticoagulant-induced coagulopathy medications is becoming increasingly complex with the introduction of various direct-acting oral anticoagulant (DOAC) agents. In recent years, DOACs such as dabigatran (a direct thrombin inhibitor) and rivaroxaban, apixaban, and edoxaban (factor Xa inhibitors, sometimes referred to as "xabans") have demonstrated improved safety in comparison to vitamin K antagonists (such as warfarin). However, detecting the presence, type, or therapeutic effect of DOACs is challenging.

There are many limitations to current laboratory testing options. Direct measurements of drug concentrations in the bloodstream are possible; however, they are typically only utilized for research purposes and are not clinically feasible at most hospitals. Assays including activated partial thromboplastin time (aPTT), prothrombin time (PT), and international normalized ratio (INR) may indicate the presence of direct thrombin inhibitors or factor Xa inhibitors but are neither sensitive nor specific for DOACs.[1-4] Thrombin time (TT), dilute thrombin time (dTT), and ecarin clotting time (ECT) are more sensitive for dabigatran, and normal values likely exclude therapeutic activity.[5-7] Anti-factor Xa (anti-Xa) activity has a linear response to increasing concentrations of rivaroxaban, apixaban, and edoxaban.[8] Many hospitals cannot perform this testing or have inadequate turnaround time for acute management. Utilizing anti-Xa testing calibrated to unfractionated heparin (UH) or low-molecular-weight heparin (LMWH) can be an acceptable alternative, as activity below the detection limit reliably excludes "xaban"-associated anticoagulation.[6]

Rapid and reliable point-of-care information capable of guiding emergent care is not widely available. Current research involves evaluations of TEG,[1,9] ROTEM,[10] and direct concentration assays[11] to fill this gap. Increased clot formation time (R time) has been noted as a sensitive indicator to the presence of DOAC activity.[1,12] However, further research is needed to validate this application of these tests in clinical practice.[1]

Delaying antidote administration until test results are available may be detrimental to patient outcomes.[2] Determining the last dose of DOAC administration is critical to determining treatment (Table 27.1). If a patient's creatinine clearance (CrCl) is normal (>60 mL/min), the half-life of any DOAC will be no longer than 12 hours and no antidote is likely necessary if

TABLE 27.1 Current DOAC-associated laboratory findings simplified to demonstrate understood effect on lab test at normal therapeutic dose

Drug	PT, INR	aPTT	TT, dTT, ECT	TEG, ROTEM	Anti-Xa
Dabigatran	No effect	May be elevated	Elevated	R time may be increased	No effect
Apixaban, rivaroxaban, edoxaban	May be elevated	May be elevated	No effect	R time may be increased	Elevated

Data from reference 13.

the last dose was taken >24 hours prior.[2] In patients without normal CrCl, drug half-life can be as long as 48 hours and clearance is less predictable.[3]

Source control is a first priority for any patient with major bleeding while on anticoagulation; those with sources that are not easily controlled should be emergently evaluated for endoscopic, endovascular, or surgical control, even if patients remain coagulopathic.[14] Reversal agents should be administered prior to invasive procedures. Patients presenting with a DOAC overdose without any clinical evidence of significant bleeding should not be treated routinely with reversal agents.[15]

If a patient presents within 2 to 4 hours of their last dose, activated charcoal (50 g enterally) should be considered.[14,16–18] Next steps depend on the type of DOAC the patient is taking, as well as the dose and time of most recent administration (Table 27.2).

Idarucizumab and andexanet alfa are designed as rapid-acting antidotes to DOACs—idarucizumab for dabigatran and andexanet alfa for factor Xa inhibitors.[14] Much like DOACs themselves, both reversal agents are relatively new and there is limited evidence to support their use. Both are recommended as first-line agents for the reversal of major or life-threatening bleeding associated with their respective DOACs.[14,15,17,19,20]

Idarucizumab is a monoclonal antibody that binds directly to dabigatran and its metabolites with a higher affinity than thrombin and irreversibly inhibits them.[14,19,22,23] Its effectiveness is dependent on the relative concentrations of both dabigatran and idarucizumab.[19] Because dabigatran is renally excreted and has a much longer half-life than its reversal agent,

TABLE 27.2 **Reversal strategies for patients taking DOACs who present with major or life-threatening hemorrhage**

Class	Direct thrombin inhibitor	Direct factor Xa inhibitor	
Drug	Dabigatran	Apixaban	Rivaroxaban
Last dose	<8–12h	8–18 hours OR ≤5 mg <8 hours or unknown time AND >5 mg	8–18 hours OR ≤10 mg <8 hours or unknown time AND >10 mg	
First-line agent	Idarucizumab, 50-g IV bolus	Andexanet alfa, 400-mg IV bolus over 30 min, then 4 mg/min gtt × 120 min Andexanet alfa, 800-mg IV bolus over 30 min, then 8 mg/min gtt × 120 min	Andexanet alfa, 400-mg IV bolus over 30 min, then 4 mg/min gtt × 120 min Andexanet alfa, 800-mg IV bolus over 30 min, then 8 mg/min gtt × 120 min	
Second-line agent	· aPCC, 25–50 units/kg · Four-factor PCC, 2,000 units · Dialysis	· Four-factor PCC, 2,000 units · aPCC, 25–50 units/kg · Four-factor PCC, 2,000 units · aPCC, 25–50 units/kg	· Four-factor PCC, 2,000 units · aPCC, 25–50 units/kg · Four-factor PCC, 2,000 units · aPCC, 25–50 units/kg	
Consider		Activated charcoal 50 g PO if last dose was <4 hours ago		

Data from references 14–23,25,30,36,37,49–51.

special care must be taken to monitor for "rebound" effect or coagulopathy after reversal.[16,20,23-25]

The RE-VERSE AD trial was a prospective, industry-sponsored cohort study that demonstrated idarucizumab was successful in correcting diluted thrombin time or ecarin clotting time in 98% of patients and in achieving hemostasis in 67.7% of patients with life-threatening bleeds, though patients with intracranial hemorrhage were excluded.[21] The risk of thrombosis with idarucizumab was reported at 6.3%. A subgroup analysis demonstrated safety and efficacy (normal hemostasis in >90%) in patients requiring reversal for urgent (<4h from reversal) surgery.[26] The findings of the RE-VERSE AD trial were larely echoed by a post-approval retrospective surveillance study (RE-VECTO) examining global use of and outcomes associated with idarucizumab.[27] Subsequent observational studies have reported success with few side effects in the use of idarucizumab for AC reversal in patients with trauma, including traumatic intracranial hemorrhage.[28]

Andexanet alfa is a recombinant human factor Xa that competitively binds to the factor Xa inhibitor at its active site with approximately the same affinity as factor Xa.[14,19,22] Unlike idarucizumab, andexanet does not permanently inactivate the receptors it binds to; it is only effective while it is taking up the active site. Because the half-life of andexanet alfa is ~1 hour, it is given as a loading dose followed by an infusion, with exact dosing dependent on the dose of factor Xa inhibitor taken and time since last dose. Although andexanet alfa is expected to interact similarly with all factor Xa inhibitors, the majority of the evidence to date has been in regard to apixaban and rivaroxaban.[29]

The ANNEXA-4 trial suggested that andexanet alfa achieved adequate hemostasis in 82% of patients.[30] A subgroup analysis of patients with traumatic or spontaneous ICH demonstrated hemostasis in 79% and 83%, respectively, after treatment with andexanet alfa.[31] Subsequent studies have shown similar effects among patients with intracranial hemorrhage specifically.[32] The associated risk of thrombosis is ~10%.[30]

If the appropriate direct reversal agent (idarucizumab or andexanet alfa) is unavailable, experts recommend treatment with four-factor prothrombin complex concentrate (PCC) or activated prothrombin complex concentrate (aPCC) in hopes of overwhelming the DOAC and lessening its resultant coagulopathy.[14,15] Four-factor PCC includes inactivated versions of all vitamin K–dependent factors, three-factor PCC includes only factors II, IX, and X, and aPCC contains activated factor VII and inactive II, IX, and X. Four-factor PCC is preferred over three-factor PCC for DOAC reversal.[14] The Anticoagulation Forum specifically recommends aPCC for reversal of dabigatran and four-factor PCC for reversal of factor Xa inhibitors, though both should be considered reasonable options if availability is limited.[16] Fresh frozen plasma (FFP) is not recommended due to its relatively low dose of factor X.[18,19,34] The recommended doses for both four-factor PCC and aPCC are weight-based, but some institutions have implemented a fixed-dose approach to minimize time and error during emergent preparation. Neither are FDA approved for DOAC reversal, though it is a common off-label use for both and is supported by many guidelines.[18]

There is currently no head-to-head comparison of idarucizumab or andexanet alfa to PCC or other reversal strategies, though randomized controlled trials are currently under way.[33] Evidence on the effectiveness of 4PCC has been mixed. [33–38] Studies comparing 4PCC and andexanet alfa are primarily observational; some have shown similar outcomes across reversal agents (in all major bleeding[39–41] and patients with ICH[38,42–44] specifically), while others have demonstrated improved outcomes with andexanet alfa in patients on direct Xa inhibitors.[45–48] Although several society guidelines recommend idarucizumab and andexanet alfa as first-line agents in the reversal of DOAC-associated hemorrhage, ongoing research is necessary.

Dabigatran can be effectively removed from the serum via hemodialysis or continuous renal replacement therapy (CRRT), though a prolonged session (>2 hours) will likely be required.[14,19,30,50,51] This approach is not recommended when other treatments (reversal agents or PCC) are available, given the risks of bleeding associated with placement of a hemodialysis catheter.[16] Apixaban and rivaroxaban are not dialyzable.[30]

KEY POINTS TO REMEMBER

· There are significant limitations in testing for DOAC activity in the emergent setting: Elevated PT, PTT, and INR values can be helpful in suggesting the presence of coagulopathy but are nonspecific to DOACs.

- Advanced coagulation testing (TT, dTT, and anti-Xa) is more helpful in excluding therapeutic levels of DOACs when levels are normal, but these tests are not widely available.
- Viscoelastic testing (e.g., TEG) suggests that prolonged clot formation (R) time should increase suspicion of DOAC activity, but further clinical research is needed.
- Timing of last known dose and expected half-life based on renal function should be used to guide reversal.
- Enteral administration of activated charcoal can reduce absorption of DOACs if taken within 2 to 4 hours of the last dose.
- The first-line reversal agents for life-threatening bleeding on a DOAC are idarucizumab for dabigatran and andexanet alfa for factor Xa inhibitors (apixaban and rivaroxaban).
- When first-line agents are not available, PCC should be used, ideally aPCC for patients on dabigatran and four-factor PCC for patients on factor Xa inhibitors.
- Dabigatran can be removed through prolonged hemodialysis. Apixaban and rivaroxaban are not dialyzable.

References

1. Dias JD, Lopez-Espina CG, Ippolito J, et al. Rapid point-of-care detection and classification of direct-acting oral anticoagulants with the TEG 6s: Implications for trauma and acute care surgery. *J Trauma Acute Care Surg*. 2019;87(2):364–370.
2. Levy JH, Ageno W, Chan NC, Crowther M, Verhamme P, Weitz JI. When and how to use antidotes for the reversal of direct oral anticoagulants: Guidance from the SSC of the ISTH. *J Thromb Haemost*. 2016;14(3):623–627.
3. Lutz J, Jurk K, Schinzel H. Direct oral anticoagulants in patients with chronic kidney disease: Patient selection and special considerations. *Int J Nephrol Renovasc Dis*. 2017;10:135–143.
4. Ebner M, Birschmann I, Peter A, et al. Emergency coagulation assessment during treatment with direct oral anticoagulants: Limitations and solutions. *Stroke*. 2017;48(9):2457–2463.
5. Peacock WF, Rafique Z, Singer AJ. Direct-acting oral anticoagulants: Practical considerations for emergency medicine physicians. *Emerg Med Int*. 2016;2016:1781684.
6. Wiegele M, Schöchl H, Haushofer A, et al. Diagnostic and therapeutic approach in adult patients with traumatic brain injury receiving oral anticoagulant therapy: An Austrian interdisciplinary consensus statement. *Crit Care*. 2019;23(1):62.

7. van Ryn J, Stangier J, Haertter S, et al. Dabigatran etexilate—a novel, reversible, oral direct thrombin inhibitor: Interpretation of coagulation assays and reversal of anticoagulant activity. *Thromb Haemost*. 2010;103(6):1116–1127.

8. Dale BJ, Chan NC, Eikelboom JW. Laboratory measurement of the direct oral anticoagulants. *Br J Haematol*. 2016;172(3):315–336.

9. Artang R, Anderson M, Nielsen JD. Fully automated thromboelastograph TEG 6s to measure anticoagulant effects of direct oral anticoagulants in healthy male volunteers. *Res Pract Thromb Haemost*. 2019;3(3):391–396.

10. Henskens YMC, Gulpen AJW, van Oerle R, et al. Detecting clinically relevant rivaroxaban or dabigatran levels by routine coagulation tests or thromboelastography in a cohort of patients with atrial fibrillation. *Thromb J*. 2018;16:3.

11. Ebner M, Birschmann I, Peter A, et al. Point-of-care testing for emergency assessment of coagulation in patients treated with direct oral anticoagulants. *Crit Care*. 2017;21(1):32.

12. Kopytek M, Zabczyk M, Natorska J, Malinowski KP, Undas A. Effects of direct oral anticoagulants on thromboelastographic parameters and fibrin clot properties in patients with venous thromboembolism. *J Physiol Pharmacol*. 2020;71(1). Epub April 27, 2020.

13. Pollack CV. Coagulation assessment with the new generation of oral anticoagulants. *Emerg Med J*. 2016;33(6):423–430.

14. Baugh CW, Levine M, Cornutt D, et al. Anticoagulant reversal strategies in the emergency department setting: Recommendations of a multidisciplinary expert panel. *Ann Emerg Med*. 2020;76(4):470–485.

15. Cuker A, Burnett A, Triller D, et al. Reversal of direct oral anticoagulants: Guidance from the Anticoagulation Forum. *Am J Hematol*. 2019;94(6):697–709.

16. Grandhi R, Newman WC, Zhang X, et al. Administration of 4-factor prothrombin complex concentrate as an antidote for intracranial bleeding in patients taking direct factor Xa inhibitors. *World Neurosurg*. 2015;84(6):1956–1961.

17. Kaatz S, Kouides PA, Garcia DA, et al. Guidance on the emergent reversal of oral thrombin and factor Xa inhibitors [published correction appears in *Am J Hematol*. 2012 Jul;87(7):748]. *Am J Hematol*. 2012;87(Suppl 1):S141–S145.

18. Frontera JA, Lewin JJ 3rd, Rabinstein AA, et al. Guideline for reversal of antithrombotics in intracranial hemorrhage: A statement for healthcare professionals from the Neurocritical Care Society and Society of Critical Care Medicine. *Neurocrit Care*. 2016;24(1):6–46.

19. Alikhan R, Rayment R, Keeling D, et al. The acute management of haemorrhage, surgery and overdose in patients receiving dabigatran. *Emerg Med J*. 2014;31(2):163–168.

20. Kustos SA, Fasinu PS. Direct-acting oral anticoagulants and their reversal agents: An update. *Medicines*. 2019;6(4):103.

21. Tomaselli GF, Mahaffey KW, Cuker A, et al. 2017 ACC Expert Consensus Decision Pathway on management of bleeding in patients on oral anticoagulants: A report of the American College of Cardiology Task Force on Expert Consensus Decision Pathways. *J Am Coll Cardiol*. 2017;70(24):3042–3067.

22. Pollack CV Jr, Reilly PA, van Ryn J, et al. Idarucizumab for dabigatran reversal— full cohort analysis. *N Engl J Med*. 2017;377(5):431–441.

23. Levy JH, Ageno W, Chan NC, et al. When and how to use antidotes for the reversal of direct oral anticoagulants: Guidance from the SSC of the ISTH. *J Thromb Haemost*. 2016;14(3):623–627.

24. Simon A, Domanovits H, Ay C, Sengoelge G, Levy JH, Spiel AO. The recommended dose of idarucizumab may not always be sufficient for sustained reversal of dabigatran. *J Thromb Haemost*. 2017;15(7):1317–1321.

25. Glund S, Moschetti V, Norris S, et al. A randomised study in healthy volunteers to investigate the safety, tolerability and pharmacokinetics of idarucizumab, a specific antidote to dabigatran. *Thromb Haemost*. 2015;113(5):943–951.

26. Levy JH, van Ryn J, Sellke FW, Reilly PA, Elsaesser A, Glund S, Kreuzer J, Weitz JI, Pollack CV Jr. Dabigatran reversal with Idarucizumab in patients requiring urgent surgery: A subanalysis of the RE-VERSE AD Study. *Ann Surg*. 2021 Sep 1;274(3):e204–e211. doi:10.1097/SLA.0000000000003638. PMID: 31599808.

27. Fanikos J, Murwin D, Gruenenfelder F, Tartakovsky I, França LR, Reilly PA, Kermer P, Wowern FV, Lane DA, Butcher K. Global use of Idarucizumab in clinical practice: Outcomes of the RE-VECTO Surveillance Program. *Thromb Haemost*. 2020 Jan;120(1):27–35. doi:10.1055/s-0039-1695771. Epub 2019 Aug 30. PMID: 31470445.

28. Oberladstätter D, Voelckel W, Bruckbauer M, Zipperle J, Grottke O, Ziegler B, Schöchl H. Idarucizumab in major trauma patients: A single centre real life experience. *Eur J Trauma Emerg Surg*. 2021 Apr;47(2):589–595. doi:10.1007/s00068-019-01233-y. Epub 2019 Sep 25. PMID: 31555877.

29. Benz AP, Xu L, Eikelboom JW, Middeldorp S, Milling TJ Jr, Crowther M, Yue P, Conley P, Lu G, Connolly SJ; ANNEXA-4 Investigators. Andexanet alfa for specific anticoagulation reversal in patients with acute bleeding during treatment with Edoxaban. *Thromb Haemost*. 2022 Jun;122(6):998–1005. doi:10.1055/s-0041-1740180. Epub 2022 Jan 7. PMID: 34996121; PMCID: PMC9251710.

30. Vílchez JA, Gallego P, Lip GY. Safety of new oral anticoagulant drugs: A perspective. *Ther Adv Drug Saf*. 2014;5(1):8–20.

31. Demchuk AM, Yue P, Zotova E, Nakamya J, Xu L, Milling TJ Jr, Ohara T, Goldstein JN, Middeldorp S, Verhamme P, Lopez-Sendon JL, Conley PB, Curnutte JT, Eikelboom JW, Crowther M, Connolly SJ; ANNEXA-4 Investigators. Hemostatic efficacy and Anti-FXa (Factor Xa) reversal with andexanet alfa in intracranial hemorrhage: ANNEXA-4 Substudy. *Stroke*. 2021 Jun;52(6):2096–2105. doi:10.1161/STROKEAHA.120.030565. Epub 2021 May 10. Erratum in: Stroke. 2021 Aug;52(8):e525. PMID: 33966491; PMCID: PMC8140631.

32. Connolly SJ, Crowther M, Eikelboom JW, et al. Full study report of andexanet alfa for bleeding associated with factor xa inhibitors. *N Engl J Med.* 2019;380(14):1326–1335.

33. Brown CS, Scott RA, Sridharan M, Rabinstein AA. Real-world utilization of andexanet alfa. *Am J Emerg Med.* 2020;38(4):810–814.

34. Panos NG, Cook AM, John S, Jones GM; Neurocritical Care Society (NCS) Pharmacy Study Group. Factor Xa inhibitor-related intracranial hemorrhage: Results from a multicenter, observational cohort receiving prothrombin complex concentrates. *Circulation.* 2020;141(21):1681–1689.

35. Schulman S, Gross PL, Ritchie B, et al. Prothrombin complex concentrate for major bleeding on factor Xa inhibitors: A prospective cohort study [published correction appears in Thromb Haemost. 2018 Dec;118(12):2188]. *Thromb Haemost.* 2018;118(5):842–851.

36. Majeed A, Ågren A, Holmström M, et al. Management of rivaroxaban- or apixaban-associated major bleeding with prothrombin complex concentrates: A cohort study. *Blood.* 2017;130(15):1706–1712.

37. Berger K, Santibañez M, Lin L, Lesch CA. A low-dose 4F-PCC protocol for DOAC-associated intracranial hemorrhage. *J Intensive Care Med.* 2020;35(11):1203–1208.

38. Gerner ST, Kuramatsu JB, Sembill JA, et al. Association of prothrombin complex concentrate administration and hematoma enlargement in non-vitamin K antagonist oral anticoagulant-related intracerebral hemorrhage. *Ann Neurol.* 2018;83(1):186–196.

39. Gómez-Outes A, Alcubilla P, Calvo-Rojas G, Terleira-Fernández AI, Suárez-Gea ML, Lecumberri R, Vargas-Castrillón E. Meta-analysis of reversal agents for severe bleeding associated with direct oral anticoagulants. *J Am Coll Cardiol.* 2021 Jun 22;*77*(24):2987–3001. doi:10.1016/j.jacc.2021.04.061. PMID: 34140101.

40. Chaudhary R, Singh A, Chaudhary R, Bashline M, Houghton DE, Rabinstein A, Adamski J, Arndt R, Ou NN, Rudis MI, Brown CS, Wieruszewski ED, Wanek M, Brinkman NJ, Linderbaum JA, Sorenson MA, Atkinson JL, Thompson KM, Aiyer AN, McBane RD 2nd. Evaluation of direct oral anticoagulant reversal agents in intracranial hemorrhage: A systematic review and meta-analysis. *JAMA Netw Open.* 2022 Nov 1;*5*(11):e2240145. doi:10.1001/jamanetworkopen.2022.40145. PMID: 36331504; PMCID: PMC9636520.

41. Nederpelt CJ, Naar L, Krijnen P, le Cessie S, Kaafarani HMA, Huisman MV, Velmahos GC, Schipper IB. Andexanet alfa or prothrombin complex concentrate for factor Xa inhibitor reversal in acute major bleeding: A systematic review and meta-analysis. *Crit Care Med.* 2021 Oct 1;49(10):e1025–e1036. doi:10.1097/ CCM.0000000000005059. PMID: 33967205.

42. Ammar AA, Ammar MA, Owusu KA, Brown SC, Kaddouh F, Elsamadicy AA, Acosta JN, Falcone GJ. Andexanet alfa versus 4-factor prothrombin complex concentrate for reversal of factor Xa inhibitors in intracranial hemorrhage.

Neurocrit Care. 2021 Aug;35(1):255–261. doi:10.1007/s12028-020-01161-5. Epub 2021 Jan 6. PMID: 33403588.

43. Pham H, Medford WG, Horst S, Levesque M, Ragoonanan D, Price C, Colbassani H, Piper K, Chastain K. Andexanet alfa versus four-factor prothrombin complex concentrate for the reversal of apixaban- or rivaroxaban-associated intracranial hemorrhages. *Am J Emerg Med*. 2022 May;*55*:38–44. doi:10.1016/j.ajem.2022.02.029. Epub 2022 Feb 24. PMID: 35272069.

44. Parsels KA, Seabury RW, Zyck S, Miller CD, Krishnamurthy S, Darko W, Probst LA, Latorre JG, Cwikla GM, Feldman EA. Andexanet alfa effectiveness and safety versus four-factor prothrombin complex concentrate (4F-PCC) in intracranial hemorrhage while on apixaban or rivaroxaban: A single-center, retrospective, matched cohort analysis. *Am J Emerg Med*. 2022 May;*55*:16–19. doi:10.1016/j.ajem.2022.02.036. Epub 2022 Feb 24. PMID: 35245776.

45. Barra ME, Das AS, Hayes BD, Rosenthal ES, Rosovsky RP, Fuh L, Patel AB, Goldstein JN, Roberts RJ. Evaluation of andexanet alfa and four-factor prothrombin complex concentrate (4F-PCC) for reversal of rivaroxaban- and apixaban-associated intracranial hemorrhages. *J Thromb Haemost*. 2020 Jul;*18*(7):1637–1647. doi:10.1111/jth.14838. Epub 2020 May 12. PMID: 32291874.

46. Vestal ML, Hodulik K, Mando-Vandrick J, James ML, Ortel TL, Fuller M, Notini M, Friedland M, Welsby IJ. Andexanet alfa and four-factor prothrombin complex concentrate for reversal of apixaban and rivaroxaban in patients diagnosed with intracranial hemorrhage. *J Thromb Thrombolysis*. 2022 Jan;*53*(1):167–175. doi:10.1007/s11239-021-02495-3. Epub 2021 Jun 8. PMID: 34101050.

47. Costa OS, Connolly SJ, Sharma M, Beyer-Westendorf J, Christoph MJ, Lovelace B, Coleman CI. Andexanet alfa versus four-factor prothrombin complex concentrate for the reversal of apixaban- or rivaroxaban-associated intracranial hemorrhage: A propensity score-overlap weighted analysis. Crit Care. 2022 Jun 16;26(1):180. doi:10.1186/s13054-022-04043-8. PMID: 35710578; PMCID: PMC9204964.

48. Cohen AT, Lewis M, Connor A, Connolly SJ, Yue P, Curnutte J, Alikhan R, MacCallum P, Tan J, Green L. Thirty-day mortality with andexanet alfa compared with prothrombin complex concentrate therapy for life-threatening direct oral anticoagulant-related bleeding. *J Am Coll Emerg Physicians Open*. 2022 Mar 5;3(2):e12655. doi:10.1002/emp2.12655. PMID: 35280921; PMCID: PMC8898077.

49. Kcentra® [package insert]. CSL Behring, Marburg, Germany; 2013. http://www.kcentra.com/docs/Kcentra_Prescribing_Information.pdf

50. Chang DN, Dager WE, Chin AI. Removal of dabigatran by hemodialysis. *Am J Kidney Dis*. 2013;61(3):487–489.

51. Peacock WF, Rafique Z, Singer AJ. Direct-acting oral anticoagulants: Practical considerations for emergency medicine physicians. *Emerg Med Int*. 2016;2016:1781684.

28 Blood from both ends: GI bleeding

Maura W. Walsh and Brian T. Wessman

A 48-year-old man presents to the ED with vomiting for 2 days. He describes the emesis as dark black and believes his stools are looking darker as well. He endorses generalized weakness, feeling lightheaded, and a poor appetite. He denies any past medical history. His wife provides additional information, including that the patient is a heavy daily drinker who does not like to frequent the doctor's office. His last drink was 2 days ago when the vomiting began. Occasionally he takes ibuprofen for musculoskeletal back pain and does not take any other daily medications. HR is 92 bpm with sinus rhythm on the bedside monitor. BP is 96/78 mmHg. He is afebrile with 95% oxygen saturation on room air. No physical abnormalities are noted on cardiac and pulmonary exams. Examination is notable for dark reddish-brown emesis in a basin he holds, but he is not currently vomiting. His abdomen is distended with a shifting fluid wave and is mildly tender to palpation, with large visible veins. He denies rebound tenderness. The patient reports his last bowel movement was while in the ED waiting room. A bedside rectal exam shows evidence of dark tarry stool around his anus (guaiac positive) with intact rectal tone. The rest of his exam is unremarkable.

What do I do now?

G I bleeding is a common ED complaint, accounting for >800,000 visits per year and >500,000 admissions.[1] As with any patient in the ED, it is important to assess the patient's stability, looking for cardiac dysrhythmias, BP abnormalities, and potential airway compromise. While tachycardia and hypotension can be poor prognostic signs for a severe GI bleed, they are nonspecific and can be misleading (e.g., a patient on a beta-blocker or a young patient with compensated shock). Key information will often be gathered from the history or by questioning corroborators.

GI bleeding can be categorized into two categories depending on the anatomic location of the bleeding source: upper or lower. For either, obtaining large-bore IV access (at least two 18G IVs in large veins like the antecubital fossa) is a critical first action to provide resuscitation as necessary. Early IV access also facilitates efficient laboratory evaluation, which includes coagulation studies, complete blood count, type and cross, and a chemistry panel. The bedside clinician should have a low threshold to request that matched blood be prepared at this time (a rate-limiting step at many institutions). In the hemodynamically unstable patient with concern for an acute GI bleed, crystalloid volume expanders or emergent uncross-matched blood can be initiated emergently. A blood urea nitrogen to creatine (BUN:Cr) ratio of >30 can be associated with upper GI bleeding.[2] It is important to note that the initial hemoglobin may be normal in an actively bleeding patient. Conversely, chronic GI bleeding can lead to hemodynamically stable patients on initial presentation who are found to have very low hemoglobin levels on laboratory evaluation. The accepted transfusion threshold is 7.0 g/dL in stable patients as more aggressive transfusion thresholds have been associated with higher mortality.[3] Another early goal in treatment management is the correction of coagulopathy and avoidance of thrombocytopenia (platelet counts <50K). Early use of fresh frozen plasma, cryoprecipitate, and protein complex concentrate (PCC) as well as platelet transfusion should be considered. Also consider chronic anticoagulant and antiplatelet usage; review the home medication list with the patient. Anticoagulation reversal agents may need to be administered early in the hospital course. Again, an early type and cross-matched blood sample becomes lifesaving for the presumed GI bleeding patient whose initial condition is stable but who subsequently decompensates in the ED.

After the patient is stabilized, it is important to determine if it is an upper or lower GI bleed, as defined by the anatomic location relative to the suspensory ligament of the duodenum (the ligament of Treitz). This step is important as it determines treatment in the ED, disposition, and subsequent management by gastroenterologists.

Obtaining a good history and physical exam can help localize the source of bleeding. A history of alcohol use, cirrhosis, NSAID use, peptic ulcer disease, or a previous upper GI bleed can all point to an upper source. Specific attention should be paid to chronic anticoagulant and antiplatelet medications. Patients should be asked about previous endoscopy or colonoscopy. Hematemesis and coffee-ground emesis are more consistent with an upper GI bleed with or without melena. However, patients with an upper GI bleed may present with melena alone. Typically, bright-red blood per rectum is more suggestive of a lower GI blood, although a brisk upper GI bleed with fast transit can cause significant hematochezia. Clots in the stool can be more suggestive of a lower GI bleed.

GI bleeding patients may present critically ill, with nonspecific complaints, or without any report of visualized bleeding. A high index of suspicion should keep GI bleeding on the differential workup. The physical exam should look for signs of active or recent bleeding, abdominal tenderness, ascites, and stigmata of chronic liver disease. Basic physical exam components should focus on HR, BP, and signs of shock (e.g., cool clammy skin or delayed capillary refill). All patients should undergo a rectal visual and physical exam and should have a developed stool sample occult guaiac test card.

UPPER GI BLEEDING

The initial management of upper GI bleeding consists of the ABCs and stabilization. Appropriate large-bore venous access needs to be placed emergently. Patients with an upper GI blood can progress from well-appearing to hemodynamic instability very quickly. The hemodynamically unstable patient should receive crystalloid volume expanders and uncrossed blood. Massive transfusion protocol should be considered in patients needing >4 units of blood to help avoid coagulopathy and thrombocytopenia. Ideally, the patient would be adequately resuscitated prior to intubation attempts. However, this is not always feasible in the unstable patient who may need emergent intervention or endoscopy. If the patient develops airway compromise, be prepared for a contaminated and difficult airway. Videolaryngoscopy is often obscured by blood and secretions, so direct laryngoscopy may provide a less obstructed view. Be prepared with multiple working suction setups and a gum elastic bougie. Rapid sequence intubation and a semi-upright position may minimize the likelihood of vomiting. If the airway cannot be visualized and attempts at intubation fail, the clinician should have a low threshold to move toward a surgical airway approach.

A nasogastric (NG) tube may be considered to aspirate and empty the stomach prior to intubation. Conversely, placement of an NG tube may lead to acute bouts of emesis, making it more difficult to secure the airway. NG tube insertion is documented as being one of the more painful procedures done to patients. Consider using topical or atomized anesthetics if NG tube placement is prioritized. Additionally, placement of an NG tube is not required to make the diagnosis of upper GI bleeding as there is a high false-negative rate due to intermittent bleeding or hemorrhage that is located past the pylorus. While a positive NG aspirate may be associated with a higher-risk lesion, there is no clear benefit of NG tube placement in terms of mortality, length of stay, or reduction in transfusion requirements.[4-6] An orogastric tube for gastric decompression can also be placed once the airway has been secured with a cuffed endotracheal tube.

Upper GI bleeding can be esophageal, gastric, or duodenal. Peptic ulcer disease due to *H. pylori* or NSAID use is the most common cause, accounting for >50% of cases.[7] Variceal bleeding should be considered and treated empirically in those with a history of alcoholism or evidence of cirrhosis on exam. Varices account for 59% of upper GI bleeds in cirrhotics.[8] Mallory–Weiss mucosal tears (caused by vomiting) and gastritis due to alcohol, NSAIDs, toxic ingestions, stress, or infection can also cause an upper GI bleed. An aorto-enteric fistula should be considered in the differential diagnosis for any patient with a history of aortic repair or grafting. While extremely rare, an aorto-enteric fistula is a life-threatening cause of upper GI bleeding that can progress quickly.

Risk assessment can be performed by calculating the Glasgow-Blatchford bleeding score (see the online medical reference MDCalc), which incorporates lab values, vital signs, physical exam findings, and historical features. Patients with a score of 0 or 1 can be discharged with outpatient follow-up.[7] The Rockall score for upper GI bleeding (see MDCalc) is another potential tool for predicting patients at risk for adverse outcomes following an acute upper GI bleed. While its convenient mnemonic of ABCDE (age, BP fall, comorbidity, diagnosis, evidence of bleeding) is easy to remember, it does require endoscopic evaluation of the potentially bleeding lesion.

Management of the patient with an upper GI bleed starts with IV administration of a proton-pump inhibitor (PPI) to neutralize the gastric pH and promote clot formation. Traditionally this was given as a bolus, then an infusion. However, studies now show that parenteral twice-daily dosing carries the same benefit of reduced high-risk stigmata and need for endoscopic therapy for the patient with an acute GI bleed.[9] The use of PPIs demonstrated no benefits on rebleeding rates, need for surgery, or mortality. If there is concern for variceal bleeding (history of varices, evidence of chronic liver disease on physical exam like ascites, report of significant alcohol abuse), patients should be started on an octreotide bolus and then an infusion (50 mcg, then 50 mcg/hour). Octreotide is a somatostatin analog to inhibit secretion of gastric acid and cause splanchnic vasoconstriction. These patients should also receive antimicrobial coverage, generally a cephalosporin (typically 1 g ceftriaxone) to mitigate the known complication of spontaneous bacterial peritonitis in GI bleed patients. Antibiotics have a demonstrated mortality benefit for patients with cirrhosis.[10] Variceal bleeding and corresponding hepatic disease is associated with higher mortality for the patient with an upper GI bleed. Massive variceal bleeds may require balloon tamponade therapy such as a Minnesota tube or a Sengstaken–Blakemore tube after intubation.

Gastroenterology should be consulted for endoscopy, which should happen ideally within 24 hours. The patient should be adequately resuscitated and optimized prior to endoscopy, given demonstrated outcome benefits. The INR should be corrected to <2.5.[7] Patients with hemodynamic instability should be admitted to the ICU for ongoing resuscitation and monitoring. Interventional radiology or surgical strategies can be considered for patients who fail to respond to medical management, blood resuscitation, and endoscopic therapies.

LOWER GI BLEEDING

Lower GI bleeding accounts for 30% to 40% of cases of GI bleeding. A directed history and physical exam should be performed while assessing the stability of the patient. Similar to patients with upper GI bleeding, large-bore IV access should be obtained early, with laboratory evaluation including type and screen as well as coagulation factors, chemistry, and blood count. Key history points include the timing of last stool output and its color and amount, symptom frequency and duration, and associated findings like pain or weight loss. While hematemesis and melena are associated with upper GI bleeding, clots and hematochezia are suggestive of lower GI bleeding. A brisk upper GI bleed or aorto-enteric pathology can cause hematochezia, and patients should be asked those historical clues as well. Anticoagulant and antiplatelet use should again be elicited and addressed.

Lower GI bleeding can be caused by diverticulosis (30–65% of cases),[10] ischemic colitis, hemorrhoids, polyps/neoplasms, angioectasias, and inflammatory bowel disease. Diverticulosis causes painless bleeding that typically self-resolves. Mesenteric ischemia due to superior mesenteric artery thrombosis/embolism or nonocclusive due to shock can be difficult to diagnose. Older patients with a history of atrial fibrillation, congestive heart failure, postprandial pain, and pain out of proportion to exam findings should raise suspicion for mesenteric ischemia.[8] Polyps and neoplasms typically present with a more indolent course of chronic anemia and weight loss. Performing a rectal exam can be helpful to evaluate for hemorrhoids or stigmata of ongoing bleeding. Hypotension, tachycardia, ongoing hematochezia, and medical comorbidities are associated with increased risk for adverse outcomes. There is not currently a well-developed risk score for lower GI bleeding.[10] Patients who are hemodynamically stable with an obvious cause of mild bleeding such as hemorrhoids or an anal fissure, or patients with normal labs and no hematochezia or melena, can be discharged with close clinic follow-up.

For the unstable or acutely anemic patient, gastroenterology should be consulted. Colonoscopy within the first 24 hours can be both diagnostic and therapeutic. A bowel preparation regimen to cleanse the distal GI tract should be discussed with gastroenterology, as this allows for proper visualization of the colon and concerning pathology. Occasionally an NG tube needs to be placed to administer the bowel preparation regimen.

It is reassuring to know that 80% of all lower GI bleeds will resolve spontaneously.[10] Computed tomography angiography (CTA) can be performed in patients with continued bleeding or if colonoscopy was nondiagnostic or unsuccessful. CTA can detect bleeding of 0.3 mL/minute and can be helpful to direct angiography. Lower GI bleeding can be intermittent, so angiography may initially be negative. The utility of technetium-99m-labeled red cell scintigraphy has been debated, but this is another investigative study often employed in the workup of lower GI bleeding.[10]

Finally, surgery may be necessary for patients who have failed endoscopic or angiographic intervention. Attempted localization of the bleed is important to prevent the morbidity of a surgical colectomy.

CASE OUTCOME

The history and physical exam findings of the patient in the case vignette are consistent with an upper GI bleed, and given the stigmata of chronic liver disease, empiric treatment of esophageal variceal bleeding is begun. Two 16G IVs are placed in the bilateral antecubital fossa. Samples for lab work, including CBC, BMP, LFTs, coagulation factors, and type and cross, are sent. He is given pantoprazole 80 mg IV, ceftriaxone 1 g, octreotide 50-mcg bolus and infusion, and 1 L lactated Ringer's. Labs demonstrate an elevated BUN of 45, Cr 1.2, elevated INR of 2.6, and hemoglobin of 8.9. His BP improves to 105/67 mmHg, and HR remains in sinus rhythm in the 80s. GI is consulted for endoscopy and the patient is admitted to medicine. Endoscopy is performed within 24 hours of admission and demonstrates esophageal varices, which are ligated. He receives 72 hours of IV PPI and octreotide as well as 7 days of antibiotics. He was discharged on an oral PPI and encouraged to abstain from alcohol.

KEY POINTS TO REMEMBER

- Obtain large-bore IV access early and send a type and screen.
- Localize the bleeding using the history and physical to direct treatment.
- Transfuse for a hemoglobin goal of >7.0 g/dL. Avoid coagulopathy and thrombocytopenia.

- Stable patients can be discharged with outpatient follow-up if low-risk features are present.
- Obtain urgent GI evaluation for endoscopy within 24 hours.

References

1. Peery AF, Crockett SD, Murphy CC, et al. Burden and cost of gastrointestinal, liver, and pancreatic diseases in the United States: Update 2018. *Gastroenterology*. 2019;156(1):254–272.
2. Witting MD, Magder L, Heins AE, Mattu A, Granja CA, Baumgarten M. Emergency department predictors of upper gastrointestinal bleeding in patients without hematemesis. *Am J Emerg Med*. 2006;24:280–285.
3. Villanueva C, Colomo A, Bosch A, et al. Transfusion strategies for acute upper gastrointestinal bleeding. *N Engl J Med*. 2013;368(1):11–21.
4. Singer A, Richman P, Kowalska A, Thode H. Comparison of patient and practitioner assessments of pain from commonly performed emergency department procedures. *Ann Emerg Med*. 1999;33(6):652–658.
5. Patreon D, Vicaut E, Debuc E, et al. Erythromycin infusion or gastric lavage for upper gastrointestinal bleeding: A multicenter randomized controlled trial. *Ann Emerg Med*. 2011;57(6):582–589.
6. Huang E, Karsan S, Kanwal F, Singh I, Makhani M, Spiegel B. Impact of nasogastric lavage on outcomes in acute GI bleeding. *Gastrointest Endosc*. 2011;74(5):971–980.
7. Stanley AJ, Laine L. Management of acute gastrointestinal bleeding. *BMJ*. 2019;364:I536.
8. Tintinalli JE, Stapczynski JS, Ma OJ, Yearly DM, Meckler GD, Cline DM, eds. *Tintinalli's Emergency Medicine: A Comprehensive Study Guide*, 8th ed. McGraw-Hill Education; 2016.
9. Sachar H, Vaidya K, Laine L. Intermittent vs continuous proton pump inhibitor therapy for high-risk bleeding ulcers: A systematic review and meta-analysis. *JAMA Intern Med*. 2014;174(11):1755–1762.
10. Gralnek IM, Neeman Z, Strate LL. Acute lower gastrointestinal bleeding. *N Engl J Med*. 2017;376(11):1054–1063.

29 I am yellow: Complications of cirrhosis

Taylor M. Douglas and Susan Cheng

A 67-year-old man is brought to the ED because his daughter was worried that he was "not acting himself." The patient lives alone and was recently widowed. EMS found him disheveled, spontaneously breathing, and confused with agitation. There were no external signs of trauma. EMS describes the scene as foul-smelling, with scattered liquor bottles. Vital signs are BP 96/60 mmHg, HR 116 bpm, rectal temperature 99.6°F, RR 22 breaths/min, SpO$_2$ 100%. Exam is significant for agitation with lethargy, icteric sclera, jaundice, regular tachycardia, a distended abdomen (tense, but not hard) with guarding on deep palpation and dilated abdominal wall veins, ecchymosis of both forearms, and bilateral pitting pedal edema. The patient's daughter reports no past medical history, medications, or allergies; she says he is a weekend drinker. You order bloodwork, an EKG, a portable CXR, and a 1-L bolus. Point-of-care ultrasound (POCUS) reveals scattered B lines with small bilateral pleural effusions, a hyperdynamic heart with adequate ejection fraction, and no pericardial effusion. As you exit the room, the lab calls to report a platelet level of 57.

What do I do now?

This middle-aged man with altered mental status necessitates consideration of a large differential diagnosis to ensure the underlying pathology is identified. In a patient without known medical problems, or consistent primary care to exclude common comorbidities, many end-stage diseases could have developed unencumbered. Therefore, the emergency physician must contemplate everything from intracranial catastrophe to dementia to intoxication (Table 29.1).

For this patient, the list of diagnoses can be narrowed based on the available collateral information and physical exam findings. The astute physician will quickly work through the differential and arrive at the most likely

TABLE 29.1 **Differential diagnosis of altered mental status**

Category	Diagnoses
Intracranial/neurologic	Ischemic cerebrovascular accident
	Subdural hemorrhage
	Intraparenchymal hemorrhage
	Neoplasm
	Normal pressure hydrocephalus
	Post-ictal state
	Nonconvulsive status epilepticus
Metabolic	Hypoglycemia
	Hyponatremia, hypernatremia
	Hypercalcemia
	Hyperosmolar hyperglycemic syndrome
	Thyroid dysfunction
	Uremic encephalopathy
	Hepatic encephalopathy
	Wernicke's encephalopathy
Infectious	Meningitis/encephalitis
	Sepsis
Cardiac	Myocardial infarction
	Pulmonary embolism
	Congestive heart failure
	CO_2 narcosis
Other	Toxidromes (alcohol, opioids, methamphetamines, synthetics)
	Drug overdose
	Polypharmacy
	Psychiatric diagnoses

diagnosis of decompensated cirrhosis, all the while eliminating other possibilities with a comprehensive workup. If this patient does indeed have hepatic encephalopathy due to his undiagnosed liver disease, the diagnostic puzzle does not end with that conclusion. Hepatic encephalopathy is the manifestation of a patient with cirrhosis unable to compensate for another insult, be it metabolic, traumatic, or infectious. This patient with decompensated cirrhosis, as defined by the presence of ascites, must be carefully evaluated for complications of his underlying disease, including gastrointestinal bleeding (see Chapter 28), spontaneous bacterial peritonitis, and superimposed fulminant liver failure (Table 29.2), as well as extrahepatic

TABLE 29.2 **Complications of cirrhosis**

Complication	Presentation	Treatment
Variceal bleeding	· Hematemesis · Melena	· Blood products · Antibiotic prophylaxis · Octreotide · EGD
Ascites	· Increasing abdominal girth · Fluid wave, shifting dullness	· Large-volume paracentesis · Ascitic fluid analysis · Oral diuretics
Sepsis	· Fever and localizing symptoms	· Antibiotics · Volume resuscitation · Ascitic fluid analysis · Source control
Spontaneous bacterial peritonitis (SBP)	· Abdominal pain and distention · Fever	· Diagnostic paracentesis · Ascitic fluid analysis · Antibiotics
Hepatic encephalopathy (HE)	· Changes in sleep pattern · Altered mental status · Asterixis	· Lactulose/rifaximin · Identify and treat trigger
Hepatorenal syndrome (HRS)	· Acute renal failure · Diagnosis of exclusion	· Albumin challenge · Vasoactive agents · Identify and treat trigger · Dialysis · Transplant evaluation

(*continued*)

TABLE 29.2 **Continued**

Complication	Presentation	Treatment
Hepatopulmonary syndrome	· Dyspnea, tachypnea, hypoxia	· Supportive care · Transplant evaluation
Umbilical hernia	· Bulge at umbilicus, can be asymptomatic	· Reduce if possible · Urgent surgery consult if incarcerated or strangulated · Outpatient referral for repair if reducible
Hepatic hydrothorax	· Dyspnea, cough, chest pain · Pleural effusion, more commonly right-sided	· Thoracentesis · Pleural fluid analysis · Treatment of ascites (as above)

insults such as myocardial infarction, sepsis, and even the relatively mundane constipation (see Table 29.1), as all can push a patient over the edge into hepatic encephalopathy.

Treatment begins for this patient as soon as he arrives despite a broad differential. Two large-bore IVs are needed given his hypotension, tachycardia, and lethargy. Implementing continuous telemetry and BP and O_2 saturation monitoring is also key. No supplemental oxygen is needed immediately, but intubation should always be considered if his mental status were to worsen with inability to protect his airway. Immediate labs include a point-of-care glucose, troponin, and venous blood gas with lactate. Initial labs include CBC, BMP, liver enzymes, ethanol level, direct/indirect bilirubin, coagulation profile, type and screen, blood cultures, TSH, and ammonia level. Also order an EKG and portable CXR, as well as a head CT without contrast as soon as the patient is clinically stable. Antibiotics should be initiated as soon as allergies can be confirmed and should cover intra-abdominal infections. Most guidelines recommend a third-generation cephalosporin such as ceftriaxone or cefotaxime, and a fluoroquinolone in patients with a penicillin allergy; however, referring to your local antibiogram is recommended due to variable resistance patterns. Begin IVF resuscitation with the recommended 30-mL/kg bolus, but closely watch for worsening respiratory status from pulmonary congestion. Volume resuscitation could then transition to albumin to minimize lung edema if the patient is hypoalbuminemic and/or blood products if the hemoglobin is <7 g/dL.

Currently, albumin infusion is recommended in patients with spontaneous bacterial peritonitis (SBP) at high risk for developing acute kidney injury and in patients with hepatorenal syndrome (HRS)-related acute kidney injury and for prevention of paracentesis-induced circulatory dysfunction (PICD). PICD includes hypotension, renal dysfunction, hypervolemic hyponatremia, and hepatic encephalopathy (HE). Human albumin is used as a plasma expander to improve intravascular volume through increased oncotic pressure. In appropriate patients, initiate albumin repletion at 1 to 1.5 g/kg body weight (up to 100 g) for the first 24 hours of treatment, usually dosed intermittently with drainage of ascites via an abdominal pigtail catheter. There is some evidence that albumin may play additional roles such as immune modulation and endothelium stabilization, with potential to improve survival in decompensated cirrhosis.

Ultrasound of the abdomen can help quantify the amount of ascites and select an appropriate access point for a diagnostic and therapeutic paracentesis. Indications for diagnostic paracentesis are evaluation of new-onset ascites and concern for peritonitis in patients with known ascites. Therapeutic paracentesis is indicated when ascites accumulation causes respiratory distress, abdominal pain or pressure, and/or concern for abdominal compartment syndrome. There is no defined limit for amount of fluid removal allowed, but the risk of PICD increases when removal exceeds 5-L.

For both procedures, informed consent should be obtained and the patient placed on continuous cardiac monitoring with repeat BP measurement every 1 to 2 minutes (or per institutional protocol). The access site identified by ultrasound is sterilized and local anesthesia provided. A diagnostic paracentesis can be performed using a large-bore needle and syringe to collect 30 mL of ascitic fluid. The Seldinger technique can be used for large-volume paracentesis. First, a needle is used to access the peritoneal cavity, then a guidewire is advanced through the access needle, the needle is removed, the catheter is threaded over the wire, the guidewire is removed, and the catheter is attached to a drainage collection system (with or without suction). Some kits utilize a catheter to be threaded directly over the access needle without the need for a guidewire. Become familiar with the kit(s) used at your institution(s). Ascitic fluid should be sent for cell count with differential, albumin, protein, glucose, LDH, Gram stain, and culture. If additional fluid is available, a sample can be sent for cytology if clinically warranted. Once the desired volume is drained, the catheter is removed and a dressing is placed at the access site.

Complications of paracentesis include bleeding, hypotension due to fluid shifts, leakage from the access site post-procedure, and infection. The initial ascitic fluid obtained may be blood-tinged, but if fluid fails to become less blood-tinged, then the procedure should be aborted. Stabilize the patient and then obtain immediate imaging of the abdomen to evaluate for signs of perforation or active hemorrhage and obtain a repeat hemoglobin level. If hypotension occurs, immediately stop any additional fluid removal and continue BP monitoring. Albumin (6–8 g per liter of ascites removed), blood product, and/or vasopressors may be considered if hypotension persists. If there is post-procedure leakage from the insertion site, a pressure dressing can be placed, or a suture can be placed if the leakage is refractory to the pressure dressing. Leakage can also be prevented by accessing the peritoneal cavity through a staggered site from the skin insertion site (Z-track technique). The skin site should be evaluated daily for any signs of erythema, swelling, or tenderness that may warrant addition or adjustment of antibiotic therapy.

In patients with end-stage liver disease, there are expected laboratory derangements as a consequence of their poor synthetic function. First, the biochemical markers AST, ALT, and alkaline phosphatase are usually normal as the inflammation seen in acute liver failure has already occurred, although there may be hyperbilirubinemia due to portal hypertension. This patient will also likely have a low albumin level, a major contributor to his pulmonary edema and ascites. As mentioned above, transition to administration of albumin as the resuscitative fluid in this patient may be beneficial due to his albumin deficiency, as would administration of albumin for large-volume paracentesis (>5-L). This dysregulated fluid balance leads to hyponatremia, similar to that seen in decompensated/end-stage congestive heart failure. As mentioned above, he also has insufficient clotting factors due to poor synthetic function, and this will be reflected by both a prolonged PT and an elevated INR. His coagulopathy is likely to be worsened due to thrombocytopenia, seen both in alcohol use due to bone marrow suppression and cirrhosis due to multiple factors.

Although these coagulopathies do not require routine intervention, there are situations in which medications or transfusions are indicated. Traditional cutoffs of <7 g/dL for hemoglobin and <10,000 for platelets, regardless of active bleeding, are still used in patients with cirrhosis. However, extra care should be taken prior to procedures in thrombocytopenic patients. There are no guidelines regarding routine transfusions before paracentesis due to insufficient evidence, but the cutoff of 10,000 or 20,000 is commonly used. In a patient with significant bleeding, the patient's coagulopathies should be treated. Transfusion of platelets to a goal of >50,000 is recommended. Vitamin K, especially in this particular patient due to his likely poor nutritional status, replenishes often-depleted stores, although the effects will not be immediately apparent as the patient must make clotting factors first. For a more immediate effect, fresh frozen plasma (FFP) should be considered, as it contains vitamin K–dependent factors (II, VII, IX, and X) as well as proteins C and S.

Direct treatment of this patient's HE must target both the underlying insult (see Table 29.1) and the clearance of the nitrogenous compounds causing his deterioration. Patients with gross disorientation, who are difficult to arouse or at risk of airway compromise, need stabilization and the early involvement of a critical care consultant. While completing the workup and treatments mentioned previously, including obtaining a serum ammonia level, HE-specific therapy can also be considered (lactulose and rifaximin). First, intubate to protect the airway if necessary. Second, if the patient is encephalopathic but does not require intubation, they are still an aspiration risk, so consider placing a nasogastric tube. Also note that a single elevated ammonia level is not diagnostic because each patient becomes encephalopathic at a different ammonia level, but levels can guide therapy over time.

Lactulose is a laxative that is metabolized into organic acids and creates an acidotic intestinal environment. This acidity facilitates peristalsis, ionizes the ammonia into ammonium excreted through stool, and helps eliminate certain ammonia-producing bacteria. Lactulose can be administered orally, through a nasogastric tube, or rectally. The preferred route is oral, dosed initially at 10 to 30 g and repeated with the goal of two or three soft bowel movements every 24 hours. If a patient is too obtunded to tolerate oral medications, a nasogastric tube should be placed or an enema (consisting of 300 mL lactulose with 700 mL water) can be used. Rifaximin is an antibiotic that is poorly absorbed and concentrates intestinally after oral ingestion. It reduces ammonia-producing bacteria in the intestine but is costly and can only be given orally. The recommended dosing is 400 mg three times a day. Other treatments are being investigated, but none have been recommended yet.

As discussed above, this patient requires ICU-level care depending on his response to resuscitative measures. A critical care consultation is indicated for patients with shock, significant gastrointestinal bleeding, and encephalopathy leading to risk of airway compromise. Consideration of ED consultation with GI/hepatology is critical to this patient's care. Any patient with liver failure who could be a potential transplant candidate should be seen by hepatology promptly and considered for transfer to a transplant center.

KEY POINTS TO REMEMBER

· Look for an inciting cause for HE as it is the consequence of another process for which a cirrhotic patient cannot compensate.

· Suspect SBP and perform a diagnostic paracentesis early in patients with new ascites or ascites with symptoms of fever, altered mental status, or abdominal pain.

· HE and HRS are both diagnoses of exclusion that require evaluation for alternative diagnoses in parallel with treatment.

Further reading

Alaniz C, Regal RE. Spontaneous bacterial peritonitis: A review of treatment options. *PT.* 2009;34(4):204–213.

Bailey C, Hern G. Hepatic failure: An evidence-based approach in the emergency department. *Emerg Med Pr.* 2010;12(4):1–22.

Biggins SW, Angeli P, Garcia-Tsao G, et al. Diagnosis, evaluation, and management of ascites and hepatorenal syndrome. *Hepatology.* 2021;74(2):1014–1048.

Chinnock B, Afarian H, Minnigan H, Butler J, Hendey GW. Physician clinical impression does not rule out spontaneous bacterial peritonitis in patients undergoing emergency department paracentesis. *Ann Emerg Med.* 2008;52(3):268–273. doi:10.1016/j.annemergmed.2008.02.016

Crabb DW, Im GY, Szabo G, Mellinger JL, Lucey MR. Diagnosis and treatment of alcohol-associated liver diseases: 2019 practice guidance from the American Association for the Study of Liver Diseases. *Hepatology*. 2020;71:306–333.

D'Amico G, Garcia-Tsao G, Pagliaro L. Natural history and prognostic indicators of survival in cirrhosis: A systematic review of 118 studies. *J Hepatol*. 2006;44(1):217–231. doi:10.1016/j.jhep.2005.10.013

Gines P, Guevara M, Arroyo V, Rodes J. Hepatorenal syndrome. *Lancet*. 2003;362:1819–1827.

Gines P, Schrier RW. Renal failure in cirrhosis. *N Engl J Med*. 2009;361(13):1279–1290. doi:10.1056/NEJMra0809139

Huff JS. Altered mental status and coma. In: Tintinalli JE, Stapczynski JS, Ma OJ, Yealy DM, Meckler GD, Cline MD, eds. *Tintinalli's Emergency Medicine*. 8th ed. McGraw-Hill Education; 2016:1156–1161.

Ichai P, Samuel D. Epidemiology of liver failure. *Clin Res Hepatol Gastroenterol*. 2011;35(10):610–617. doi:10.1016/j.clinre.2011.03.010

Khungar V, Poordad F. Hepatic encephalopathy. *Clin Liver Dis*. 2012;16(2):301–320. doi:10.1016/j.cld.2012.03.009

Long B, Koyfman A. The emergency medicine evaluation and management of the patient with cirrhosis. *Am J Emerg Med*. 2018;36(4):689–698. doi:10.1016/j.ajem.2017.12.047

O'Mara SR, Gebreyes K. Hepatic disorders. In: Tintinalli JE, Stapczynski JS, Ma OJ, Yealy DM, Meckler GD, Cline MD, eds. *Tintinalli's Emergency Medicine*. 8th ed. McGraw-Hill Education; 2016:525–532.

Prat LI, Wilson P, Freeman SC, et al. Antibiotic treatment for spontaneous bacterial peritonitis in people with decompensated liver cirrhosis: A network meta-analysis. *Cochrane Database Syst Rev*. 2019;9(9):CD013120. doi:10.1002/14651858.CD013120.pub2

Runyon BA. Management of adult patients with ascites due to cirrhosis: Update 2012. *AASLD Practice Guideline*. 2012;1–96.

Tufoni M, Zaccherini G, Caraceni P, Bernardi M. Albumin: Indications in chronic liver disease. *United European Gastroenterol J*. 2020;8(5):528–535. doi:10.1177/2050640620910339

Vilstrup H, Amodio P, Bajaj J, et al. Hepatic encephalopathy in chronic liver disease: 2014 practice guideline by the American Association for the Study of Liver Diseases and the European Association for the Study of the Liver. *Hepatology*. 2014;60(2):715–735. doi:10.1002/hep.27210

30 I can't pee: Acute renal failure

Joseph Nobile, Sagar B. Dave, and
Daniel Haase

A 59-year-old man is brought to the ED by EMS for
confusion. His vital signs are temperature 36.5°C,
BP 110/65 mmHg, HR 92 bpm, RR 26 breaths/min, and
SpO_2 92% on room air. Fingerstick glucose is 98. On
examination, the patient is lethargic and unable to
provide any history. He moans to deep sternal rub but
does not open his eyes. His pupils are midrange and
reactive. He withdraws all four extremities to pain. When
auscultating his heart, you hear a normal S1 and S2 as
well as an intermittent scratching sound. His pulmonary
exam reveals bibasilar crackles. His abdominal exam is
unremarkable and his extremities are warm and well
perfused with trace pedal edema. His wife arrives and
relates that his mental status has been worsening over
the past 2 days to the point where she had difficulty
awakening him this morning. He has no medical history
other than osteoarthritis. He takes no prescription
medications but she relates that he has been training
for a half-marathon and has been taking ibuprofen
regularly. She denies any toxic habits. His laboratory
results are Na 136, K 6.9, Cl 108, HCO_3 10, BUN 138, and
Cr 6.9. His VBG pH is 7.15 with a $PvCO_2$ of 28.

What do I do now?

Acute kidney injury (AKI) is a common and serious problem encountered in critically ill patients in the ED. Its prevalence has been difficult to measure due to the various definitions and classifications.[1] AKI has been estimated to account for 5% of hospital admissions and to affect 3% to 18% of hospitalized patients.[2,3] Although only 1% to 5% of patients affected will require renal replacement therapy (RRT), a single episode of AKI has been correlated with an increased risk of hospital mortality, and 13% of critically ill patients with AKI who survive to hospital discharge go on to require long-term RRT.[3,4] In critically ill patients with AKI, mortality has been estimated anywhere from 15% to 80%.[5] Not only are there devastating short- and long-term clinical effects of AKI, but it is also associated with longer ICU length of stay, hospital admission, and overall cost of care.

Renal function is defined by three processes: (1) blood flow into the glomeruli, (2) ultrafiltrate forming and transitioning into the renal tubules. with subsequent reabsorption or secretion of solutes and water, and (3) tubular fluid, now called urine, drained from renal tubules through the ureters into the bladder and expelled via urethra. An insult that interferes with any of these functions or structures can lead to AKI or acute renal failure. Each kidney is composed of millions of nephrons that collectively contribute to the overall glomerular filtration rate (GFR), which represents the volume of fluid filtrated over time. Serum creatinine (Cr) is derived from the metabolism of creatinine phosphate in muscle tissue that is filtrated by the glomerulus and is used as a surrogate for GFR. An overall decrease in hourly urine output is considered the earliest indicator of AKI, yet this can be difficult to assess during an ED evaluation. All of these can be used in conjunction and separately to evaluate overall renal function.

AKI is a syndrome defined by a rapid (hours to days) decline of kidney function. Definitions of AKI have changed over the years, and the Risk, Injury, Failure, Loss, End-stage (RIFLE) criteria in 2004 and the AKI network (AKIN) staging in 2009 merged in 2012 to create the Kidney Disease Improving Global Outcomes (KDIGO) classifications. By these criteria, AKI is defined by an increase in Cr of 0.3 mg/dL over 48 hours; an increase in Cr to 1.5 times the patient's baseline, presumed to have occurred over the past 7 days; or a decrease in urine output to <0.5 mL/kg/hour for 6 hours.[6] KDIGO further separates AKI into three escalating stages defined by Cr and urine output.

It is important to recognize that AKI is a syndrome that can result from different underlying etiologies and associated conditions. AKI also encompasses a spectrum of severities, ranging from incidental and mild to severe with life-threatening metabolic derangements. Patients can be asymptomatic in mild forms of AKI but may present with various signs and symptoms as their kidney function declines. They can have subjective or objective evidence of decreased urine output and subsequent volume overload, such as dyspnea, peripheral edema, or pulmonary edema. Patients may also have stigmata of uremia, such as encephalopathy or pericarditis.

The different causes of AKI can be roughly divided into four large categories, based upon where the problem is occurring in relation to the kidney: pre-renal, intrinsic renal, post-renal, or vascular. Pre-renal etiologies are caused by a decrease in renal blood flow, leading to a decrease in GFR. This can be caused by decreased circulating blood volume, such as in hypovolemic states, or by a decrease in effective renal blood flow, which itself may have a myriad of causes. In hepatorenal syndrome, splanchnic vasodilation shunts blood flow away from the kidneys. In cardiorenal syndrome, increased central venous pressure causes an increase in renal venous pressure, which will decrease blood flow across the kidney. A similar increase in venous pressure and resistance is the cause of AKI in abdominal compartment syndrome. Finally, several medications can lead to a decrease in renal blood flow by vasoconstriction of afferent arterioles, most notably ACE inhibitors.

Intrinsic renal injuries can be further broken up depending on the specific part of the nephron that is being affected. The tubulointerstitial space can be injured in a number of ways, the most common of which is acute tubular necrosis (ATN). The prevalence of ATN has been estimated to be ~45% among hospitalized patients with AKI.[7] ATN occurs from three major causes: ischemia, sepsis, or exposure to nephrotoxins.[8] Contrast-induced nephropathy has also been a traditionally well-known cause of AKI. However, studies have shown that the risk is greatest with diagnostic angiography and high-osmotic contrast agents, which are being utilized much less frequently for conventional CT imaging.[9]

Acute interstitial nephritis (AIN) occurs secondary to infiltration of the interstitial space of the kidney by inflammatory cells. This is typically secondary to medications, most commonly NSAIDs but also certain antibiotics such as penicillins, cephalosporins, and trimethoprim–sulfamethoxazole. It can less commonly be caused by autoimmune conditions such as systemic lupus erythematosus or sarcoidosis. It takes 10 days, on average, for AIN to develop after a new medication is started, so a thorough medication history is essential in any patient presenting with AKI.[10] Other common tubulointerstitial causes of AKI include multiple myeloma, tumor lysis syndrome, and rhabdomyolysis.

Glomerular diseases are typically associated with the nephritic syndrome and nephrotic syndrome. Nephritic syndrome, which is characterized by AKI, hematuria, and hypertension, can be caused by post-streptococcal glomerulonephritis, anti–basement membrane diseases, cryoglobulinemia, and vasculitides such as granulomatosis with polyangiitis, IgA vasculitis, and lupus nephritis. Prompt recognition of the nephritic syndrome is important as these conditions carry higher risk of rapid progression to kidney failure. These patients will often require immunosuppressive therapy to prevent worsening of their condition. Nephrotic syndrome, which is described by profound proteinuria, fat cells in urine, and overall edema, can be caused by membranous nephropathy, focal segmental glomerulosclerosis, diabetes mellitus, and, similar to nephritic syndrome, by autoimmune processes and infection. Fluid management becomes the focus of management for these patients.

Post-renal AKI is caused by obstruction to the urinary tract that leads to an increase in tubular pressure and depressed renal function. This is most commonly due to prostatic hypertrophy; however, it may also be caused by bilateral ureteral compression in the setting of abdominal tumor burden or fibrinous adhesion, lack of detrusor muscle contraction in the setting of neurogenic shock or spinal cord injury, traumatic transection in the setting of girdle injuries, or urinary retention secondary to medications. Finally, systemic diseases affecting the renal vascular system can lead to reduction in glomerular filtration. These include cases of thrombotic microangiopathy, such as in malignant hypertension, thrombotic thrombocytopenic purpura/ hemolytic uremic syndrome, sickle cell vasculopathy, thromboembolic disease leading to renal artery occlusion, or scleroderma renal crisis.

As noted above, AKI can be readily diagnosed via the KDIGO criteria, requiring a thorough clinical history and physical exam, and Cr from a basic metabolic panel (BMP). The BMP will also show evidence of any metabolic derangements, such as hyperkalemia, acidosis, or uremia. Performing a further laboratory and radiologic workup can be helpful for ED providers, particularly with undifferentiated AKI. A bedside ultrasound of the kidneys and bladder can quickly diagnose urinary retention and hydronephrosis as well as assess volume status. Adjuncts such as chest x-ray to further assess volume status or a CT scan to evaluate for obstruction can be helpful to guide management. A urinalysis with urine microscopy can also be helpful in suggesting specific etiologies. For example, the presence of blood on dipstick analysis with a lack of microscopic hematuria can suggest myoglobinuria and rhabdomyolysis. The presence of red and white cell casts can point to a glomerular or interstitial process, respectively, whereas hyaline casts can be seen in tubular injuries.

Obtaining urine electrolyte concentrations and calculating the fractional excretion of sodium (FENa) has been classically utilized to differentiate between pre-renal causes of AKI and intrinsic renal etiologies, specifically ATN. Traditionally, an FENa of <1% has been associated with pre-renal etiologies, while higher FENa percentages are due to other causes of AKI. Although 1% is typically used as a cutpoint, there is no value that truly represents the demarcation between these categories. The calculation has been shown to be more accurate and beneficial in patients with severely reduced GFR. Additionally, the excretion of sodium is altered by diuretics, although in these circumstances, a fractional excretion of urea can be calculated alternatively.[11]

If the cause of AKI remains unclear, other laboratory tests, such as complement levels, anti-nuclear antibodies, ANCA levels, serum protein electrophoresis, etc., can be useful. However, these lab results will not come back in a timely matter and need not be ordered on ED patients unless specifically requested by consultants.

ED management of AKI is rooted in recognition and stabilization with a focus on treating any readily reversible causes as well as treatment of any life-threatening metabolic derangements. Pre-renal disease is often reversible, and the mainstay of therapy is fluid management. If a patient is clinically hypovolemic, an infusion of isotonic crystalloid should be administered.[12] Conversely, diuresis and optimizing cardiac output should be considered in patients with signs of clinical hypervolemia to decrease central venous pressure and improve renal perfusion. It is worth noting that patients in renal failure typically require higher doses of diuretics to overcome their decrease in GFR.[13] Literature does not support treatment with medications such as dopamine and fenoldopam aimed at increasing renal perfusion, and these medications are not primary therapies in the ED. For patients with signs of post-renal nephropathy due to urethral obstruction, insertion of an indwelling urinary catheter can rapidly decompress the bladder and improve the AKI. If urethral catheterization is not feasible, then suprapubic catheterization may need to be performed. For proximal obstruction, a nephrostomy tube may be necessary. Intrinsic renal disease can be difficult to manage in the ED. Regardless of therapy, the goal should be achieve euvolemia in patients and avoid hypovolemia. Strict monitoring of volume status and urine output should be initiated immediately to assess response to treatment and guide further resuscitation.

Equally important is the treatment of the metabolic derangements that can occur in the setting of severe AKI. Hyperkalemia can be temporized with IV calcium agents (calcium gluconate or calcium chloride), which work to stabilize the myocardial membrane. Insulin works to drive serum potassium into the cell by enhancing the activity of the Na-K-ATPase pump, primarily located on skeletal muscle. Insulin should typically be given with dextrose infusion. In patients with severe hyperkalemia, inhaled beta-2 agonists, such as albuterol, should be considered. Beta-2 agonists, much like insulin, work by enhancing the Na-K-ATPase on skeletal muscle. Sodium bicarbonate administration causes the release of H^+ from the cell, resulting in intracellular movement of potassium. Severe uncompensated metabolic acidosis (usually defined as a pH of <7.2) can be treated with an isotonic bicarbonate infusion. The BiCAR-ICU trial has shown this approach to be effective in reducing RRT rates in patients with severe AKI and acidemia.[14] All of these treatments are temporizing agents; they do not eliminate potassium from the body but allow for other treatments to work.

Elimination of potassium from the body can be achieved in several ways. Kaliuresis can be attempted with diuretics, although this may prove ineffective depending on the severity of the patient's AKI. Patiromer, a GI cation exchanger, has been used for chronic hyperkalemia, though its role in acute hyperkalemia has not been extensively studied. Sodium polystyrene sulfate had been used previously to promote GI excretion; however, it has not been shown to be particularly effective and may cause intestinal ischemia in rare cases.

RRT must be considered if these medical therapies prove ineffective, although there is no consensus on the absolute values that should prompt emergent initiation. In general, patients with worsening acidosis, severe hyperkalemia, refractory hypoxemia secondary to pulmonary edema, severe uremia, or clinical toxicity, especially when coupled with oliguria or anuria, should be discussed with a nephrologist.[15] Toxins that may need emergent RRT include but are not limited to salicylates, lithium, toxic alcohols (such as ethanol or methanol), valproic acid, vancomycin, metformin, carbamazepine, baclofen, and certain cases of acetaminophen toxicity. The Extracorporeal Treatments in Poisoning (ExTRIP) workgroup has reviews to evaluate which toxins can be treated with RRT, and your local poison control center should be contacted to guide management.[16] A temporary dialysis catheter can be rapidly inserted in the jugular or femoral vein at bedside using Seldinger technique, allowing prompt initiation of RRT. Although only a minority of patients will require emergent RRT, it can be a lifesaving procedure when employed in the proper circumstances.

In conclusion, AKI is a prevalent and dangerous diagnosis. AKI may present with rising Cr, decrease in GFR, and diminished urine output. Diagnosis by an emergency medicine physician is crucial in care, along with evaluating causes. Management includes optimizing fluid status, stabilizing metabolic derangements, and identifying early need for RRT. Vigilance in recognition and executing appropriate management is the pivotal role of an emergency medicine physician.

KEY POINTS TO REMEMBER

- AKI is most commonly defined as an acute increase in creatinine of 0.3 mg/dL, increase in creatine to 1.5 times baseline, or decrease in urine output to <0.5 mL/kg/hr over 6 hours.
- AKI is a syndrome that can be caused by a multitude of different etiologies and can present on wide spectrum of disease severity.

- Initial management should focus on treating reversible causes of AKI such as hypo- or hypervolemia and post-obstructive uropathy.
- AKI can cause lethal complications such as hyperkalemia, acidemia, or hypoxemia from fluid overload and should be treated aggressively.
- Refractory hyperkalemia, acidemia, hypervolemia with hypoxemia, complications of uremia such as severe encephalopathy or pericarditis, or certain toxicities should prompt emergent RRT.

References

1. Hoste E, Kellum J, Selby N, et al. Global epidemiology and outcomes of acute kidney injury. *Nature Rev Nephrol.* 2018;14:607–625. doi:10.1038/s41581-018-0052-0

2. Challiner R, Ritchie J, Fullwood C, Loughnan P, Hutchison A. Incidence and consequence of acute kidney injury in unselected emergency admissions to a large acute UK hospital trust. *BMC Nephrol.* 2014;15:84. doi:10.1186/1471-2369-15-84

3. Selby N, Crowley L, Fluck R, et al. Use of electronic results reporting to diagnose and monitor AKI in hospitalized patients. *Clin J Am Soc Nephrol.* 2012;7(4):533–540. doi:10.2215/cjn.08970911

4. Luo X, Jiang L, Du B, Wen Y, Wang M, Xi X. A comparison of different diagnostic criteria of acute kidney injury in critically ill patients. *Critical Care.* 2014;18(4):R144. doi:10.1186/cc13977

5. Co I, Gunnerson K. Emergency department management of acute kidney injury, electrolyte abnormalities, and renal replacement therapy in the critically ill. *Emerg Med Clin North Am.* 2019;37(3):459–471. doi:10.1016/j.emc.2019.04.006

6. KDIGO clinical practice guideline for acute kidney injury. *Kidney Int Suppl.* 2012;2(1):1–138. doi:10.1038/kisup.2012.1

7. Bouchard J, Acharya A, Cerda J, et al. A prospective international multicenter study of AKI in the intensive care unit. *Clin J Am Soc Nephrol.* 2015;10(8):1324–1331. doi:10.2215/cjn.04360514

8. Luther M, Caffrey A, Dosa D, Lodise T, Laplante K. Vancomycin plus piperacillin/tazobactam and acute kidney injury in adults: A systematic review and meta-analysis. *Open Forum Infect Dis.* 2016;3(suppl_1). doi:10.1093/ofid/ofw172.1353

9. Luk L, Steinman J, Newhouse J. Intravenous contrast-induced nephropathy—the rise and fall of a threatening edea. *Adv Chronic Kidney Dis.* 2017;24(3):169–175. doi:10.1053/j.ackd.2017.03.001

10. Praga M, González E. Acute interstitial nephritis. *Kidney Int.* 2010;77(11):956–961. doi:10.1038/ki.2010.89

11. Diskin C, Stokes T, Dansby L, Radcliff L, Carter T. Toward the optimal clinical use of the fraction excretion of solutes in oliguric azotemia. *Ren Fail.* 2010;32(10):1245–1254. doi:10.3109/0886022x.2010.517353

12. McGee S. Is this patient hypovolemic? *JAMA.* 1999;281(11):1022. doi:10.1001/jama.281.11.1022

13. Chawla L, Davison D, Brasha-Mitchell E et al. Development and standardization of a furosemide stress test to predict the severity of acute kidney injury. *Critical Care.* 2013;17(5):R207. doi:10.1186/cc13015

14. Jaber S, Paugam C, Futier E et al. Sodium bicarbonate therapy for patients with severe metabolic acidaemia in the intensive care unit (BICAR-ICU): A multicentre, open-label, randomised controlled, phase 3 trial. *Lancet.* 2018;392(10141):31–40. doi:10.1016/s0140-6736(18)31080-8

15. Ronco C, Ricci Z, De Backer D, et al. Renal replacement therapy in acute kidney injury: Controversy and consensus. *Critical Care.* 2015;19(1):146. doi:10.1186/s13054-015-0850-8

16. The Extracorporeal Treatments in Poisoning Workgroup. EXTRIP. Blood Purification in Toxicology: Reviewing the Evidence and Providing Recommendations. https://extrip-workgroup.org/recommendations. Last accessed: March 23, 2023.

Further reading

Allen JC, Gardner DS, Skinner H, Harvey D, Sharman A, Devonald MAJ. Definition of hourly urine output influences reported incidence and staging of acute kidney injury. *BMC Nephrol.* 2020;21(1):19. doi:10.1186/s12882-019-1678-2

Co I, Gunnerson K. Emergency department management of acute kidney injury, electrolyte abnormalities, and renal replacement therapy in the critically ill. *Emerg Med Clin North Am.* 2019;37(3):459–471. doi:10.1016/j.emc.2019.04.006

Foxwell DA, Pradhan S, Zouwail S, Rainer TH, Phillips AO. Epidemiology of emergency department acute kidney injury. *Nephrology.* 2020;25(6):457–466. doi:10.1111/nep.13672

Hudson KB, Sinert R. Renal failure: Emergency evaluation and management. *Emerg Med Clin North Am.* 2011;29(3):569–585. doi:10.1016/j.emc.2011.04.005

Makris K, Spanou L. Acute kidney injury: Definition, pathophysiology and clinical phenotypes. *Clin Biochem Rev.* 2016;37(2):85–98.

Mirrakhimov AE, Barbaryan A, Gray A, Ayach T. The role of renal replacement therapy in the management of pharmacologic poisonings. *Int J Nephrol*. 2016;2016:3047329. doi:10.1155/2016/3047329

Ostermann M, Joannidis M. Acute kidney injury 2016: Diagnosis and diagnostic workup. *Crit Care*. 2016;20(1):299. doi:10.1186/s13054-016-1478-z

Petejova N, Martinek A. Acute kidney injury due to rhabdomyolysis and renal replacement therapy: A critical review. *Crit Care*. 2014;18(3):224. doi:10.1186/cc13897

31 Electrolyte emergencies

Russell A. Trigonis and Timothy J. Ellender

A 49-year-old male with a history of hypertension, diabetes, and chronic kidney disease presents to the ED with generalized weakness and "just not feeling like myself, doc." He states that his symptoms have been slowly progressive over the last few days. His only other complaint is some back pain after doing yard work yesterday, for which he has been treating with ibuprofen. The patient's prescribed home medications include metoprolol, lisinopril, metformin, and furosemide, all of which he has been taking as prescribed. His notable vital signs include HR 65 bpm, BP 110/76 mmHg, and RR 20 breaths/min, with oxygen saturations of 97% on room air. His physical exam is unremarkable other than mild pretibial pitting edema. Triage laboratory studies are notable for a potassium [K] of 6.6 mEq/L and a creatinine of 4.1 mg/dL from a baseline 2 months prior of 1.4 mg/dL. His initial EKG shows peaked T-waves.

What do I do now?

yperkalemia is a classic case that is seen in almost every emergency medicine training simulation session and has a known treatment algorithm that is frequently rehearsed. Despite this, its presentation does not always fall into a cookie-cutter template. In addition, though its treatments are well known, the rationale behind the agents and appropriate dosing is less often discussed. The importance of good understanding of both the diagnosis and treatment of hyperkalemia cannot be understated as even a mildly elevated potassium level (K 4.5–5.0 mEq/L) is associated with a 25% increase in 30-day mortality, and patients with severely elevated levels (K > 6.5 mEq/L) are 75% more likely to die.

Hyperkalemia is fortunately not particularly difficult to diagnose. Given the ubiquity of laboratory studies ordered in the ED, we often have a potassium value early in a patient's evaluation. In interpreting elevated potassium levels, our first question should be: Is it valid? It is well known that hemolyzed lab samples show elevated levels of potassium as intracellular K is released. While most samples do note if they are hemolyzed, some, including point-of-care testing, do not. In order to differentiate "pseudohyperkalemia" or hemolyzed hyperkalemia from the true pathologic state, context is key.

Patients with a history of renal dysfunction are by their nature more likely to have elevated potassium levels as their organs most responsible for clearing the cation are diseased. In addition, several common medications can lead to decreased potassium clearance, with or without associated renal dysfunction. Angiotensin-converting enzyme inhibitors and angiotensinogen II receptor blockers (ACEi/ARBs) are classically blamed, but potassium-sparing diuretics, NSAIDs, antibiotics (including trimethoprim), and even beta-blockers can affect our normal potassium homeostasis. Many patients with chronic diuretic use are even prescribed supplemental potassium to take daily. In addition to renal impairments, cellular lysis from hemolysis, rhabdomyolysis, or even significant tissue necrosis following trauma or ischemia can pour potassium into the extracellular milieu. Large transfusions of packed red blood cells also contain high potassium loads from hemolyzed cells. Even without tissue damage, the faulty regulation of cellular shifting seen in diabetic ketoacidosis (DKA) can also lead to a mass exodus of potassium from inside the safety of the cell's phospholipid walls.

While sometimes a clear antagonist is driving the hyperkalemia, it is more often a multifactorial etiology. Take for example our patient: history of chronic kidney disease exacerbated by dehydration associated with his yard work, ongoing diuretic use, NSAIDs for muscle pain, and possibly even a component of rhabdomyolysis. He is also on metoprolol and has a history of diabetes with unknown glycemic control, a perfect combination for developing hyperkalemia.

Once the diagnosis is established with an abnormal laboratory value and a clinical context, the provider's first step should be to obtain an initial EKG. While the hyperkalemia changes on EKGs are well documented, it is important to remember that the classical textbook progression as the potassium increases is not reliable. A patient can degenerate directly from a sinus rhythm with peaked T-waves to a sinusoidal rhythm, skipping right over the widening intervals. Regardless of the morphology, the finding of EKG changes associated with hyperkalemia should trigger an immediate reflex to initiate continuous cardiac telemetry and treat emergently. The treatment approach is threefold: Stabilize, shift, and excrete.

Stabilization refers to stabilization of the cardiac myocytes to prevent the heart from degrading to an unstable rhythm. Here, the agent of choice is IV calcium. Ionized or active calcium can help decrease the heart's proclivity to fire ectopic beats. Hyperkalemia increases our heart's resting potential, bringing it closer to its threshold or firing potential. Increasing calcium, in turn, increases that firing potential, normalizing the gap between the resting and threshold levels. IV calcium can be given in two formulations, as calcium gluconate or calcium chloride. The difference between these two compounds is the concentration of the calcium in each. Calcium gluconate contains 4.5 mEq of calcium in each gram. Calcium chloride contains a more robust 14 mEq of calcium in the same volume. Calcium chloride, remembered as "CC" or "Code Calcium," is classically used during cardiac arrest. Its use is often limited outside of arrest due to the risk of severe skin and tissue necrosis if it extravasates. It can be safe if administered via central access. Calcium gluconate, on the other hand, is safe for peripheral administration. Importantly, it should be given in larger doses (2–3 g) due to its lower calcium content. The overall dosing of calcium is not based on trying to obtain a certain therapeutic level; rather, it is targeting normalization of the EKG. Calcium should act within 1 to 3 minutes and should be re-dosed until EKG changes are seen. Even after reaching an effective level, it should also be re-dosed every 30 to 60 minutes due to its overall short duration of action. This is very important to remember as patients may board for long periods in the ED while awaiting final disposition.

After stabilization, the next intervention is targeted to shift the potassium into the intracellular space. The primary agents here are insulin and beta-agonists. Insulin is administered concomitantly with dextrose to drive potassium intracellularly. A common regimen is 10 units regular insulin administered via IV push as well as 50 mL of 50% dextrose (1 ampule of D_{50}). The IV insulin bolus drives the potassium in while the dextrose protects from associated hypoglycemia. However, given that many patients with hyperkalemia have renal dysfunction, the decreased clearance of insulin may lead to significant hypoglycemia despite treating with dextrose. It has actually been found that 5 units may have a similar efficacy as 10 units with fewer adverse events. In addition, treating with multiple doses of D_{50} (2 ampules, 50 g) or starting a dextrose infusion may also mitigate this risk. Overall, dosing with insulin and dextrose should drop the patient's potassium level 0.6 to 1.1 mEq/L. Once administered, you should check glucose levels hourly and aggressively treat any hypoglycemia. The insulin should act for 4 to 6 hours, whereas the glucose may be metabolized in just an hour.

Shifting of potassium can also be achieved with beta-agonists, namely inhaled albuterol. Albuterol acts via multiple mechanisms to drive potassium intracellularly. In fact, it can drop potassium levels by up to 1 mEq/L in 30 minutes. However, it is ineffective in patients taking nonselective beta-blockers, and even up to 40% of people not on beta-blockers also show some resistance through unknown mechanisms. Given this, while albuterol is a potent agent, it should never be used alone. To get these effects, it also must be dosed at high levels, normally ordered as 10 to 20 mg as a continuous nebulized treatment, four to eight times what is normally used for bronchodilation.

Sodium bicarbonate is another often-quoted agent for shifting potassium, but its efficacy in hyperkalemia has come into question recently. The thought process is valid: Acidosis causes potassium to shift out of cells; therefore, inducing an alkalosis should reverse this change. The problem lies not in the theory, but in the practice. First, this physiology only holds true if the patient is acidotic. If the patient has a normal pH, there is limited benefit in this treatment. Second, sodium bicarbonate is normally administered in the ED as a hypertonic bolus (8.4% sodium bicarbonate, or 1 mEq/mL in a 50-mL ampule). While this does increase the pH, the hypertonic nature also drags some potassium from the intracellular space, leading to a minimal effect on overall serum potassium concentration. On the other hand, isotonic sodium bicarbonate (150 mEq/L or 3 ampules 8.4% sodium bicarbonate in 1 L sterile water or D_5W) does help with the acidosis and does not have the osmotic effect of drawing out potassium, giving it a net effect of decreasing K. However, these patients often cannot tolerate the volume required to achieve the benefit of bicarbonate therapy. Overall, this leaves sodium bicarbonate as an agent with limited utility for treatment of hyperkalemia in the ED.

With the cardiac membranes stabilized and the potassium shifted intracellularly, the final step is to eliminate the potassium. Everything to this point is a temporizing measure; excretion is the definitive therapy. Here, we have three avenues to pursue, colloquially summarized as "pee it out, poop it out, or bleed (dialyze) it out." Diuresing is dependent on the patient's ability to produce urine. If the patient is anuric with end-stage renal disease and dialysis dependent, diuresis is clearly not an option. However, if the patient does make some urine, this approach should be embraced first. Diuresis is most effective with a loop diuretic such as furosemide. This should be dosed appropriately, especially in the setting of renal dysfunction. Aim for higher doses such as furosemide 60 to 120 mg as an IV push. If the patient is over-diuresed with this regimen and becomes hypovolemic, we can easily replace losses with IV fluids such as isotonic bicarbonate solution as noted above or another balanced crystalloid like lactated Ringer's. Sodium chloride or normal saline infusions should be avoided because they generate a metabolic acidosis that can in fact worsen hyperkalemia. In addition to furosemide, thiazide diuretics such as chlorothiazide also enhance potassium excretion and may be given. Fludrocortisone may also have a role in helping to stimulate additional potassium excretion in patients on ACEi/ARBs.

Using the GI system for potassium elimination is currently controversial with respect to its overall efficacy as well as even its safety. Classically sodium polystyrene sulfonate or even newer agents such as sodium zirconium cyclosilicate have been used to help bowel elimination of potassium. However, none of these strategies work in an acute fashion, and therefore they should not be pursued in an emergent situation.

Finally, elimination of potassium occurs most rapidly and definitively through hemodialysis. For patients with truly life-threatening hyperkalemia, all of the above treatments should be performed while simultaneously contacting a nephrology team to arrange for hemodialysis. Dialysis can clear potassium at a rate of 1 mEq/hour depending on the dialysate used in the treatment. Following dialysis, there may be a rebound seen as potassium redistributes from the intracellular space, but the overall total-body potassium will be less and more easily managed.

In summary, hyperkalemia is a life-threatening pathology seen not infrequently in the ED. Though its diagnosis and management are taught to all levels of emergency medicine providers, its prevalence demands that we stay educated and vigilant toward it. The interventions presented here provide emergency physicians with the tools to stabilize and treat this critically ill patient population. Additional electrolyte emergencies commonly encountered in emergency medicine are summarized in Table 31.1.

TABLE 31.1 **Electrolyte emergencies**

Electrolyte emergency	Symptoms/ presentation feature	Treatment	Special considerations
Hypokalemia	Weakness, cramping, EKG changes (QT prolongation, U-waves, T-wave flattening/ inversion)	Oral and parenteral repletion. IV repletion must be performed slowly.	Concurrent hypomagnesemia is common in hypokalemic patients. Treatment of low Mg may be required to effectively treat hypokalemia.
Hypocalcemia	Paresthesias, hyperreflexia, muscle fasciculations, EKG changes (ST prolongation), hypotension, bradycardia, seizures	IV calcium gluconate via peripheral line or IV calcium chloride if central access available	May develop during massive transfusions as the citrate in blood products will bind free calcium

TABLE 31.1 **Continued**

Electrolyte emergency	Symptoms/ presentation feature	Treatment	Special considerations
Hypercalcemia	Delirium, abdominal pain, hyporeflexia, nephrolithiasis	IV fluid if hypovolemic, IV bisphosphonate (zoledronic acid)	Most common cause of severe hypercalcemia is malignancy, either through production of PTHrH or bone invasion by osteolytic lesions.
Hypophosphatemia	Weakness, poor nutrition, DKA	Oral or IV phosphate either as K-Phos or Na-Phos depending on potassium levels	Patients with poor nutrition or uncontrolled diabetes may have initially normal phosphate levels but can develop severe hypophosphatemia as resuscitation or feeding begins.
Hyperphosphatemia	Symptoms of hypocalcemia (phosphate binds free calcium), calciphylaxis	Volume resuscitate, consider forced diuresis (IV fluids + furosemide)	Most commonly occurs in setting of acute or chronic renal failure. Unlikely to be an isolated finding without renal dysfunction.
Hypomagnesemia	Tetany, seizures, arrhythmias (prolonged QT interval that may progress to torsades de pointes)	IV magnesium as slow bolus	Fast administration may cause bradycardia or hypotension. Only bolus quickly in life-threatening arrythmias.

- Hyperkalemia is a common but life-threatening finding in the ED.
- Clinical context is necessary to confirm the laboratory findings, with the etiology often being multifactorial.
- An EKG is an essential step after recognition of hyperkalemia, and the patient should be placed on cardiac telemetry.
- The treatment approach is threefold: Stabilize, shift, and eliminate.
- Stabilize cardiac membranes with 1g calcium chloride or 3 g calcium gluconate.
- Shift with IV insulin, IV glucose, and continuous inhaled albuterol. Never use albuterol as monotherapy.
- Eliminate with aggressive diuresis in non-anuric patients. If they become hypovolemic, resuscitate with balanced crystalloids. GI elimination is not beneficial in the acute setting.
- If anuric or not responding to above treatments, involve nephrology early and arrange for emergent dialysis.

Further reading

Ahee P, Crowe AV. The management of hyperkalaemia in the emergency department. *Emerg Med J*. 2000;17(3):188–191. doi:10.1136/emj.17.3.188

Blumberg A, Weidmann P, Shaw S, Gnädinger M. Effect of various therapeutic approaches on plasma potassium and major regulating factors in terminal renal failure. *Am J Med*. 1988;85(4):507–512. doi:10.1016/s0002-9343(88)80086-x

Lindner G, Burdmann EA, Clase CM, et al. Acute hyperkalemia in the emergency department: A summary from a Kidney Disease: Improving Global Outcomes conference. *Eur J Emerg Med*. 2020;27(5):329–337. doi:10.1097/MEJ.0000000000000691

Mahoney BA, Smith WAD, Lo DS, Tsoi K, Tonelli M, Clase CM. Emergency interventions for hyperkalaemia. *Cochrane Database Syst Rev*. 2005;(2):CD003235. doi:10.1002/14651858.CD003235.pub2

McMahon GM, Mendu ML, Gibbons FK, Christopher KB. Association between hyperkalemia at critical care initiation and mortality. *Intensive Care Med*. 2012;38(11):1834–1842. doi:10.1007/s00134-012-2636-7

Moussavi K, Fitter S, Gabrielson SW, Koyfman A, Long B. Management of hyperkalemia with insulin and glucose: Pearls for the emergency clinician. *J Emerg Med*. 2019;57(1):36–42. doi:10.1016/j.jemermed.2019.03.043

Pun PH, Middleton JP. Dialysate potassium, dialysate magnesium, and hemodialysis risk. *J Am Soc Nephrol*. 2017;28(12):3441–3451. doi:10.1681/ASN.2017060640

Daniel Holt and Timothy J. Ellender

A 22-year-old male presents to the ED with
nausea and vomiting for 2 days. His nausea
has been persistent and worsening and he has
vomited approximately five times in the past
24 hours. He also endorses diffuse abdominal
cramping that is worsening, generalized
weakness and malaise, as well as thirst and
frequent urination. He has been unable to
tolerate drinking water due to his nausea,
despite his thirst. His past medical history is
significant for diabetes mellitus type 1, for which
he is prescribed insulin. Of note, he is recently
unemployed and has been unable to afford his
home insulin. HR is 115 bpm and regular, BP is
90/58 mmHg, temperature is 37.6°C, and oxygen
saturation is 92% on 4 L/min flow through a
nasal cannula. He is tachypneic, taking labored,
deep breaths. His exam is notable for an ill-
appearing young male, with diffuse abdominal
pain, without any rebound tenderness or
guarding as well as dry mucous membranes.

What do I do now?

This case, a young diabetic unable to comply with home medications, with features concerning for diabetic ketoacidosis (DKA), is a common emergency medicine presentation. Improved understanding of DKA and protocolized treatments have significantly reduced the mortality of this complication.[1] However, given the prevalence of diabetes and the myriad of causes that may precipitate this complication, it is imperative that emergency physicians are experts in understanding and managing this process.

DKA occurs most frequently in those under 30 and in those with type 1 diabetes, although it may occur in type 2 diabetes as well.[2] DKA can occur at any age; elderly patients have higher mortality rates given the range of complications associated with it. DKA is often contrasted with hyperosmolar hyperglycemic state (HHS), another potentially fatal condition, more frequently associated with type 2 diabetes and older adults, although with an increasing prevalence in children.[3]

Relative insulin deficiency is the underlying cause of DKA, as the body is unable to utilize glucose as an energy source. In turn, proteins and lipids are catabolized for fuel; these processes generate a state of hyperglycemia and ketonemia. This hyperglycemia leads to osmotic shifts and diuresis, producing symptoms of polyuria and polydipsia, leading to profound hypovolemia. Ketone build up, and electrolyte disturbances from osmotic changes lead to acidosis, which may worsen volume depletion as well as stimulate hyperventilation and respiratory distress, as described in the case.[4,5] In contrast, patients with HHS also suffer insulin deficiency leading to profound hyperglycemia (>600 mg/dL), however with a more gradual onset in symptoms and enough insulin present to suppress ketogenesis.[6] Patients experiencing these metabolic and electrolyte derangements may experience nausea, vomiting, abdominal pain, as well as altered mental status.

While this case does not appear to offer any diagnostic uncertainty, we must consider other diseases in our differential, including other forms of ketoacidosis (starvation and/or alcoholic), HHS, renal failure, and/or lactic acidosis.[5] In addition, in managing DKA, it is important to work to identify the precipitating factor. The most common is improper insulin dosing or noncompliance, as well as infection.[7] Numerous other causes exist, including but not limited to pregnancy, substance abuse, medications, myocardial infarction, cerebrovascular accident, gastrointestinal hemorrhage, pancreatitis, trauma, and/or surgery. Physicians should be diligent in their history and exam, and the workup should be sufficient to rule out these underlying factors.

Initial evaluation should focus on identifying significant electrolyte and metabolic derangements and potential precipitating factors, as well as evaluating for common sources of infection. In patients with features concerning for DKA, check electrolytes (including phosphorus and calcium), obtain a complete blood count, and perform a general diagnostic workup for common sources of infection (e.g., CXR, blood cultures, urinalysis screen). It should be noted that DKA itself may cause a leukocytosis, although a left shift or neutrophil predominance should increase the level of suspicion for an underlying infection. An ECG should be obtained to evaluate for myocardial infarction and to screen for profound electrolyte disturbances. Troponin levels should not be obtained unless the ECG, history, or exam findings are concerning for myocardial infarction, as elevated troponin levels in patients with no coronary disease have been reported in 27% of patients in DKA.[8] Urinalysis is beneficial in evaluating for ketonuria as well as infection.

Abdominal pain and alterations in mental status often lead to difficult clinical decisions on whether to pursue workup for intra-abdominal pathology, as these are common symptoms of DKA. Patients with abdominal pain out of proportion to their acidosis are more likely to have underlying abdominal pathology, and early imaging can be beneficial.[9] Evaluation for pancreatitis, while prudent, is with the caveat that DKA itself may cause elevations in lipase levels.[10] In cases of uncertainty, it is reasonable to aggressively resuscitate patients, obtaining advanced imaging in patients whose symptoms do not improve.[11] Alterations in mental status are more common when serum osmolality is >320.[4] Therefore, further neurologic evaluation may be warranted in patients with serum osmolality under this threshold or in those whose neurologic symptoms do not improve with resuscitation and treatment.

Diagnostic definitions of DKA vary, although most include a blood glucose level of >250 mg/dL, an elevated anion gap, a decreased plasma bicarbonate level (thresholds vary), and evidence of ketonuria or ketonemia.[1,12] Rarely, in 2.6% to 3.2% of admissions for DKA, patients may present with glucose levels <250, a state known as euglycemic diabetic ketoacidosis (EDKA).[13] Risk factors for EDKA include starvation, pregnancy, chronic liver disease, and use of sodium-glucose-cotransporter-2 (SGLT-2) inhibitors.[14] Although most definitions include a depressed pH, it should be noted that concurrent metabolic alkalosis processes may occur (i.e., vomiting), leading to a normalized pH in a small portion of patients with DKA. Routine blood gas analysis may not be necessary in the evaluation and treatment of patients with DKA, although many centers utilize pH for patient triage.

Fluid resuscitation, insulin replacement, management of electrolytes (especially potassium), and supportive care are the cornerstones of treatment. Volume repletion should be started immediately to improve perfusion and lower glucose and ketone levels. Furthermore, insulin responsiveness is improved after volume restoration.[1] Initial fluid resuscitation should consist of 15 to 20 mL/kg/hr of an isotonic crystalloid solution, or approximately 2 L in the first 2 hours.[15] The type of crystalloid solution to be used is debated, as traditional teaching and guidelines recommend the use of isotonic saline, which is known to cause hyperchloremic metabolic acidosis itself. Accordingly, clinicians may prefer balanced crystalloid solutions such as Lactated Ringer's or PlasmaLyte. Further fluid management following this initial bolus should be guided by hemodynamics, urine output, respiratory function, and repeated laboratory values, with a goal of full volume restoration in 24 hours. A standard approach includes a maintenance infusion of 0.45% saline at 250 to 500 cc/hr; however, rates and fluid choice should be evaluated on an individual basis, given differences in patient comorbidities as well as variances in sodium levels.[11] Careful monitoring of glucose levels must occur throughout, and dextrose should be added to these fluids when the blood glucose level is <250 mg/dL.[5,16]

Of note, these pillars of treatment also apply to patients experiencing HHS, and treatment algorithms often combine the two processes. However, as previously noted, pathophysiologic differences exist between DKA and HHS, with the onset of HHS occurring over many days. Therefore, early and gradual fluid resuscitation should be emphasized in treating HHS to avoid excessive decreases in serum osmolality, which may lead to devastating neurologic injury due to either cerebral edema or central pontine myelinolysis. While practice patterns vary, some guidelines advocate holding insulin therapy until fluid resuscitation alone is no longer sufficient for lowering blood glucose levels.[17]

Prior to initiating insulin therapy, serum potassium levels should be obtained as patients in DKA have decreased total-body potassium levels due to their acidosis and volume loss via diuresis and vomiting. The initiation of insulin therapy and fluid resuscitation will further provoke hypokalemia, and electrolytes must be frequently monitored with a goal serum potassium of 4 to 5 mmol/L targeted. If initial serum potassium levels are <3.3 mmol/L, supplemental potassium should be administered prior to insulin infusion. In patients with initial serum potassium levels of 3.3 to 5.2 mmol/L, 20 to 30 mEq/L of potassium should be included in the fluid resuscitation of these patients.[12]

When potassium levels are confirmed to be >3.3 mEq/L, low-dose regular insulin should be administered via continuous infusion. High-dose regimens have been shown to lead to increased episodes of hypoglycemia and hypokalemia.[18] Many hospitals have protocolized insulin administration in patients with DKA. A standard approach includes administration of regular insulin at 0.1 to 0.14 units/kg/hr, decreasing this rate to 0.05 units/kg/hr when blood glucose levels fall to <200 mg/dL. Generally, bolus dosing should be avoided given increased risk in hypoglycemic events and concern that large osmotic shifts may lead to cerebral edema, especially in younger patients.[19] However, in cases of refractory hyperglycemia, a bolus dose of 0.1 to 0.14 units/kg of insulin may be needed.

Intubation of patients in DKA should be performed only in the most extreme circumstances and with utmost caution. Most often, symptoms of DKA resolve following adequate resuscitation and advanced airway management is not needed. Furthermore, patients with profound metabolic acidosis from DKA typically present with a compensatory respiratory alkalosis, with minute ventilations that can be difficult to match on a ventilator. Withholding this physiologic compensatory mechanism from patients may worsen their acidosis.

Similarly, judicious use of bicarbonate in the resuscitation of DKA should be exercised. Some advocate for its use when serum pH is <6.9; however, the benefits of improved myocardial contraction, improved catecholamine response, and decreased work of breathing should be weighed against harms such as worsening hypokalemia, hypertonicity, lactic acidosis, and even possible cerebral edema.[5] Patients generally respond favorably to early and aggressive resuscitative measures as previously discussed without the need for supplemental bicarbonate.

Patients with prolonged ED stays will need repeated physical examinations and careful monitoring of hemodynamics, glucose, and electrolytes. Glucose levels should be monitored hourly at minimum and more frequently if significant insulin/dextrose adjustments are made. Electrolytes, including but not limited to potassium, bicarbonate, and the anion gap, should be monitored every 2 hours during the initial resuscitation of DKA. Severe hypokalemia during the treatment of DKA can be life-threatening and electrolyte as well as osmotic shifts are typical. Gradual correction of these osmotic and electrolyte abnormalities may lessen the risk of cerebral edema, a feared complication in the management of young patients with DKA. Any deterioration in mental status during treatment should be promptly evaluated via neuroimaging and treated with IV mannitol (1–2 g/kg).[19] Persistent acidosis and/or a persistent anion gap despite treatment and resuscitative measures may be indicative of an underlying infectious process and further evaluation, including repeated examination, laboratory evaluation, and advanced imaging, may be needed. Overly aggressive fluid resuscitation may lead to the development of pulmonary edema in elderly patients or those with underlying cardiac dysfunction, so respiratory function should be closely monitored.

Patients presenting in DKA should be admitted for inpatient management. Level of care will vary by hospital-specific policies regarding hemodynamics, oxygen requirements, nursing management of insulin infusions, and monitoring frequency. Patients with hemodynamic instability and profound/persistent acidosis are likely best managed in an ICU setting given the need for extensive nursing care as well as frequent reassessment and management. Site-specific guidelines and protocols should be reviewed and observed.

Given the increasing prevalence of diabetes and the potential mortality of DKA, proper evaluation and management by emergency medicine providers is essential. Providers will also be responsible for the care of patients presenting with other endocrine diseases and complications, such as hyperosmolar hyperglycemic state, myxedema coma, thyrotoxicosis, and adrenal crisis. A summary of these presentations is outlined in Table 32.1.

TABLE 32.1 **Select endocrine disorders**

Disorder	Symptoms/exam	Treatment	Special considerations
Hyperosmolar hyperglycemic state	· Tachycardia · Hypotension · Altered mental status · Dry mucous membranes	· Fluid resuscitation · Insulin · Electrolyte repletion	Differs from DKA in that: · Typically patient with diabetes mellitus type 2 · Blood glucose markedly elevated (>600) · No profound acidemia or anion gap · Minimal ketones · Marked serum osmolality
Myxedema coma	· Hypotension · Bradycardia · Hypothermia · Altered mental status · Signs of hypothyroidism	· Thyroid hormone replacement · Hydrocortisone	· Like DKA, must identify precipitating factors · Steroids should be given as treatment may precipitate adrenal insufficiency.
Thyrotoxicosis	· Tachycardia · Hypertension · Fever · Agitation · Signs of hyperthyroidism	· PTU or methimazole · Beta-blocker · Inorganic iodine · Steroids	· Give iodine >1 hour after PTU or methimazole. · Methimazole is teratogenic in first trimester.
Adrenal crisis	· Refractory hypotension · Altered mental status	· Steroids · Vasopressors if unresponsive to fluids	Primary adrenal insufficiency · Hyperkalemia · Hyponatremia · Skin pigmentation Secondary adrenal insufficiency · Hypokalemia · Cushingoid

- Identification of precipitating factors in DKA is critical to evaluation and management.
- Fluid resuscitation, insulin repletion, and close electrolyte monitoring are the cornerstones of therapy for DKA.
- Repeated evaluation and laboratory monitoring should be utilized in patients with prolonged ED boarding times.
- A variety of other endocrine disorders exist, each with different presentations, requiring varying evaluations and management strategies.

References

1. Kitabchi AE, Umpierrez GE, Miles JM, et al. Hyperglycemic crises in adult patients with diabetes. *Diabetes Care*. 2009;32:1335.
2. Henriksen OM, Røder ME, Prahl JB, Svendsen OL. Diabetic ketoacidosis in Denmark: Incidence and mortality estimated from public health registries. *Diabetes Res Clin Pract*. 2007;76(1):51–56.
3. Bagdure D, Rewers A, Campagna E, Sills MR. Epidemiology of hyperglycemic hyperosmolar syndrome in children hospitalized in USA. *Pediatr Diabetes*. 2013;14(1):18–24.
4. Gomez-Diaz RA, Rivera-Moscoso R, Ramos-Rodriguez R, et al. Diabetic ketoacidosis in adults: Clinical and laboratory features. *Arch Med Res*. 1996;27:177.
5. Nyce AL, Lubkin CL, Chansky ME. Diabetic ketoacidosis. In: Cydulka RK, Fitch MT, Joing SA, Wang VJ, Cline DM, Ma OJ, eds. *Tintinalli's Emergency Medicine Manual*. 8th ed. McGraw-Hill Education; 2016:1457–1464.
6. Stoner GD. Hyperosmolar hyperglycemic state. *Am Fam Physician*. 2017;96(11):729–736.
7. AlMallah M, Zuberi O, Arida M, Kim HE. Positive troponin in diabetic ketoacidosis without evident acute coronary syndrome predicts adverse cardiac events. *Clin Cardiol*. 2008;31:67–71.
8. Umpierrez G, Freire A. Abdominal pain in patients with hyperglycemic crises. *J Crit Care*. 2002;17(1):63–67.
9. Rizvi A. Serum amylase and lipase in diabetic ketoacidosis. *Diabetes Care*. 2003;26(11):3193–3194.
10. Farkas J. Anatomy of a DKA resuscitation. *Internet Book of Critical Care*. https://emcrit.org/ibcc/dka/
11. Wilson JF. Diabetic ketoacidosis in the clinic. *Ann Intern Med*. 2010;152:ITC1-1–ITC1-16.

12. Nyenwe EA, Kitabchi AE. Evidence-based management of hyperglycemic emergencies in diabetes mellitus. *Diabetes Res Clin Pract*. 2011;94(3):340–351.

13. Nasa P, Chaudhary S, Shrivastava PK, Singh A. Euglycemic diabetic ketoacidosis: A missed diagnosis. *World J Diabetes*. 2021;12(5):514–523. doi:10.4239/wjd.v12.i5.514

14. Long B, Lentz S, Koyfman A, Gottlieb M. Euglycemic diabetic ketoacidosis: Etiologies, evaluation, and management. *Am J Emerg Med*. 2021;44:157–160.

15. Marino PL. Organic acidoses. In: Marino PL, ed. *The ICU Book*. 4th ed. Wolters Kluwer Health/Lippincott Williams & Wilkins; 2014:610–613.

16. Kitabchi AE, Ayyagari V, Guerra SM. The efficacy of low-dose versus conventional therapy of insulin for treatment of diabetic ketoacidosis. *Ann Intern Med*. 1976;84(6):633–638.

17. Scott AR; Joint British Diabetes Societies (JBDS) for Inpatient Care; JBDS Hyperosmolar Hyperglycaemic Guidelines Group. Management of hyperosmolar hyperglycaemic state in adults with diabetes. *Diabet Med*. 2015;32(6):714–724.

18. Butkiewicz EK, Leibson CL, O'Brien PC, Palumbo PJ, Rizza RA. Insulin therapy for diabetic ketoacidosis: Bolus insulin injection versus continuous insulin infusion. *Diabetes Care*. 1995;18(8):1187–1190.

19. Hale PM, Rezvani I, Braunstein AW, et al. Factors predicting cerebral edema in young children with diabetic ketoacidosis and new-onset type I diabetes. *Acta Paediatr*. 1997;86:626.

Further reading

Nyenwe EA, Kitabchi AE. Evidence-based management of hyperglycemic emergencies in diabetes mellitus. *Diabetes Res Clin Pract*. 2011;94(3):340–351.

Scott AR; Joint British Diabetes Societies (JBDS) for Inpatient Care; JBDS Hyperosmolar Hyperglycaemic Guidelines Group. Management of hyperosmolar hyperglycaemic state in adults with diabetes. *Diabet Med*. 2015;32(6):714–724.

Westerberg DP. Diabetic ketoacidosis: Evaluation and treatment. *Am Fam Physician*. 2013;87(5):337–346.

33 Transplant troubles: Managing post-transplant complications

Shyam Murali and Clark G. Owyang

A 52-year-old woman presents via EMS to your ED with a 3-day history of nausea, vomiting, and abdominal pain. The pain is in her epigastric region and she describes it as a dull ache. She has also had fevers, chills, fatigue, and decreased appetite. Her initial vitals are HR 115 bpm, RR 22 breaths/min, SpO_2 97%, temperature 38.2°C, BP 108/47 mmHg. A point-of-care blood glucose is 230 mg/dL. She appears ill and uncomfortable with dry mucous membranes and has no focal neurologic deficits. Aside from tachycardia and tachypnea, her cardiopulmonary exam is unremarkable. On abdominal exam, she has moderate tenderness to palpation in the upper abdomen, without peritoneal signs. Large-bore IVs are established, blood is drawn for labs, and you initiate fluid resuscitation with lactated Ringer's. She states that she has a history of type 2 diabetes mellitus, hypertension, and hepatitis C. The patient also mentions to you that she had a liver transplant 5 months ago.

What do I do now?

With nearly 40,000 transplant surgeries being performed in the United States each year, all emergency physicians should be trained to handle life-threatening complications associated with transplants. Long-term outcomes are often influenced by chronic immunosuppression, high rates of complications, and frequent hospital admissions. While immuno-suppressive drugs have allowed transplant recipients to survive longer with lower risk of transplant rejection, these medications depress the recipient's ability to fight severe infections. In addition to the medical complications, patients are at risk for surgical complications, including hernias, bowel obstructions, anastomotic strictures, and vascular abnormalities. We will review the most common complications based on organ and time since transplant (Table 33.1).

TABLE 33.1 **Common infections by time post-transplant**

Time since transplant	Common infections

Early (<1 month)	• Hospital-associated infections
	  • Vascular-catheter infections
	  • Healthcare-associated pneumonia
	  • *Clostridium difficile* colitis
	• Surgical-site infections
	• Donor-originated infections
	• Pneumonia or CNS infections due to Candida and Aspergillus species
	• Reactivated varicella zoster infection

Intermediate (1–6 months)	• Viral
	  • Cytomegalovirus
	  • BK polyomavirus
	  • Hepatitis
	  • EBV
	• Fungal
	  • *Pneumocystis jirovecii*
	  • *Histoplasma*
	  • *Coccidioides*
	  • *Cryptococcus*
	  • Tuberculosis
	• Other opportunistic infections
	  • *Toxoplasma gondii*
	  • *Nocardia*

TABLE 33.1 **Continued**

Late (>6 months)	· Community-acquired infections
	· Typical respiratory viruses
	· *Pneumococcus*
	· *Legionella*
	· *Listeria*
	· Post-transplant lymphoproliferative disorder associated with EBV infection

The most common complaints of ED visits for solid organ transplant patients are abdominal pain and GI symptoms (nausea, vomiting, and diarrhea). The admission rate for transplant patients ranges from 30% to 74%. Common admission diagnoses are organ-specific and include infections, complications of the implant or graft (including rejection), fluid and electrolyte disorders, and acute renal failure.

Infection is a common complication within the first year post-transplant. Complex physiology and medication regimens make recognizing infections challenging, and identification of an infection requires a high level of clinical suspicion. While immunosuppressive drugs can increase the risk of infections, they also blunt the inflammatory response. Fever is the most common sign.

The time since transplantation also plays an important role in identifying the type of infection. Within the first month after transplant, infections are typically hospital-associated infections, surgical site infections, or from the donor organ. During this time, Candida or Aspergillus species can present as pneumonia or CNS infections; reactivated varicella zoster infection can also be common.

Intermediate infections (1–6 months post-transplant) are mostly opportunistic organisms that take advantage of an immunosuppressed host. During this period, viral (cytomegalovirus, BK polyomavirus, hepatitis, Epstein–Barr virus [EBV]) and fungal *(Pneumocystis jirovecii, Histoplasma, Coccidioides, Cryptococcus,* tuberculosis) pathogens are key microbes to consider, in addition to opportunistic bacterial infections. Patients may be on prophylactic antimicrobials during this period.

Infections >6 months from transplantation will more likely be community-acquired infections. During this time, typical respiratory viruses and *Pneumococcus, Legionella,* and *Listeria* predominate. A severe post-transplant complication associated with EBV infection is post-transplant lymphoproliferative disorder (PTLD), and the diagnosis may be challenging because it is usually not associated with a positive Monospot test, splenomegaly, or pharyngitis in the transplant patient. Furthermore, the pathogenesis is a complicated imbalance of the immune system marked by decreased T-cell surveillance allowing lymphoid or plasmacytic proliferation. Ultimately, prompt involvement with the transplant team will expedite the treatments of reduction in immunosuppression or consideration of rituximab.

Primary varicella zoster infections can rapidly disseminate and lead to severe illness due to pneumonia, encephalitis, pancreatitis, hepatitis, and DIC. Patients who are exposed to chicken pox should receive varicella zoster immune globulin post-exposure prophylaxis. Of note, solid organ transplant is a specific risk factor for developing extended-spectrum beta-lactamase (ESBL)-producing Enterobacteriaceae infections, which should prompt emergency physicians to administer broader-spectrum antibiotics than their usual regimen.

As with the general population, transplant patients who present with sepsis or septic shock should be immediately treated with early broad-spectrum antibiotics and IV fluid resuscitation. If a fungal infection is suspected, amphotericin B can also be given, along with ganciclovir for presumed viral infections. Serum and urine testing should be tailored to the patient's presentation and the history and physical exam findings. Consider imaging as appropriate to determine the source of the infection. In all cases, speak with the patient's transplant physician, and consultation to infectious disease specialists may improve outcomes for these patients.

Transplant rejection occurs when the recipient's immune system destroys the transplanted tissue. Though variable by allograft type, the risk of acute rejection and graft loss is highest in the first 3 months post-transplantation. Transplant patients are closely followed by their transplant center during this period, and unplanned ED visits are rare. At the time of transplant and for a short time afterwards, patients are placed on induction therapy with the aim of depleting or inactivating T cells. This is followed by maintenance therapy with immunosuppressants, where the agents are titrated to the lowest acceptable doses that prevent allograft rejection.

Rejection, which should be considered after ruling out infections and surgical complications (described below in the organ-specific discussion), is divided into three categories: hyperacute, acute, and chronic:

Hyperacute rejection occurs within minutes after revascularization in the operating room, typically due to preexisting recipient antibodies that react to the donor antigens. The treatment is immediate removal of the transplanted organ.

Acute rejection occurs within weeks to months after transplant due to T cells attacking donor major histocompatibility complex (MHC). This reaction can cause vasculitis and can be prevented with immunosuppression.

Chronic rejection takes months to years to develop and is caused by both humoral and cell-mediated processes. Again, this causes intimal thickening and fibrosis of the graft vessels leading to ischemia.

Symptoms during an acute rejection episode are nonspecific and depend on the transplanted organ. Patients most frequently present with fever, abdominal pain, graft tenderness, nausea, vomiting, changes in urination or bowel movements, shortness of breath, and/or altered hemodynamics. In renal transplant patients, rejection is diagnosed by a new increase in creatinine >25% from baseline, worsening hypertension, proteinuria >1 g/day, or elevated levels of donor-derived cell-free DNA (dd-cfDNA; released into bloodstream from dead cells in the injured allograft). Liver transplant rejection may present with jaundice, elevated liver function tests, or decreased synthetic capability (decreased albumin, elevated PT/PTT). Acute heart transplant rejection often presents with decompensated heart failure, frequently associated with dysrhythmias, pulmonary edema, renal failure, chest pain, and even sudden cardiac death. Rejection in lung transplant patients can present with pleural effusion, pulmonary edema, cough, or hypoxemia.

To prevent acute and chronic rejection, patients take multiple daily immunosuppressive medications (Table 33.2). These therapies also often worsen or cause cardiovascular disease, renal tubular damage, encephalopathy, seizure, stroke, neutropenia, malignancy, and musculoskeletal disorders. Furthermore, adverse events may be potentiated when these medications are combined with other chronic medications due to cytochrome P-450

TABLE 33.2 **Immunosuppressive medications**

Class	Medications	Toxicity
Calcineurin inhibitors	Cyclosporin	Nephrotoxicity (due to renal vasoconstriction), hepatotoxicity, neurotoxicity, hyperkalemia, hypertension, dyslipidemia, gingival hyperplasia, hypertrichosis, malignancies
	Tacrolimus	Acute renal failure, tremors, electrolyte disturbances, headaches
	Pimecrolimus	Infections, lymphoma, skin malignancies (risk correlates with dosage and duration of treatment)
Anti-proliferatives	Azathioprine	Leukopenia, hepatotoxicity, systemic reactions (fever, abdominal pain, nausea, vomiting, anorexia), malignancies (hematologic, skin)
	Mycophenolate mofetil	GI symptoms (diarrhea, esophagitis, gastritis, GI hemorrhages, etc.), anemia, hypertension,
	Methotrexate	GI symptoms, hepatotoxicity, CNS symptoms (headache, fatigue, malaise), fever, macrocytosis
mTOR receptor inhibitors	Sirolimus	CNS symptoms, GI symptoms, hypertension, anemia, thrombocytopenia, hypercholesterolemia, pulmonary toxicity, skin malignancies, lymphoma, stomatitis
	Everolimus	GI symptoms, stomatitis, hypercholesterolemia, hyperglycemia, anemia, lymphopenia,
Monoclonal and polyclonal antibodies	Rituximab	Thrombocytopenia, GI perforation, pulmonary toxicity, serum sickness
Corticosteroids	Methylprednisolone Prednisone	Iatrogenic Cushing's syndrome, neurotoxicity, hyperglycemia, immune suppression, gastritis, GI hemorrhage, premature atherosclerotic disease

interactions and other direct interactions. For example, diltiazem, verapamil, and amiodarone increase concentrations of cyclosporin and tacrolimus. Conversely, concurrent use of phenytoin causes decreased levels of cyclosporin and tacrolimus and increased levels of phenytoin. For certain medications, drug levels may be obtained to ensure a therapeutic window. Any suspected adverse effect warrants consultation with the transplant physician to discuss potential dosing or regimen changes.

Treatment in the ED for acute rejection episodes consists of pulse corticosteroids (typically methylprednisolone 3–5 mg/kg daily for three to five doses; typically the maximum dose is 500 mg, but some regimens include doses up to 1,000 mg). Contact the patient's transplant physician to discuss augmenting the dose of other immunosuppressants in the patient's regimen. If there is any concern about acute rejection, the patient should be transferred to a facility staffed with transplant specialists.

Graft-versus-host disease (GVHD) is a rare but potentially life-threatening disorder seen in solid organ transplant patients. Though more commonly associated with hematopoietic stem cell transplantation, the incidence of GVHD with solid organ transplant varies by organ and is most common with transplant of small intestine and liver. Skin rash and diarrhea are often the initial symptoms, followed by rapid multisystem disease affecting the bone marrow and other nontransplanted organs. It has a mortality of 30% to 75%. A high degree of suspicion is required to diagnose this problem early, and treatment is the same as that of acute transplant rejection.

Kidney transplants are typically placed extraperitoneally in the iliac fossa due to the proximity to major vessels and the bladder. For renal transplant patients who present to the ED, the differential diagnosis for acute allograft dysfunction is broad, and the presence of a prerenal origin of the symptoms does not absolve the clinician from further investigation. In fact, complications of the device, implant, or graft represent the most common reason for hospital admission. Of note, patients can have recurrence of their initial glomerular disease process that created the need for transplant; recurrence rates can be as high as 50%.

Urinary tract infections (UTIs) carry significant risk and should be treated regardless of severity, because all infections are considered complicated in renal transplant patients. Reflux into the renal cavity can profoundly increase the risk of progression to pyelonephritis. Patients with lower UTIs should be treated for at least 7 days and patients with upper UTIs should be treated for 2 to 3 weeks. Local and patient-specific susceptibility data should be used with close attention paid to the potential drug interactions. The Infectious Diseases Society of America does not recommend routine screening for asymptomatic bacteriuria beyond the first month post-transplant.

Surgical complications can include ureteral stenosis, fistula, or necrosis, stent obstruction, arterial or venous thrombosis or stenosis, hematoma, renal infarct, arterial aneurysm or dissection, or nephrolithiasis or ureterolithiasis.

The physical exam should evaluate for volume status, vital signs, graft tenderness, and other signs of urinary pathology. In addition to serum renal function tests, assessment for urinary infection, proteinuria, and hematuria should be performed with urinalysis with microscopy and urine culture. Plasma levels of dd-cfDNA may be elevated (>1%) in patients with acute rejection. Renal ultrasound with Doppler should also be performed to evaluate for hydronephrosis or vascular compromise (stenosis, thrombosis, etc.).

In contrast to kidney transplantation, orthotopic liver transplants involve the removal of the recipient's native liver prior to placement of the donor liver. Liver transplant patients most commonly present to the ED with abdominal pain and/or fever. Infections are a major source of morbidity and mortality in liver transplant patients, accounting for >50% of early post-transplant deaths. Gram-negative bacteria cause a significant proportion of deaths related to infections, which can present as intra-abdominal abscesses, bacterial pneumonia, cholangitis, peritonitis, bacteremia, and others. Gram-positive and anaerobic organisms also contribute to serious complications post-transplant. Broad-spectrum empiric antibiotics should be given early to patients with potentially serious infections.

Infections are less common in the late post-transplant period, and most occur in patients who require stronger immunosuppression regimens to prevent episodes of chronic rejection. The most common causes of late deaths are chronic rejection and new malignancy. Liver transplant recipients are at higher risk than the general population for the development of cutaneous carcinomas, lymphomas, and lymphoproliferative disorders, likely due to immunodysregulation. These disorders often regress in response to reduction or discontinuation of the immunosuppressive regimen.

The most common late surgical complications include incisional hernias and biliary strictures. Interestingly, anastomotic biliary strictures rarely need surgical intervention and may be amenable to endoscopic evaluation and intervention. The presence of a biliary stricture does warrant evaluation of the patency of the hepatic artery as ischemic-type intrahepatic strictures are common indications for retransplantation. Other surgical complications include biliary stones, biliary sludge, bilomas, hepatic arterial thrombosis, aneurysm, or stenosis, portal vein thrombosis or stenosis, and hepatic vein thrombosis or stenosis.

Signs of acute liver transplant rejection include progressive jaundice, scleral icterus, abdominal pain, fever, malaise, generalized weakness, dark urine, and light-colored stools. Early elevations of alkaline phosphatase and bilirubin are followed by a rise in AST and ALT; however, these elevations are nonspecific and can also occur with other complications such as cholestasis, cholangitis, and drug toxicity.

Heart transplants are typically performed for severe cardiogenic shock with reversible end-organ dysfunction. The donor heart is completely denervated, resulting in loss of sympathetic, parasympathetic, and sensory innervation; this is especially important and may be associated with arrhythmias, painless myocardial infarction, and other atypical presentations. However, many studies show that reinnervation can take place over the first few years post-transplant.

Mortality rates are highest in the first 6 months post-transplant, primarily caused by non-CMV infections, graft failure, and rejection. Beyond the first year, cardiac allograft vasculopathy, due to rapid atherosclerosis, is a main cause of graft failure. Sudden cardiac death is strongly associated with cardiac allograft vasculopathy and is responsible for ~10% of all post-transplant deaths. Cardiac arrhythmias are common, with premature ventricular contractions (PVCs) seen in up to 100% of cardiac transplant patients. Frequent premature atrial contractions (PACs) and atrial flutter have been associated with allograft rejection.

Unlike in kidney transplant rejection, which can be managed with supportive measures such as hemodialysis, cardiac allograft dysfunction can be quickly fatal. These patients should be evaluated quickly, and their care should include a multidisciplinary approach to streamline management, irrespective of stable vital signs. Laboratory evaluation should include troponin, brain natriuretic peptide, and C-reactive protein to evaluate for rejection and signs of heart failure. Point-of-care cardiac ultrasound (POCUS) can be used to evaluate for wall-motion abnormalities, right or left ventricular failure, pericardial fluid, and valve abnormalities. Unstable dysrhythmias should be treated with prompt cardioversion, while stable patients can receive a beta-blocker for rate control. In addition, management of heart failure in transplant patients is similar to management in nontransplant patients: supplemental oxygen, short-term positive-pressure ventilation, diuretics, vasodilators, and inotropic support.

For heart transplant patients who present to the ED with shortness of breath, it is important to consider cardiac (allograft dysfunction, pericardial effusion and tamponade, constrictive pericarditis, arrhythmias), pulmonary (infections, tumors, drug toxicity such as sirolimus-associated interstitial pneumonitis), renal (calcineurin inhibitor–induced nephrotoxicity, nephropathy secondary to steroid-induced diabetes, hypertensive renal disease), and hematologic (anemia of chronic disease) diagnoses.

The transplanted lung is unique in that it is constantly exposed to the environment and at risk of infections. Furthermore, bronchial arterial circulation can take up to 4 weeks to be re-established, causing delayed return of arterial systemic blood supply. Acute cellular rejection is prevalent within the first year, and because patients may be asymptomatic, spirometry is used to monitor lung function. Other symptoms may include fever, dyspnea, malaise, cough, and hypoxemia, with or without radiologic airspace opacities. After the first year, chronic dysfunction can manifest as obliterative bronchiolitis causing physiologic obstruction and is a leading cause of morbidity.

The airway anastomoses are the most vulnerable site for complications and most often occur in the first year. These airway complications have an incidence of ~2% to 33% and include bronchial stenosis, dehiscence, exophytic granulation tissue formation, bronchomalacia, bronchovascular fistulas, and endobronchial infections.

CMV, EBV, and HHV-6 commonly affect lung transplant patients in the first 6 months post-transplant. With higher levels of immunosuppression, opportunistic infections can cause severe disease, even with minimal exposure. *P. aeruginosa* and *S. aureus* are fatal causes of pneumonia in the early postoperative period. Valganciclovir and trimethoprim–sulfamethoxazole prophylaxis can reduce the risk of CMV and Pneumocystis infection, respectively. Fungal infections, most often due to Candida and Aspergillus, are more common in lung transplant patients than other solid organ transplants. Inhaled amphotericin prophylaxis can be used to prevent Aspergillus infections, and first-line treatment for suspected infections is voriconazole.

POCUS can reveal right heart strain and RV dilatation. Patients can also have pleural lining complications, such as pneumothorax, hemothorax, and chylothorax. Effusions can present secondary to infections, rejection, or malignancy, and further characterization with aspiration may be needed for diagnosis.

The presence of metabolic syndromes, including diabetes and dyslipidemia, portends worse outcomes in lung transplant patients. The risk of lung cancer is increased by sixfold compared to the general population. Sirolimus and everolimus can impair wound healing and cause interstitial pneumonitis.

The care of solid organ transplant patients is complex with a multitude of factors that can affect a fine-tuned balance of immunosuppression. Infectious risks, anatomic complications, and timeline post-transplant are important consideration for the emergency physician; early and intermediate complications of transplant should prompt timely involvement of the transplant team.

KEY POINTS TO REMEMBER

- Acute rejection episodes can be treated with high-dose methylprednisolone.
- Infections are common due to immunosuppression and must be rapidly recognized and treated with broad-spectrum antibiotics, antifungals, and antivirals.
- Immunosuppressive medications prevent transplant rejection but increase the risk for serious infections, cardiovascular disorders, malignancy, and organ damage.
- Involve the patient's transplant physician, transplant surgeon, and specific organ consultant early during the patient's care and consider transfer to a transplant center if needed.

Further reading

Adegunsoye A, Strek ME, Garrity E, Guzy R, Bag R. Comprehensive care of the lung transplant patient. *Chest.* 2017;152(1):150–164. doi:10.1016/j.chest.2016.10.001

Assi MA, Pulido JS, Peters SG, McCannel CA, Razonable RR. Graft-vs.-host disease in lung and other solid organ transplant recipients. *Clin Transplant.* 2007;21(1):1–6. doi:10.1111/j.1399-0012.2006.00573.x

Boitard C, Bach JF. Long-term complications of conventional immunosuppressive treatment. *Adv Nephrol Necker Hosp.* 1989;18:335–354.

Chacko P, Philip S. Emergency department presentation of heart transplant recipients with acute heart failure. *Heart Fail Clin.* 2009;5(1):129–143. doi:10.1016/j.hfc.2008.08.011

Chiu LM, Domagala BM, Park JM. Management of opportunistic infections in solid-organ transplantation. *Prog Transplant.* 2004;14(2):114–129. doi:10.7182/prtr.14.2.d8526452qt422v52

Choudhary NS, Saigal S, Bansal RK, Saraf N, Gautam D, Soin AS. Acute and chronic rejection after liver transplantation: What a clinician needs to know. *J Clin Exp Hepatol.* 2017;7(4):358–366. doi:10.1016/j.jceh.2017.10.003

Cozzi E, Colpo A, De Silvestro G. The mechanisms of rejection in solid organ transplantation. *Transfus Apher Sci.* 2017;56(4):498–505. doi:10.1016/j.transci.2017.07.005

Engels EA, Pfeiffer RM, Fraumeni JF Jr, et al. Spectrum of cancer risk among US solid organ transplant recipients. *JAMA.* 2011;306(17):1891–1901. doi:10.1001/jama.2011.1592

Ergin M, Dal Ü, Granit D, Aslay S, Selhanoğlu M. Management of renal transplant patients in the emergency department. *Eurasian J Emerg Med.* 2015;14:83–87.

Eskander MA, Adler E, Hoffmayer KS. Arrhythmias and sudden cardiac death in post-cardiac transplant patients. *Curr Opin Cardiol.* 2020;35(3):308–311. doi:10.1097/HCO.0000000000000731

Eufrásio P, Parada B, Moreira P, et al. Surgical complications in 2000 renal transplants. *Transplant Proc.* 2011;43(1):142–144. doi:10.1016/j.transproceed.2010.12.009

Freeman L, Awad Sh. Evaluation and management of solid organ transplant patients in the emergency department. *Emergency Medicine Reports.* 2004;25(2).

Gatz JD, Spangler R. Evaluation of the renal transplant recipient in the emergency department. *Emerg Med Clin North Am.* 2019;37(4):679–705. doi:10.1016/j.emc.2019.07.008

Iwatsuki S, Starzl TE, Gordon RD, et al. Late mortality and morbidity after liver transplantation. *Transplant Proc.* 1987;19(1 Pt 3):2373–2377.

Long B, Koyfman A. The emergency medicine approach to transplant complications. *Am J Emerg Med.* 2016;34(11):2200–2208. doi:10.1016/j.ajem.2016.08.049

Lovasik BP, Zhang R, Hockenberry JM, et al. Emergency department use among kidney transplant recipients in the United States. *Am J Transplant.* 2018;18(4):868–880. doi:10.1111/ajt.14578

Machuzak M, Santacruz JF, Gildea T, Murthy SC. Airway complications after lung transplantation. *Thorac Surg Clin*. 2015;25(1):55–75. doi:10.1016/j.thorsurg.2014.09.008

McElroy LM, Schmidt KA, Richards CT, et al. Early postoperative emergency department care of abdominal transplant recipients. *Transplantation*. 2015;99(8):1652–1657. doi:10.1097/TP.0000000000000781

Mıhçıokur S, Doğan G, Kocalar G, Erdal R, Haberal M. Emergency department visits after kidney, liver, and heart transplantation in a hospital of a university in Turkey: A retrospective study. *Exp Clin Transplant*. 2019;17(Suppl 1):264–269. doi:10.6002/ect.MESOT2018.P120

Mohseni MM, Li Z, Simon LV. Emergency department visits among lung transplant patients: a 4-year experience. *J Emerg Med*. 2021;60(2):150–157. doi:10.1016/j.jemermed.2020.10.005

Patchell RA. Neurological complications of organ transplantation. *Ann Neurol*. 1994;36(5):688–703. doi:10.1002/ana.410360503

Porrett PM, Hsu J, Shaked A. Late surgical complications following liver transplantation. *Liver Transpl*. 2009;15(Suppl 2):S12–S18. doi:10.1002/lt.21893

Santacruz JF, Mehta AC. Airway complications and management after lung transplantation: Ischemia, dehiscence, and stenosis. *Proc Am Thorac Soc*. 2009;6(1):79–93. doi:10.1513/pats.200808-094GO

Savitsky EA, Uner AB, Votey SR. Evaluation of orthotopic liver transplant recipients presenting to the emergency department. *Ann Emerg Med*. 1998;31(4):507–517.

Schold JD, Elfadawy N, Buccini LD, et al. Emergency department visits after kidney transplantation. *Clin J Am Soc Nephrol*. 2016;11(4):674–683. doi:10.2215/CJN.07950715

Schuurmans MM, Tini GM, Zuercher A, Hofer M, Benden C, Boehler A. Practical approach to emergencies in lung transplant recipients: How we do it. *Respiration*. 2012;84(2):163–175. doi:10.1159/000339345

Scott CD, Dark JH, McComb JM. Arrhythmias after cardiac transplantation. *Am J Cardiol*. 1992;70(11):1061–1063. doi:10.1016/0002-9149(92)90361-2

Sia IG, Paya CV. Infectious complications following renal transplantation. *Surg Clin North Am*. 1998;78(1):95–112. doi:10.1016/s0039-6109(05)70637-x

Sternbach GL, Varon J, Hunt SA. Emergency department presentation and care of heart and heart/lung transplant recipients. *Ann Emerg Med*. 1992;21(9):1140–1144. doi:10.1016/s0196-0644(05)80661-4

Trzeciak S, Sharer R, Piper D, et al. Infections and severe sepsis in solid-organ transplant patients admitted from a university-based ED. *Am J Emerg Med*. 2004;22(7):530–533. doi:10.1016/j.ajem.2004.09.010

Turtay MG, Oguzturk H, Aydin C, Colak C, Isik B, Yilmaz S. A descriptive analysis of 188 liver transplant patient visits to an emergency department. *Eur Rev Med Pharmacol Sci*. 2012;16 Suppl 1:3–7.

UNOS. Organ transplant trends: More transplants than ever. https://unos.org/data/transplant-trends/. Published December 23, 2020. Accessed January 9, 2021.

Unterman S, Zimmerman M, Tyo C, et al. A descriptive analysis of 1251 solid
    organ transplant visits to the emergency department. *West J Emerg Med.*
    2009;10(1):48–54.

Van De Wauwer C, Van Raemdonck D, Verleden GM, et al. Risk factors for airway
    complications within the first year after lung transplantation. *Eur J Cardiothorac
    Surg.* 2007;31(4):703–710. doi:10.1016/j.ejcts.2007.01.025

Zhang Y, Ruiz P. Solid organ transplant-associated acute graft-versus-host disease.
    Arch Pathol Lab Med. 2010;134(8):1220–1224. doi:10.1043/2008-0679-RS.1

34 Cancer alphabet soup: Oncology complications

Clark G. Owyang and Shyam Murali

A 72-year-old man with a history of acute myeloid leukemia (AML), having attained first complete remission, presented to the ED with altered mental status, generalized weakness, and spontaneous epistaxis. He was febrile, tachycardic, and hypoxemic. Laboratory values showed a hemoglobin of 4 g/dL, platelets of 59,000/μL, and WBC count of 110,000/μL with 90% blasts. LDH activity was profoundly elevated, and coagulopathy was evident with elevated PT/INR, elevated D-dimer, and decreased fibrinogen. Chemistry revealed elevated phosphorous, potassium, and uric acid levels with a decreased calcium level. Creatinine was elevated to 2.6 mg/dL. B-type natriuretic peptide was elevated to >10,000 pg/mL. He was intubated and a central line, was placed with oozing noted from puncture sites.

What do I do now?

A side from the obvious multiorgan system involvement of this critically ill patient, the patient's profound leukocytosis and history of AML highlight the likely relapsed state of his leukemia. Specifically, the high WBC count (hyperleukocytosis) of his relapsed AML is a marker of his high risk for three complications: disseminated intravascular coagulation (DIC), hyperviscosity syndrome (HVS), and tumor lysis syndrome (TLS). These conditions associated with hyperleukocytosis will be the focus of this chapter as they are significant oncologic complications faced in acute care medicine. Hyperleukocytosis is defined variably with a range of total leukemic blood cell counts >50,000/μL or 100,000/μL; it is seen in both acute and chronic leukemias, with the risk of complications higher in the acute leukemias.[1] Additionally, the elevated LDH activity serves as a poor prognostic factor and as a general indicator of the tumor burden activity of the patient's AML. Using this AML case vignette as context, this chapter will focus on the definitions, risk stratification, and interventions in acute care medicine expected in the ED/ICU interface.

DISSEMINATED INTRAVASCULAR COAGULATION

A well-known physiologic derangement in critical care, DIC is generally considered a consumptive coagulopathy associated with various malignancies, as well as other broad etiologies (sepsis, trauma, toxicology) seen in critically ill populations. In short, DIC is due to an activation of the tissue factor–dependent coagulation pathway, suppression of fibrinolysis, and the loss of anticoagulation pathways (Table 34.1).[2] While diagnostic

TABLE 34.1 **Thrombotic and coagulopathic mechanisms of DIC**

Thrombosis	Coagulopathy/bleeding
Fibrinogen → fibrin	Coagulation factor depletion
Platelet activation	Fibrinogen depletion
Tissue factor expression	Lysis of thrombi
	Thrombocytopenia
	Activation of protein C

scoring algorithms have been created, there is no gold standard or single diagnostic test for confirmation of DIC. It remains a clinical diagnosis with support from laboratory assays.[3,4] The International Society on Thrombosis and Haemostasis has accurate diagnostic and prognostic criteria for DIC incorporating decreased platelet level and fibrinogen with increased PT and fibrin degradation products.[2] While elevated coagulation assays are nonspecific and present in many critically ill patients, the increased fibrin degradation products and D-dimer levels more specifically reflect an abnormal elevation of thrombin in the clotting cascade.[5] Specific to this case of oncologic complications (i.e., relapsed AML), DIC can be seen in both solid and liquid malignancies with an incidence of ~7% in solid tumors and 15% to 20% in leukemia/lymphoma patients.[6–8] While the specific mechanisms have yet to be fully elucidated and vary among different malignancies, DIC in cancer appears to result from direct expression of tissue factor and activator of factor X.[5] Many patients present with bleeding syndrome, though interestingly some present with thrombosis.

Current guidelines for DIC treatment are structured around clinical bleeding to drive transfusion thresholds.[9] Previously, blood product transfusion for the low fibrinogen, elevated coagulation assays, and low platelets was thought to be contraindicated as it would "feed the fire." However, current guidelines for the non-bleeding patient are as follows: Hemoglobin should be maintained >7 g/dL and platelets kept >10,000/μL. A more conservative platelet threshold of >50,000/μL should be pursued in the hemorrhaging patient along with the administration of cryoprecipitate, targeting fibrinogen ≥100 g/dL. Fresh frozen plasma is recommended for INR >1.5 despite unclear benefits with INR <1.85.[9] Further coagulopathy should be addressed by targeting an activated partial thromboplastin time (aPTT) of <1.5 times normal.[5] An international consensus paper showed the variation in expert opinion and limited randomized controlled trial data available to guide DIC management.[10] For thrombosis associated with DIC, the treatment approaches are heterogenous but favor low-molecular-weight heparin or novel oral anticoagulants (NOACs). Of note, heparin therapy in acute promyelocytic leukemia remains controversial as this subtype often has a high prevalence of hemorrhagic complications and deaths.[5,6] The cornerstone of DIC treatment remains addressing the underlying cause.

HYPERVISCOSITY SYNDROME

Concomitant with the coagulopathy noted in the DIC scenario above, the markedly elevated WBC count puts the patient at risk for hypoperfusion and organ failure (specifically, neurologic and respiratory) due to increased blood viscosity. HVS is a constellation of symptoms reflecting increased internal resistance to flow in the serum, due to the rise in either cellular or acellular blood components. Blood viscosity is normally between 1.4 and 1.8 centipoise, with symptoms manifesting usually >3.0 centipoise; importantly, the clinical presentation is more useful than viscosity measurement as these measurements are inaccurate in hyperleukocytosis.[11] The causes and specific organ system involvement are heterogenous; death (often secondary to bleeding), neurologic complications, and pulmonary complications are common.[1,12] Diseases of pathologic elevation in acellular components include myeloma, Waldenström's macroglobulinemia, cryoglobulinemia, and other causes of hyperglobulinemia. Rarely, infusions of intravenous immunoglobulin (IVIG) have been reported to produce transient hyperviscosity by a similar mechanism of acellular components.[13] Cellular component elevation may be seen in the broad categories of leukemia, polycythemia vera, and thrombocytosis. While clinical presentation of acute lymphoblastic leukemia (ALL) often has higher WBC counts, AML more commonly has leukostasis that results in end-organ damage.[11]

The increased internal resistance to blood flow causes hypoperfusion, decreased microvascular circulation, and coagulation derangements. There is no strict laboratory cutoff for blood viscosity, though common cutoffs for cellular and acellular components of blood have been defined (Table 34.2). Different patients will manifest symptoms and organ system involvement at different viscosity levels. The clinical manifestations show the classic triad of mucosal bleeding, visual abnormalities, and neurologic abnormalities. However, end-organ manifestations can also involve cardiovascular and pulmonary systems with hypervolemia and cardiac failure. While the laboratory signs associated with hematologic malignancies leading to hyperleukocytosis vary, the risk for hyperviscosity or leukostasis has been cited to occur with leukocyte counts between 100,000/μL and 250,000/μL.[11]

TABLE 34.2 **Common laboratory values for HVS**

Paraproteinemia	IgM	>3 g/dL
	IgA	>10 g/dL
	IgG	>15 g/dL
Cellular components	AML	>300 × 10³/dL
	ALL	>600 × 10³/dL
	CML, blast phase	>100 × 10³/dL
	CML, accelerated phase	>100 × 10³/dL
	CML, chronic phase	>100 × 10³/dL
	Essential thrombosis	>1,000 × 10³/dL

Ig, immunoglobulin; AML, acute myeloid leukemia; ALL, acute lymphoblastic leukemia; CML, chronic myeloid leukemia

Treatment options for HVS include cytoreductive therapies to decrease the peripheral WBC count via hydroxyurea or emergent induction chemotherapy. Plasmapheresis is another option that is recommended when leukemic counts are >50,000/μL and there are symptoms of end-organ involvement. However, there is risk for significant coagulopathy and bleeding specific to using leukapheresis in acute promyelocytic leukemia.[14] Plasmapheresis removes whole plasma and replaces it typically with either 4% to 6% albumin or fresh frozen plasma.[11] Similar to DIC, patients with HVS should be maintained with an adequate platelet count to prevent intracranial hemorrhage—sources cite goal levels of 20,000/μL to 30,000/μL.[15] Transfusions during the hyperleukocytosis period should be judicious as there is risk for potentiating HVS. Patients with HVS often have a dilutional anemia due to plasma volume expansion driven by the tumor burden and expanded acellular components of blood (i.e., immunoglobulins). IV fluids (free of calcium and potassium) should be administered at roughly two to five times the normal maintenance rate; use caution in those with heart failure and those at risk for congestion.

TUMOR LYSIS SYNDROME

TLS is defined by derangements in phosphate, potassium, calcium, and uric acid levels, reflecting the cellular breakdown of tumor burden. TLS most commonly arises after the start of initial chemotherapy and has been reported with every type of tumor. Risk factors are bulky, rapidly proliferating, treatment-responsive tumors (acute leukemias [AML and ALL], high-grade non-Hodgkin lymphomas [Burkitt lymphoma]). The breakdown of the purine nucleotides from cells releases nephrotoxins, such as uric acid and xanthine, causing urate nephropathy. The two manifestations of TLS that drive treatment are renal injury and electrolyte derangements.

Treatment options for TLS are a combination of oncologic-specific medications as well as interventions to address the underlying metabolic derangements. Traditionally, allopurinol and rasburicase are the two interventions to address the nephrotoxic effects of cellular breakdown. Allopurinol enzymatically inhibits the production of xanthine and uric acid while rasburicase prevents uric acid buildup by converting it to the harmless allantoin. While adult data are limited, one of the few randomized clinical trials on rasburicase found it to be more effective than allopurinol in reducing uric acid levels in a population at high risk for TLS.[16] However, it should not be used in patients with G6PD deficiency. As there may be concomitant risk for HVS depending on tumor burden, the TLS patient should be volume resuscitated with fluids low in potassium and calcium similar to HVS treatment.[17]

The consequences of missing the diagnosis of TLS is renal injury, which has important associations in critical care. Mechanistically, the TLS-mediated uric acid crystals and calcium–phosphate deposition lead to acute kidney injury (AKI), which is associated with increased mortality—both from an oncologic perspective (the chemotherapy effectiveness and chances for complete remission are decreased)[18] and in the context of critical care (AKI is associated with higher mortality).[19] Early consultation with nephrology for early initiation of dialytic therapy is key in addition to fluid resuscitation, as severe cases rapidly cause metabolic acidosis and hyperkalemia. It is common on presentation to the ED to meet criterion for emergent dialysis. Serial assessment of uric acid and electrolytes, including phosphorus and calcium, will be necessary depending on the length of time spent in the ED.[20]

- Hyperleukocytosis is caused by leukemic cell proliferation (seen in both acute and chronic) and has critical care complications of DIC, HVS, and TLS.
- Data are limited for many of the interventions for DIC; however, coagulation factors should be replaced and platelets repleted if <50,000/μL in the context of serious bleeding, despite the previously held fear of "fueling the fire."
- HVS/leukostasis can be present in a variety of malignancies of cellular and acellular components and should be considered with CNS and pulmonary dysfunction.
- Treatments of choice for HVS are cytoreductive therapies: induction chemotherapy (if the patient is able to tolerate it), hydroxyurea, and plasmapheresis (except for acute promyelocytic leukemia).
- TLS prophylaxis can be performed with allopurinol; however, rasburicase is more effective for renal and uric acid level outcomes and should be used (except in G6PD deficiency).

References
1. Rollig C, Ehninger G. How I treat hyperleukocytosis in acute myeloid leukemia. *Blood*. 2015;125(21):3246–3252.
2. Gando S, Meziani F, Levi M. What's new in the diagnostic criteria of disseminated intravascular coagulation? *Intensive Care Med*. 2016;42(6):1062–1064.
3. Levi M. Disseminated intravascular coagulation in cancer: An update. *Semin Thromb Hemost*. 2019;45(4):342–347.
4. Toh CH, Hoots WK. The scoring system of the Scientific and Standardisation Committee on Disseminated Intravascular Coagulation of the International Society on Thrombosis and Haemostasis: A 5-year overview. *J Thromb Haemost*. 2007;5(3):604–606.
5. DeLoughery TG. Disseminated intravascular coagulation. In: DeLoughery TG, ed. *Hemostasis and Thrombosis*. Springer International Publishing; 2019:55–59.
6. Barbui T, Falanga A. Disseminated intravascular coagulation in acute leukemia. *Semin Thromb Hemost*. 2001;27(6):593–604.
7. Sallah S, Wan JY, Nguyen NP, Hanrahan LR, Sigounas G. Disseminated intravascular coagulation in solid tumors: Clinical and pathologic study. *Thromb Haemost*. 2001;86(3):828–833.

8. Chi S, Ikezoe T. Disseminated intravascular coagulation in non-Hodgkin lymphoma. *Int J Hematol.* 2015;102(4):413–419.

9. Fusaro MV, Netzer G. Disseminated intravascular coagulation. In: Hyzy RC, ed. *Evidence-Based Critical Care: A Case Study Approach.* Springer International Publishing; 2017:619–624.

10. Squizzato A, Hunt BJ, Kinasewitz GT, et al. Supportive management strategies for disseminated intravascular coagulation: An international consensus. *Thromb Haemost.* 2016;115(5):896–904.

11. O'Connor BP, Subramanian IM. Management of hyperviscosity syndromes. In: Hyzy RC, ed. *Evidence-Based Critical Care: A Case Study Approach.* Springer International Publishing; 2017:647–653.

12. Porcu P, Cripe LD, Ng EW, et al. Hyperleukocytic leukemias and leukostasis: A review of pathophysiology, clinical presentation and management. *Leuk Lymphoma.* 2000;39(1–2):1–18.

13. Gertz MA. Acute hyperviscosity: Syndromes and management. *Blood.* 2018;132(13):1379–1385.

14. Blum W, Porcu P. Therapeutic apheresis in hyperleukocytosis and hyperviscosity syndrome. *Semin Thromb Hemost.* 2007;33(4):350–354.

15. Kaide CG, Emerson G. Acute blast crisis/hyperviscosity syndrome: Blasting off! In: Kaide CG, San Miguel CE, eds. *Case Studies in Emergency Medicine: LEARNing Rounds: Learn, Evaluate, Adopt, Right Now.* Springer International Publishing; 2020:31–39.

16. Cortes J, Moore JO, Maziarz RT, et al. Control of plasma uric acid in adults at risk for tumor lysis syndrome: Efficacy and safety of rasburicase alone and rasburicase followed by allopurinol compared with allopurinol alone—results of a multicenter phase III study. *J Clin Oncol.* 2010;28(27):4207–4213.

17. Koneru H, Bozyk PD. Tumor lysis syndrome. In: Hyzy RC, ed. *Evidence-Based Critical Care: A Case Study Approach.* Springer International Publishing; 2017:641–645.

18. Zafrani L, Canet E, Darmon M. Understanding tumor lysis syndrome. *Intensive Care Med.* 2019;45(11):1608–1611.

19. Fortrie G, de Geus HRH, Betjes MGH. The aftermath of acute kidney injury: A narrative review of long-term mortality and renal function. *Crit Care.* 2019;23(1):24.

20. Wilson FP, Berns JS. Tumor lysis syndrome: New challenges and recent advances. *Adv Chronic Kidney Dis.* 2014;21(1):18–26.

35 Hot as a hare: Critically ill toxidromes

Samuel Garcia and Aaron Skolnik

A 16-year-old young woman is brought into the ED by EMS after being found unresponsive in her bedroom by her father. She is obtunded and taken directly to the resuscitation room on arrival. Her father notes that she seemed to be in her usual state of health and was last seen well 2 hours prior to presentation. He heard a loud "thud" in her room and found her unresponsive on the floor, next to empty pill bottles labeled as an over-the-counter sleep aid containing diphenhydramine. The patient had previously expressed passive death wish but has never attempted suicide before and has never been on psychiatric medication. Her father notes she has seemed increasingly depressed after the recent start of the school year and is concerned that she may have intentionally overdosed. He reports she otherwise only has access to acetaminophen at home and denies any history of illicit drug use. On the cardiac monitor, her HR is 140 bpm and the rhythm is regular with a wide QRS complex. Her BP is 150/90 mmHg, RR is 22 breaths/min, pulse oximetry reads 100% on room air, and point-of-care glucose is 120 mg/dL. Her rectal temperature is 39°C and her skin is flushed and dry. Neurologic examination is otherwise significant for bilateral equal and minimally reactive pupils at 5 mm and hyperreflexic deep tendon reflexes with 6 beats of clonus at the ankles bilaterally. As you continue to examine her, she has a generalized tonic-clonic seizure.

What do I do now?

This patient presents to the ED in extremis with a history of an acute ingestion of diphenhydramine. She is tachycardic, hypertensive, hyperthermic, and anhidrotic and has altered mentation. The differential diagnosis for this presentation includes anticholinergic poisoning, sympathomimetic toxicity, sedative–hypnotic withdrawal, serotonin syndrome, neuroleptic malignant syndrome, malignant hyperthermia, heat stroke, sepsis, and thyrotoxicosis, among others.

The first priority is the initial resuscitation and stabilization of this critically poisoned patient. This includes airway assessment and management if required, obtaining venous access, and placing the patient on continuous cardiac and pulse oximetry monitoring. Hypotension should be managed with balanced crystalloid administration and direct-acting vasopressors (i.e., norepinephrine) as needed. In the altered patient, point-of-care glucose should be checked or empiric IV dextrose given. Based on the clinical presentation, specific toxidromes can be identified and any drug-specific antidotes implemented.

There are five classic toxidromes: opioid, sedative–hypnotic, sympathomimetic, cholinergic, and anticholinergic (Table 35.1). These toxidromes are important as they permit initiation of empiric treatment based on the clinical presentation alone, prior to the establishment of a definitive diagnosis. It is also important to remember that co-ingestions may occur and the patient's clinical presentation may involve features of more than one toxidrome.

The opioid toxidrome is characterized by miosis, bradypnea, and depressed mental status. It results from the stimulation of μ-opioid receptors resulting in generalized depression of autonomic activity. This can also lead to bradycardia, hypotension, hypoactive bowel sounds, and hypothermia. The sedative–hypnotic toxidrome is most often caused by γ-aminobutyric acid (GABA) receptor agonists such as benzodiazepines, barbiturates, and ethanol, leading to CNS depression. This results in anxiolysis, modest respiratory depression, bradycardia, hypotension, and hypothermia. In contrast, cholinergic toxicity is caused by excessive accumulation of acetylcholine at the neuromuscular junctions and synapses. It is classically caused by organophosphate insecticide or nerve agent poisoning but can be caused by anticholinesterase prescription medications, such as physostigmine. It is characterized by miosis, sialorrhea, lacrimation, bronchorrhea, bradycardia,

TABLE 35.1 Signs and symptoms of classic toxidromes

	Toxidrome				
	Opioid	Sedative–hypnotic	Sympathomimetic	Cholinergic	Anticholinergic
Level of consciousness	Depressed	Depressed	Agitation, delirium	Variable	Variable, delirium
Skin	Variable	Variable	Diaphoretic	Diaphoretic	Dry
Pupils	Miotic	Variable	Mydriatic	Miotic	Mydriatic
Reflexes	Variable	Variable	Hyperreflexic	Variable	Hyperreflexic
Temperature	Normal to decreased	Normal to decreased	Hyperthermic	Variable	Hyperthermic
Heart rate	Normal or decreased	Normal or decreased	Tachycardic	Variable	Tachycardic
Respiratory rate	Decreased	Normal or decreased	Tachypneic	Variable	Variable
Blood pressure	Normal or hypotensive	Normal or hypotensive	Hypertensive	Variable	Normal or hypertensive

and urinary and fecal incontinence. Sympathomimetic toxicity is caused by stimulants such as cocaine and methamphetamines, which increase sympathetic neurotransmission by several molecular mechanisms. Classic signs include reactive mydriasis, psychomotor agitation, tachycardia, hypertension, hyperthermia, tachypnea, and diaphoresis.

The case presented above is classic for anticholinergic toxicity given the reported use of diphenhydramine, an antihistamine with well-described antimuscarinic properties, and the clinical features consistent with an anticholinergic toxidrome. It is important to differentiate anticholinergic toxicity from other etiologies, as each toxidrome will require a unique set of antidotes and treatments. The traditional mnemonic for the signs present in anticholinergic toxicity is:

"**Mad as a hatter**": anxiety, agitation, confusion, dysarthria, carphologia, delirium, visual hallucinosis, coma, and seizures
"**Hot as a hare**": hyperthermia
"**Dry as a bone**": anhidrosis
"**Red as a beet**": skin hyperemia
"**Blind as a bat**": non-reactive mydriasis, and
"**Full as a flask**": urinary retention.

The antagonism of muscarinic receptors in the CNS results in alterations in mental status, whereas the antagonism in the peripheral nervous system results in all the other symptoms described above.

One of the earliest and most frequently encountered signs in an anticholinergic overdose is tachycardia. The distinguishing feature of this toxidrome, however, is dry axillary skin due to the antimuscarinic inhibition of apocrine sweat glands. The "toxicologist's handshake" consists of placing one's hand into the axilla of the patient to determine if anhidrosis is present, a feature that would distinguish anticholinergic from sympathomimetic toxicity, for example. Other signs include urinary retention and the absence of bowel sounds secondary to decreased GI motility. Decreased GI motility may result in delayed absorption of the ingested agents, further prolonging their effects.

Medications commonly associated with anticholinergic toxicity include antihistamines, cyclic antidepressants, some antipsychotics (olanzapine, quetiapine, clozapine, chlorpromazine), antiparkinsonian drugs (benztropine), and antispasmodics (dicyclomine, hyoscyamine), among others. It is important to remember that anticholinergic toxicity can also be caused by botanicals and other natural sources. The most common plants and mushrooms containing anticholinergic alkaloids include jimsonweed (*Datura stramonium*), deadly nightshade (*Atropa belladonna*), mandrake (*Mandragora officinarum*), and fly agaric (*Amanita muscaria*) mushrooms. Anticholinergic symptoms typically begin within 1 hour of ingestion and may continue for days. Severe toxicity, although rare, can be fatal and may result from rhabdomyolysis-induced kidney injury, disseminated intravascular coagulation, dysrhythmias, or complications of uncontrolled seizures.

The diagnostic evaluation should include obtaining basic laboratory work such as a point-of-care glucose, a complete blood count, and a comprehensive metabolic panel including serum electrolyte levels such as potassium and magnesium. Serum salicylate, acetaminophen, and ethanol levels may also be useful as co-ingestion is common in intentional overdoses. Urine screens for drugs of abuse are of limited utility but may inform psychiatric disposition after critical illness has resolved. All poisoned patients should have an immediate ECG obtained to evaluate for signs of cardiotoxicity.

Activated charcoal decontamination is only indicated for patients who arrive within 1 hour after ingestion and are able to protect their airway. Benzodiazepines are indicated for treating seizures in these patients. They have been recommended to decrease the risk of hyperthermia and rhabdomyolysis and to increase the seizure threshold. In patients presenting with intraventricular conduction abnormalities, a sign of sodium channel blockade, serum alkalinization with sodium bicarbonate may be effective in narrowing of the QRS and preventing dysrhythmias.

Physostigmine, a reversible acetylcholinesterase inhibitor, is a direct antidote for anticholinergic toxicity and is indicated for severe agitation or delirium. It works by allowing acetylcholine to build up at neuronal synapses and overcome cholinergic blockade. It has been underutilized in the past due to concerns about its safety after cases were published where patients with severe tricyclic antidepressant (TCA) toxicity experienced sudden cardiac arrest soon after the administration of physostigmine.

It has since been relatively contraindicated in TCA toxicity, presence of intraventricular conduction delays (PR > 200 or QRS > 100), history of seizures, and asthma, and in suspected mechanical GI obstruction. In the absence of these features, physostigmine has been demonstrated to be safe and effective in treating central anticholinergic syndrome. Studies have supported its efficacy as both a diagnostic and a therapeutic tool. It has been proven to overall decrease the rate of invasive testing and complications when compared with benzodiazepines alone. If no contraindications are present, consider using physostigmine in consultation with a poison control center. The dosing of physostigmine for adults is 0.5 mg infused over 2 to 5 minutes. In children, the dose is 0.02 mg/kg (maximum of 0.5 mg). The onset of action is within 3 to 8 minutes. It is important that the patient be on continuous cardiac monitoring during and after its administration. Physostigmine may be re-dosed every 5 to 10 minutes for a maximum dose of 2 mg over the first hour. Important side effects to consider are bradycardia, dysrhythmias, seizures, and cholinergic toxicity. It is important to note that the half-life of physostigmine is often shorter than that of the ingested drug; therefore, physostigmine will often need to be re-administered. It is prudent to have atropine or glycopyrrolate at the bedside for bradycardia or severe cholinergic excess caused by physostigmine.

The disposition of a patient presenting in an anticholinergic toxidrome is based on the type of ingestion, the quantity ingested, and signs and symptoms in the ED. Patients who ingested long-acting agents or a large quantity may require extended observation as they can experience delayed sequelae due to decreased GI motility, as previously described. If physostigmine is administered, the patient should be admitted for further monitoring.

KEY POINTS TO REMEMBER

- Anticholinergic toxicity is a clinical diagnosis.
- The first priority in a critically ill toxicology patient is immediate resuscitation and stabilization, followed by rapid diagnostic evaluation and application of drug-specific antidotes.

- Obtain an ECG on any patient presenting with signs or symptoms of anticholinergic toxicity to evaluate the QRS interval.
- Prior to administering physostigmine, determine any contraindications and administer in consultation with a poison control center.
- If physostigmine will be administered, the patient must be on continuous cardiac monitoring to evaluate for adverse effects.
- All patients who receive physostigmine should be admitted for observation.

Further reading

Arens A, Kearney T. Adverse effects of physostigmine. *J Med Toxicol*. 2019;15(3):184–191.

Boley S, Stellpflug S. A comparison of resource utilization in the management of anticholinergic delirium between physostigmine and nonantidote therapy. *Ann Pharmacother*. 2019;53(10):1026–1032.

Burns M, Linden C, Graudins A, Brown R, Fletcher K. A comparison of physostigmine and benzodiazepines for the treatment of anticholinergic poisoning. *Ann Emerg Med*. 2000;35(4):374–381.

Ceha L, Presperin C, Young E, Allswede M, Erickson T. Anticholinergic toxicity from nightshade berry poisoning responsive to physostigmine. *J Emerg Med*. 1997;15(1):65–69.

Chadwick A, Ash A, Day J, Borthwick M. Accidental overdose in the deep shade of night: A warning on the assumed safety of "natural substances." *BMJ Case Reports*. 2015;bcr2015209333.

Glatstein M, Alabdulrazzaq F, Scolnik D. Belladonna alkaloid intoxication: The 10-year experience of a large tertiary care pediatric hospital. *Am J Ther*. 2016;23(1):e74–e77. 10.1097/01.mjt.0000433940.91996.16

Kimlin E, Easter J, Ganetsky M. A 46-year-old woman with altered mental status and garbled speech. *J Emerg Med*. 2009;37(1):69–74.

Levine M, Brooks D, Truitt C, Wolk B, Boyer E, Ruha A. Toxicology in the ICU. *Chest*. 2011;140(3):795–806.

Morton H. Atropine intoxication. *J Pediatr*. 1939;14(6):755–760.

Oerther S, Behrman A, Ketcham S. Herbal hallucinations: Common abuse situations seen in the emergency department. *J Emerg Nurs*. 2010;36(6):594–596.

Pentel P, Peterson C. Asystole complicating physostigmine treatment of tricyclic antidepressant overdose. *Ann Emerg Med*. 1980;9(11):588–590.

Schneir A. Complications of diagnostic physostigmine administration to emergency department patients. *Acad Emerg Med*. 2003;42(1):14–19.

Skolnik A, Wilcox S. General toxicology and toxidromes. *Critical Care Secrets*. 2013;545–551. doi:10.1016/B978-0-323-08500-7.00093-X

Suchard J. Assessing physostigmine's contraindication in cyclic antidepressant ingestions. *J Emerg Med*. 2003;25(2):185–191.

Watkins J, Schwarz E, Arroyo-Plasencia A, Mullins M. The use of physostigmine by toxicologists in anticholinergic toxicity. *J Med Toxicol*. 2014;11(2):179–184.

36 Dying in the Emergency Department: Death trajectories and palliative care in the emergency department

April Jessica Pinto and
Marie-Carmelle Elie

A 74-year-old woman presents to the ED via emergency medical services with shortness of breath. At the bedside, her daughter shares that the patient has a history of metastatic breast cancer, chronic obstructive pulmonary disease (COPD), congestive heart failure (CHF), and stage 3 chronic kidney disease. The patient's initial vital signs include a regular heart rate of 120 bpm, a respiratory rate of 22 breaths/min, a blood pressure of 128/84 mmHg, and an O_2 level of 88%. The blood glucose level is 103 mg/dl. She is tachypneic, has rales bilaterally, has interrupted speech limited to 5–6 word phrases and you begin noninvasive positive pressure ventilation (NIPPV) and administer intravenous (IV) furosemide, and nebulized albuterol. The creatinine level is 7.6 mg/dl, and her potassium level is 6.7 mmol/dl. She becomes increasingly altered and is no longer able to participate in discussions. You inform her daughter of your concerns that her condition is deteriorating and that emergent dialysis and intubation will need to be considered. Her daughter states she is an only child and wants everything done for the patient to keep her alive. The patient is married but has been estranged from her husband for one year. In your state, the legal next of kin assigns primary decision-making to the spouse. You call the spouse, and he wishes that she have a do-not-resuscitate (DNR) order instituted, as he understands that she would want comfort care.

What do I do now?

Advance directives are written wishes documented by a patient describing their preferences regarding medical treatments, resuscitation, and life-prolonging efforts. Advance directives may be used in the event that the patient is unable to make their own decisions, due to either a life-limiting illness or a temporary condition. Often, advance directives include the patient's personal philosophy, religious preferences, directions on interventions such as nutrition and placement of a feeding tube, mechanical ventilation, and surgeries. Documents may also include the wish to be fully resuscitated or not (DNR) in the event of cardiac or respiratory arrest. These directives also serve as comprehensive documents that include information on whom the patient has designated as their healthcare proxy or decision maker. The absence of an advance directive that provides guidance to providers is a prevalent public health concern for the geriatric population and for those with serious or advanced illness.[1] Recent evidence demonstrates that whereas only 46% of Americans over the age of 65 years have advance directives, only 7% report discussing these wishes with their physician, and <50% have had such discussions with their loved ones.[7] In the ED, the deterioration of the patient's clinical state with the consequent loss of capacity to make decisions is a common occurrence. Ideally, all patients at risk for experiencing a serious health event would have robust goals-of-care discussions well in advance of a decline in health. These discussions should include end-of-life preferences regarding "code" or resuscitation status with their healthcare providers, family members (next of kin), or healthcare surrogates. However, these discussions frequently occur in the ED at a time of medical crisis when the patient has lost the ability to express their wishes directly.

Best practices include the discussion of code status during the initial encounter and assessment of the patient. As an example, patients presenting with shortness of breath with a history of advanced stages of their disease including CHF COPD, or metastatic cancer have a potential to decompensate quickly. Deferring discussions regarding code status and end-of-life care may introduce challenges if the patient becomes incapacitated; thus, it is best to have these discussions early, while the patient is able to participate.

If the patient arrives to the ED altered or unable to participate in goals-of-care discussions, it is imperative to engage the patient's next of kin or healthcare surrogate. While there are details specific to each state, in the

United States, the generally accepted order of next of kin is spouse, adult children, parents, and siblings. If adult children or siblings represent the next of kin and there are multiple adult children or multiple siblings, then they must reach a majority consensus. For example, for an incapacitated patient with five children, if two children wish full resuscitation and three wish comfort measures, the majority's desire to proceed with comfort measures would prevail by law. If a legally married patient is separated or otherwise estranged from a spouse, local statutes may still recognize that individual as the primary next of kin. Additional distinctions in next-of-kin order and designation may vary by state. Providers should refer to their respective local statutory guidance to best understand state-specific variations. Importantly, even for an incapacitated patient, the patient's known preferences for their care, even if undocumented, should guide the shared medical decisions of the clinician and family. Arguably, the known preferences of the incapacitated patient should supersede the order of kinship and surrogacy, constructs designed to advocate for the patient's wishes.

A timely assessment is indispensable in emergency medicine, specifically in life-limiting situations. When an ED physician believes a patient is likely to die within the next month, that patient is 2.4 times more likely to do so compared with patients whom the ED physician does not expect to experience 1-month mortality.[5] The ED physician assessment, while limited from the perspective of the primary provider or specialist familiar with the patient, likely confers a level of objectivity that improves short-term prognostication. When limited by time and the busy ED environment, one can conduct a conversation defining discrete goals of care and code status in minutes. Table 36.1 provides guidance on the SPIKES (Setting up, Perception, Invitation, Knowledge, Empathy, and Strategy or Summary) rubric for communication of difficult news.[2] Strong emotions are often present by the family and patient when hearing difficult news and responding non-verbally and verbally with empathic communication is crucial. Table 36.2 provides a framework NURSE (Name, Understand, Respect, Support, Explore) for responding to strong emotions with empathy.[6]

It is important that the preferences and goals inform any recommendations extended by the clinical team of care expressed or pre-defined by the patient. It is also appropriate and ethical to ensure that recommendations are weighed against medical indications and the risks and benefits afforded

TABLE 36.1 **SPIKES rubric for delivering bad news**[2]

S	Setting up	• Set up and prepare the environment in which you will be having the discussion. • Minimize distractions and ensure privacy in the space. • Ensure that the correct individuals will be present for the discussion, as directed by the patient or healthcare surrogate. • Prepare information to share and communicate with team members who may be involved so that they are aware of the anticipated dialogue.	• *"Whom would you wish to be present when we discuss your diagnosis?"* • *"What time can you and your loved ones set aside for us to discuss your care?"*
P	Perception	• Assess the patient's perception and understanding of their current situation; begin with open-ended questions.	• *"What is your understanding of what has happened today?"* • *"What have your physicians told you about your condition?"*
I	Invite	• Request permission from the patient to discuss a serious matter. • This may also be an appropriate time to invite other pertinent decision-makers, as deemed by the patient, to attend the conversation. • It is the patient's choice to engage in the conversation or elect for someone else to receive the difficult information.	• *"I have some difficult news to share with you; would this be a good time?"* • *"Who would you prefer to have this conversation and make decisions regarding your care?"*

TABLE 36.1 **Continued**

K	Knowledge	· Inform the patient with appropriate terminology of events leading up to the patient's current condition. · Speak factually, avoid euphemisms, and provide the big picture. · Allow for silence and response. · Ask if there are any questions you may answer.	· *"The cancer has returned, and there are no further treatments. I wish things were different."* · *"She has bled into her brain, and there is irreversible swelling and damage. I am concerned that she may not survive this event."*
E	Empathy	· Validate the emotions of those in the room. · Use vocabulary aligning with what is witnessed or verbalized. · Employ empathetic statements. (see Table 36.2) · Allow for open-ended responses when communication is unclear.	· *"I can see how shocking this is for you and your family."* · *"I can't imagine what this must be like for your family."* · *"Tell me more about that."*
S	Summary and Strategy	· Use this time to summarize what has occurred, support that can be offered, and reasonable expectations of the next steps.	· *"I hope I have helped answer your questions and provided guidance regarding the options available."* · *"When would you like to schedule our next meeting?"*

TABLE 36.2 NURSE mnemonic for communicating with empathy[6]

N	Name	• Naming the emotion that you can identify acknowledges and allows the patient/ surrogate to be seen • State what you can see	• *"It sounds like you are frustrated.* • *"This situation seems very overwhelming."*
U	Understand	• Acknowledge that it is normal to have strong feelings, thoughts, or emotions	• *"This helps me understand what you might be feeling."* • *"I can only imagine what feelings or thoughts you must be having."*
R	Respect	• Commend the surrogate and family for their work in being a patient and caregiver • Praise surrogate and family for their role in supporting patient	• *"I can see that you have been really trying to follow the instructions your doctor provided."* • *"You are a great job being his/her/ their advocate."*
S	Support	• Offer support on behalf of yourself or your team • Speak of non-abandonment by the medical team	• *"We will be with you every step of the way. Please let us know what you need."* • *"Our team is here to help support you through this."*
E	Explore	• When an emotional response is not expected or differences exist, open-ended non-judgemental exploration of emotion might be warranted • Be curious!	• *"Tell me more about what you are thinking."* • *"Could you say more about what you mean when you say . . . ?."*

to the patient.[3] Specifically, consider the older patient living independently with co-morbidities, who wishes to retain his independence and has expressed an unwillingness to be admitted to a skilled nursing facility or accept artificial nutrition. Following the cardiopulmonary resuscitation of patients > 65 years for cardiac arrest, survival is typically associated with nursing facility discharge, and the risk of long-term cognitive deficit is high. Sharing this information may help direct the decision to opt against CPR in patients who are unwilling to reside in a nursing facility.

Palliative care includes aggressive therapies and treatments, such as radiation therapy, chemotherapy, pleural catheterization, and other interventions and treatments aimed at reducing pain and discomfort or improving the quality of life. Palliative care may be provided to patients who have serious or advanced illness, and may be appropriate at any point in the illness trajectory, especially when the desired outcome is symptom management or relief.[4]

Hospice is provided to patients with serious life-limiting conditions whose life expectancy is anticipated to be <6 months if the disease were to take its natural course.[4] For patients in hospice, the focus is on quality of life and comfort; however, hospice patients may choose to be full code. This approach may be appropriate for patients who have a high functional baseline and have a goal aligned with a specific timeframe. For example, a 45-year-old woman on hospice with metastatic cancer living independently at home may choose to be full code and accept advanced therapies to survive to her daughter's wedding day, anticipated in 2 weeks. Consultation with palliative care or hospice may be appropriate in the emergency department based on the preferences of the family and patient and when there are unclear goals of care or conflict.

When a patient is incapacitated with no written advance directives, discussions with the next of kin regarding goals of care should focus on a best understanding of what the patient would want done. While some patients have previously broached this discussion with their providers, close family members or next of kin, there are times when this is not the case or these individuals are unable to serve as proxy for the patient's wishes. In those instances, prior court cases have set a precedent that "clear and convincing evidence" of the patient's wishes that can be recited by those with whom it was shared may serve as surrogates. As in the case presented, if the estranged husband had not had discussions with the patient regarding her wishes, but the patient had shared these beliefs with her daughter, it would be the responsibility of the physician to elicit this information and act in accordance with the patients's known wishes.

When the shared decision is to transition to comfort care, or the discontinuation or withdrawal of non-palliative interventions, it may be appropriate to begin the process while the patient is in the ED. Benefits of this approach include timely execution of the preferences of the patient and family, a reduction of distressing symptoms (i.e., pain, anxiety, nausea, delirium), and appropriate alignment of institutional resources to the patient's healthcare needs. It is important that the physician document the discussion, including the decision-makers engaged, the values and preferences expressed, the shared decisions and goals of the palliative interventions.

The discussion that follows will be specifically designed to address the management of the actively dying patient in the ED.

Low dose parenteral opiates are preferred for the management of severe dyspnea and pain symptoms as they have a quick onset of action and may be titrated to patient comfort. If the control of symptoms have been achieved, scheduled dosing with oral medications may be administered, if tolerated. In patients that exhibit severe signs of distress, frequent administration, or escalation of dosing, an infusion of opiate medications may be considered.

Parenteral benzodiazepines are also effective in the management of severe dyspnea and may be used in conjunction with or instead of opiates for control of refractory symptoms. Benzodiazepines have the added benefit of managing terminal delirium, agitation, or seizures. Whenever opiates or benzodiazepines are administered, it is important to educate family members about the level of sedation and coma that may incur. This may be very distressing to families that struggle with reconciling the goal of symptom optimization against that of maintaining a level of consciousness to participate in meaningful communication with loved ones.

For those on mechanical ventilation, either the patient may be fully extubated and the endotracheal tube removed after appropriate suctioning or the ventilator may simply be turned to a set rate with an FiO_2 of 21%

(same as room O_2) and room settings, with the endotracheal tube left in place.

Prior to the removal or withdrawal of mechanical ventilation, it is important to counsel the family regarding anticipated clinical changes, such as gasping and increased work of breathing. It is also important to provide guidance on the anticipated amount of time patients may be expected to survive upon extubation. While most patients will expire within minutes to hours, upon extubation, some patients can survive for several days. Be sure to turn off monitors and alarms at the bedside and do your best to establish adequate symptom control prior to extubation to allow for a peaceful, disruption-free transition. Prior to extubation, the provider should stop and ensure reversal of paralytic medications, which do not contribute to achieving comfort measures in care withdrawal. IV access should be maintained to allow the provision of comfort-based therapies. Glycopyrrolate (0.2–0.4 mg IV) can be helpful to minimize secretions, given 20–30 min before a patient is extubated or for any end-of-life patient who may be struggling with swallowing secretions. We recommend the parenteral administration of an opioid, such as 2–10 mg of morphine, prior to extubation to control dyspnea and pain. Consider adding a benzodiazepine, such as 1–2 mg of IV lorazepam, if the patient appears anxious. If symptoms require more frequent dosing, you may consider placing the patient on a continuous infusion of sedative or opiate medications to optimize comfort.

Regardless of whether the patient's care involves a ventilator, during the process of medical de-escalation, it is of utmost importance to titrate medications to the patient's symptoms and comfort. In the final stages of life, not all patients will be able to verbalize their pain and discomfort. It will become increasingly important to look for nonverbal signs of discomfort in these patients, such as tachycardia, labored respirations, grimacing, and writhing. Titrate medications with a respiratory rate goal of <30 breaths/min and eliminate grimacing, labored breathing, and other nonverbal signs of discomfort. Infusions may have delayed efficacy, so a strategy to immediately address symptoms may be to use bolus dosages until comfort is achieved. It is important to highlight that families and loved ones may experience emotional distress as patients transition and to maintain communication about the process to ensure clarity on the goals of the care provided.

- The next of kin or healthcare proxy is dictated by statute. It provides the order in which family members and others can assume responsibility for making healthcare decisions if the patient lacks capacity. Unless a court has appointed a legal guardian, in most cases, the order of assignment is the patient's spouse, followed by adult children, parents, siblings, and relatives. If there are multiple children, siblings, etc., a majority consensus will be employed. Any state-specific variations should be referenced depending on your area of practice.[3]
- Consider using a communication rubric such as the SPIKES for difficult conversations: Set up, Perception, Information, Knowledge, Empathy, Summary, and Strategy. Respond with empathic language: Name, Understand, Respect, Support, Explore.
- Palliative care may be provided to patients who have serious or advanced illness and may be appropriate at any stage of the disease trajectory. The goal of palliative care is to relieve and manage physical, emotional, and spiritual symptoms and distress experienced as a consequence of the disease process.
- Hospice is provided to patients with serious life-limiting conditions with an anticipated life expectancy of <6 months if the disease were to take its natural course. Patients can be full code while on hospice.
- When de-escalating or withdrawing care, the provider should plan for the optimization of comfort. Opioids and benzodiazepines are useful in treating symptoms of pain and dyspnea. When actively managing symptoms, these drugs are preferably administered as a bolus rather than an infusion and should be titrated to effect (i.e., comfort) rather than a scheduled prespecified dosage.

References

1. California Health Care Foundation. Poll finds wide gap between the care patients want and receive at end of life. https://www.chcf.org/press-release/poll-finds-wide-gap-between-the-care-patients-want-and-receive-at-end-of-life/. Published August 30, 2018. Accessed December 28, 2020.

2. Kaplan M. SPIKES: A framework for breaking bad news to patients with cancer. *Clin J Oncol Nurs.* 2010;14(4):514–516. doi:10.1188/10.CJON.514-516

3. Luce J, Alpers A. Legal aspects of withholding and withdrawing life support from critically ill patients in the United States and providing palliative care to them. *Am J Respir Crit Care Med.* 2000;162:2029–2032.

4. National Institute on Aging. *What are palliative care and hospice care?* https://www.nia.nih.gov/health/what-are-palliative-care-and-hospice-care. Published 2020. Accessed November 3, 2020.

5. Ouchi K, Strout T, Haydar S, et al. Association of emergency clinicians' assessment of mortality risk with actual 1-month mortality among older adults admitted to the hospital. *JAMA Netw Open.* 2019;2(9):e1911139. doi:10.1001/jamanetworkopen.2019.11139

6. VitalTalk. Responding to Emotion: Respecting. https://www.vitaltalk.org/guides/responding-to-emotion-respecting/. Last accessed: March 22, 2023.

7. Yadav KN, Gabler NB, Cooney E, et al. Approximately one in three US adults completes any type of advance directive for end-of-life care. *Health Aff.* 2017;36(7):1244–1251.

Further reading

Palliative Care Network of Wisconsin. Delivering bad news, part 1. https://www.mypcnow.org/fast-fact/delivering-bad-news-part-1/. Published 2020. Accessed November 3, 2020.

Palliative Care Network of Wisconsin. Delivering bad news, part 2. https://www.mypcnow.org/fast-fact/delivering-bad-news-part-2/. Published 2020. Accessed November 3, 2020.

Palliative Care Network of Wisconsin. Fast facts. https://www.mypcnow.org/fast-facts/. Published 2020.

Palliative Care Network of Wisconsin; Von Gunten C, Weissman D. *Symptom control for ventilator withdrawal in the dying patient.* https://www.mypcnow.org/fast-fact/symptom-control-for-ventilator-withdrawal-in-the-dying-patient/. Published 2020. Accessed November 3, 2020.

Palliative Care Network of Wisconsin; Von Gunten C, Weissman D. *Ventilator withdrawal protocol.* https://www.mypcnow.org/fast-fact/ventilator-withdrawal-protocol/. Published 2020. Accessed November 3, 2020.

Index

glomerular diseases, 288, 319
glucocorticoids, 98–99
glycopyrrolate
    airway topicalization and, 6, 11
    awake fiberoptic intubation, 6
    ketamine and, 8
    subglottic stenosis, 26
goals-of-care discussions, 344–45
graft-versus-host disease (GVHD), 319
Guérin, C., 99–101
Guillain–Barré syndrome (GBS), 233, 235, 237

healthcare surrogates, 344–45, 349–50
heated high-flow nasal cannulas, 27–28
Heimlich valves, 55
heliox, 27–28
hemodialysis, 260
hemoptysis, 41–46
    anticoagulants and, 43
    bronchial artery embolization, 44–45
    bronchoscopy, 44–45
    case example, 41
    causes of, 42*b*
    chest imaging, 43, 44
    cough reflex and, 43–44
    direct laryngoscopy, 43–44
    endotracheal tubes, 44
    focused history, 43
    focused physical examination, 43
    initial management of, 43
    intubation, 43–44
    laboratory evaluation, 43
    large-bore suction catheters, 44
    laryngeal mask airway, 43–44
    localizing source of, 44
    multidisciplinary approach to, 44–45
    nebulized tranexamic acid, 43
    noninvasive positive-pressure
        ventilation, 43
    patient disposition, 45–46
    positive end-expiratory pressure and, 43
    safety precautions when treating, 42
    temporizing measures, 45

videolaryngoscopy, 43–44
Yankauer suction catheters, 44
hemorrhagic resuscitation, 247–54
    case example, 247
    classifications of hemorrhagic shock, 248
    overview, 252–53
    transfusion of blood products, 249–50
hemorrhagic stroke
    first hours of management, 212–13
    general discussion, 202
hemorrhoids, 272
hemostatic control, 239–46
    case example, 239
    Minnesota tube placement, 243*b*
    overview, 240, 244–45
hepatic encephalopathy, 276–78
HHS (hyperosmolar hyperglycemic state), 304–5, 306
high-flow nasal cannula (HFNC), 68
    contraindications to, 67–68
    COVID-19 and, 68
    fraction of inspired oxygen, 65–67
    hypoxemic respiratory failure, 67
    liter flow, 65–66
    overview, 65–66
    physiologically difficult airways, 34–35, 37–38, 39
    positive end-expiratory pressure and, 66
    ROX index, 66–67
hospice, 349
H. pylori, 270
HTS (hypertonic saline), 197
Hunt and Hess grading scale, 219*t*
HVS (hyperviscosity syndrome), 330–31
hydrocephalus
    aneurysmal SAHs and, 226
    intracerebral hemorrhage and, 213
hyperacute rejection, 317
hyperglycemia, 304
hyperkalemia, 295–302
    case example, 295
    diagnosis of, 296–97

melena, 269

membrane oxygenator, 109f

mental status, 276t, 305

mesenteric ischemia, 272

methicillin-resistant *Staphylococcus aureus* (MRSA), 119

methylprednisolone, 318t

MG (myasthenia gravis), 232–33, 235–37, 238. *See also* neuromuscular emergencies

midazolam
    awake fiberoptic intubation, 8–9
    mechanical ventilator and, 80
    physiologically difficult airways, 37–38
    subglottic stenosis, 26

Minnesota tube, 242, 243b, 271

minute ventilation (MV), 72

MIST2 trial, 56

modified Fisher grading scale, 226t

Montgomery T-Tubes, 29f, 29–30

mortality rates
    proning and, 99–101
    tracheo-innominate artery fistula hemorrhages, 17

MRSA (methicillin-resistant *Staphylococcus aureus*), 119

mucosal atomization, 7

MV (minute ventilation), 72

myasthenia gravis (MG), 232–33, 235–37, 238. *See also* neuromuscular emergencies

nasal approach, AFOI, 7, 9–10, 11

nasal masks, 62

nasogastric (NG) tube, 270, 281–82

National Institutes of Health Stroke Scale (NIHSS), 202, 204t, 207

needle thoracostomy, 57–58

negative pressure ventilation (NPV), 235–36

neoplasms, 272

nephritic syndrome, 288

nephrotic syndrome, 288

neurogenic pulmonary edema, 226

neuromuscular blockade
    acute respiratory distress syndrome, 93, 98–99
    myasthenia gravis, 235–36

neuromuscular emergencies, 231–38
    anticholinesterases, 236–37
    case example, 231
    differential diagnosis and presentation, 232–34
    Guillain–Barré syndrome, 233, 235, 237
    immunosuppressants, 236–37
    intravenous immune globulin, 236–37
    Lambert–Eaton myasthenic syndrome, 232–33, 235
    myasthenia gravis, 232–33, 235
    negative pressure ventilation, 235–36
    neuromuscular blockers, 235–36
    plasma exchange, 236–37
    spinal cord ischemia and cord compression, 233–34
    treatment, 235–37
    workup, 234–35

neuromuscular junction (NMJ)
    botulism, 233
    Lambert–Eaton myasthenic syndrome, 232–33, 235
    myasthenia gravis, 232–33, 235–37, 238
    organophosphate toxicity, 233

New England Journal of Medicine, 99–101

NG (nasogastric) tube, 270, 281–82

NIHSS (National Institutes of Health Stroke Scale), 202, 204t, 207

nimodipine, 225–26

non-aneurysmal SAHs, 218

nonconvulsive status epilepticus (SE), 185

noninvasive positive-pressure ventilation (NIPPV)
    hemoptysis, 43
    physiologically difficult airways, 35–36, 39

post-transplant lymphoproliferative disorder (PTLD), 315–16

potassium. *See also* hyperkalemia
   diabetic ketoacidosis and, 307
   eliminating, 299–300
   shifting of, 298–99

pregnancy, status epilepticus and, 188

pressure-control ventilation, 73

pressure targets. *See also* positive end-expiratory pressure and
   lung-protective ventilation, 75–77
   peak inspiratory pressure, 75

pressure ulcers, 99–101, 102

primary PTX, 57

prone positioning (proning), 97–103
   acute respiratory distress syndrome, 92–93, 94
   adverse effects and limitations, 99–101
   back compressions and, 99–101
   benefits of, 99
   "burrito" approach, 100*t*
   de-proning trial, 99
   head and neck positioning, 100*t*
   mortality rates and, 99–101
   placement of IV tubing and arterial monitoring, 100*t*, 102
   pre-procedure checklist, 99–101, 100*t*
   pressure ulcers, 99–101, 102
   prophylactic hydrocolloid dressings, 99–101
   refractory ARDS, 106
   sedation and, 102
   swimming positions, 100*t*, 102

prophylactic hydrocolloid dressings, 99–101

propofol, 8, 80

prothrombin complex concentrate (PCC), 213, 259–60, 268

proximal plugging, subglottic stenosis, 29–30

psuedochylothorax, 51–52

PTLD (post-transplant lymphoproliferative disorder), 315–16

PTX (pneumothorax), 55, 56–58, 59

pulmonary arterial hypertension (PAH), 33–34

pulmonary hypertension, 141–47

pyridoxine (vitamin B6) deficiency, 188

RA (rheumatoid arthritis), 51–52

rapid sequence induction/intubation (RSI), 37–38

REBOA (resuscitative endovascular balloon occlusion of the aorta), 244

re-expansion pulmonary edema (REPE), 54

refractory ARDS, 105–14
   case example, 105–6
   clinical and historical context, 106–7
   clinical outcomes, 112
   prone positioning, 106
   venovenous extracorporeal membrane oxygenation, 107–13, 108*f*, 109*f*, 111*b*

refractory status epilepticus (RSE), 184

rejection, transplant, 316–19

remifentanil, 26

renal replacement therapy (RRT), 286, 291

REPE (re-expansion pulmonary edema), 54

RESCUEicp trial, 195

respiratory rate (RR), 72

respiratory viruses, 315–16

resuscitative endovascular balloon occlusion of the aorta (REBOA), 244

RE-VERSE AD trial, 259

rheumatoid arthritis (RA), 51–52

RIFLE (Risk, Injury, Failure, Loss, End-stage) criteria, 286

right ventricle (RV) function, 36

right ventricular dysfunction
   ARDS, 141–47
   case example, 141
   diagnosis, 142–43
   diagnostic testing, 143
   imaging, 142*f*, 142–43
   pharmacotherapy, 144–45, 144*t*
   pulmonary hypertension and, 141–47
   reducing RV afterload and PVR, 143–44
   vasoactive therapy, 145